MW01231387

Nutritional Care

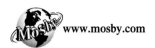 www.mosby.com

POCKET GUIDE TO

Nutritional Care

Mary Courtney Moore, RN, RD, PhD
Clarksville, Tennessee

Fourth Edition

with 29 illustrations

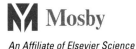

Mosby

An Affiliate of Elsevier Science

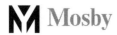

An Affiliate of Elsevier Science

Vice-President, Nursing Editorial Director: Sally Schrefer
Editor: Yvonne Alexopoulos
Developmental Editor: Melissa K. Boyle
Project Manager: Linda McKinley
Senior Production Editor: Jennifer Furey
Designer: Amy Buxton
Cover Photo: PhotoDisc

FOURTH EDITION

NOTICE

Pharmacology is an ever-changing field. Standard safety percautions must be
followed, but as new research and clinical experience broaden our
knowledge, changes in treatment and drug therapy may become necessary or
appropriate. Readers are advised to check the most current product
information provided by the manufacturer of each drug to be administered to
verify the recommended dose, the method and duration of administration,
and contraindications. It is the responsibility of the treating physician, relying
on experience and knowledge of the patient, to determine dosages and the
best treatment for each individual patient. Neither the Publisher nor the editor
assumes any liability for any injury and/or damage to persons or property
arising from this publication.

Mosby, Inc.
An Affiliate of Elsevier Science
11830 Westline Industrial Drive
St. Louis, Missouri 63146

Printed in China

Library of Congress Cataloging-in-Publication Data

Moore, Mary Courtney.
    Pocket guide to nutritional care / Mary Courtney Moore.—4th ed.
      p. ; cm.
    Includes bibliographical references and index.
    ISBN 0-323-00843-7
    1. Diet therapy—Handbooks, manuals, etc. 2. Nutrition—Handbooks,
manuals, etc. 3. Diet to disease—Handbooks, manuals, etc.
    [DNLM: 1. Diet Therapy—Handbooks. 2. Nutrition—Handbooks. WB
39 M823p 2001] I. Title: Nutritional care. II. Title.
RM217.2.M66 2001
615.8'54—dc21   00-045244

03 04 GW/QBC 9 8 7 6 5 4

To
Bill and Evan,
the best family anywhere

*"I was hungry and you fed me,
thirsty and you gave me a drink; . . .
sick and you took care of me. . . ."*

Matthew 25:35-36

Reviewers

Preface

This *Pocket Guide to Nutritional Care* is designed to be a brief, yet comprehensive resource that can easily be carried to inpatient or outpatient settings and consulted as needed. Many of the features of previous editions have been retained, including the emphasis on performing a thorough nutrition assessment as a basis for planning nutrition interventions and teaching, an overview of cultural impacts on nutrition, an emphasis on the importance of weight control and physical activity in the maintenance of good health, and the application of enteral and parenteral nutrition support wherever appropriate.

This edition of the book has been extensively revised to bring it up-to-date and to make it more user-friendly. It incorporates recent changes in the field of nutrition, including the replacement of the Recommended Dietary Allowances with Dietary Reference Intakes, the new *Dietary Guidelines for Americans,* and the development of new growth charts. An important new feature in this edition is the inclusion of a glossary, printed on shaded pages at the back of this text to make this useful information easy to access. Several content areas have been significantly expanded to reflect their importance in nutritional care and/or new information available since the publication of the previous edition. These subjects include alcohol-related disorders (Chapter 19); sources of caffeine in foods and beverages (Appendix G); food-borne illnesses and food safety (Appendix K); and resources for nutrition intervention, referral, and teaching (Appendix I).

My hope is that this fourth edition of the *Pocket Guide to Nutritional Care* will be an up-to-date and useful reference for health professionals and that it will serve to improve the care of their patients.

Mary Courtney Moore

Contents

NUTRITION FOR HEALTH PROMOTION

I

The following chapters introduce normal nutrition. Included in the discussion are a summary of the required nutrients, an explanation of nutritional guidelines, an overview of digestion and absorption, a description of the process of nutritional assessment, and a discussion of nutritional needs and concerns throughout the life cycle. These chapters provide a basis for understanding the role of nutrition in health promotion and prevention of disease.

Nutrition and Health: Overview

1

More than 40 nutrients are known to be essential for human health. All of these nutrients are found in foods and beverages, but some skill and planning may be required to choose a diet adequate in all nutrients. Appendix A summarizes the roles, major food sources, and symptoms of deficiency of nutrients known to be essential.

Healthy People Initiative

Healthy People is an ongoing project aimed at increasing the years of healthy life and decreasing disparities in health care among Americans. The initiative identifies the most significant and controllable health issues for Americans and focuses on public and private sector attempts to address them. In the current summary (*Healthy People 2010;* available at www.health.gov/healthypeople/), all of the top four leading contributors to health impairments—cigarette smoking, prevalence of overweight, prevalence of sedentary lifestyles, and alcohol misuse—are closely related to nutritional status. Thus, the need for education about nutrition and healthful changes in lifestyle is a high priority among Americans.

Dietary Reference Intakes

In every country it is necessary to have a careful estimate of the nutrient needs of the population in order to provide a basis for setting nutrition policy, monitoring the adequacy of the food supply, and educating the public about proper diet. In the United States, the **Recommended Dietary Allowances (RDAs)** have been used since the 1940s, with periodic revisions. Other countries have established their own guidelines. In the past, much of the focus of the RDAs has been on prevention of nutritional deficiencies. Prompted by the growing recognition of the role of nutrition in health promotion and prevention of chronic diseases, U.S. and Canadian nutritionists are developing new guidelines, called the **Dietary Reference Intakes (DRIs).** The DRIs will be used in the same manner as the RDAs were, in regulating the fortification of foods (addition of nutrients, as in vitamin D fortification of milk) and the composition of diet supplements; setting goals and budgets for food assistance programs for low-income families, schools, and the elderly; planning menus for individuals in the military and in many institutions; determining what nutrition information should be supplied on food labels; and similar purposes.

Currently, DRIs are available for the B vitamins and for the nutrients involved in bone formation and maintenance (calcium, phosphorus, magnesium, vitamin D, and fluoride). The DRIs include two sets of guidelines: first, either an RDA (which retains the former name) or an **Adequate Intake (AI)** is specified, and second, a **Tolerable Upper Intake Level (UL)** is given for most nutrients. The RDA, which is estimated to meet the needs of almost all (97% to 98%) of the healthy population, is assigned where nutrient needs are well established. An AI is assigned when nutrient needs cannot be quantified as precisely, but the recommendation is believed to cover the needs of the population. The UL is defined as the upper limit of intake associated with a low risk of adverse effects in almost all members of a population. The DRIs for some nutrients are higher than the old RDAs. For instance, inadequate calcium intake increases the risk of developing osteoporosis. Therefore, the DRI for calcium for nonpregnant adults between 19 and 50 years of age has been set at 1,000 mg/day, an increase of 25% over the most recent RDA. Table 1-1 lists the DRIs that have been released to date. For nutrients for which no DRIs have been published yet, such as protein and vitamin A, this book uses the most recent edition of the RDAs (1989).

Guides for Wise Food Choices

The DRIs are useful for health care professionals, the food industry, and government agencies involved in food and health policy, but most individuals would find them hard to translate into appropriate food choices. The *Dietary Guidelines for Americans* and the **Food Guide Pyramid** have been developed to help the public choose foods wisely. Nutritional labeling on foods is designed to make it easier to know what nutrients are in foods.

Dietary Guidelines for Americans

The *Dietary Guidelines for Americans* (2000) are intended to help Americans optimize their health and reduce nutrition-related health risks. The guidelines are summarized as follows.

Aim for fitness

Aim for a healthy weight

Numerous health problems, including hypertension, heart disease, stroke, type 2 diabetes, arthritis, pulmonary problems, and breast cancer and certain other cancers, are associated with being over-weight. Avoiding weight gain or losing excess weight involves lifestyle changes that require specific choices, such as increasing physical activity and choosing a variety of healthful foods low in fat and added sugars.

Individuals who are overweight need to lose the excess weight gradually. A loss of 5% to 15% of body weight, even if that does not make the individual normal weight, may improve his or her health, functional ability, and quality of life. An increasing number of children are overweight. Children need to be encouraged to choose from a variety of low-fat foods from the Food Guide Pyramid (described later in this chapter), and they should be provided only rarely with foods high in fats and added sugars.

Individuals with eating disorders attempt to control their weight in unhealthful ways. Frequent binge eating, with or without periods of food restriction, preoccupation with body weight or food, dramatic weight loss, excessive exercise, self-induced vomiting, and laxative abuse are signs of eating disorders.

Be physically active every day

Physical activity reduces the risk of heart disease, colon cancer, and type 2 diabetes (see Chapter 18). In addition, it strengthens muscles, bones, and joints; improves psychological well-being; and helps to control high blood pressure and body weight. Adults need at least 30 minutes of moderate physical activity daily, and children need at least 60 minutes. A regular exercise program is one way to be physically active, but it is also possible to incorporate an adequate amount of physical activity into the daily routine (e.g.,

Table 1-1A   Dietary Reference Intakes

Life-Stage Group	Thiamin (mg/d)	Riboflavin (mg/d)	Niacin (mg/d)[a]	Vitamin B₆ (mg/d)	Folate (µg/d)[b]	Vitamin B₁₂ (µg/d)	Pantothenic Acid (mg/d)	Biotin (µg/d)	Choline (mg/d)[c]	Vitamin D₃ (µg/d)	Calcium (mg/d)	Phosphorus (mg/d)	Magnesium (mg/d)	Fluoride (mg/d)	Vitamin C (mg/d)	Vitamin E (mg/d)	Selenium (µg/d)
Infants																	
0-6 mo	0.2*	0.3*	2*	0.1*	65*	0.4*	1.7*	5*	125*	5*	210*	100*	30*	0.01*	40*	4*	15*
6-12 mo	0.3*	0.4*	3*	0.3*	80*	0.5*	1.8*	6*	150*	5*	270*	275*	75*	0.5*	50*	6*	20*
Children																	
1-3 yr	0.5	0.5	6	0.5	150	0.9	2*	8*	200*	5*	500*	460	80	0.7*	15	6	20
4-8 yr	0.6	0.6	8	0.6	200	1.2	3*	12*	250*	5*	800*	500	130	1.1*	25	7	30
9-13 yr	0.9	0.9	12	1.0	300	1.8	4*	20*	375*	5*	1300*	1250	240	2.0*	45	11	40
Males																	
14-18 yr	1.2	1.3	16	1.3	400	2.4	5*	25*	550*	5*	1300*	1250	410	3.2*	75	15	55
19-30 yr	1.2	1.3	16	1.3	400	2.4	5*	30*	550*	5*	1000*	700	400	3.8*	90	15	55
31-50 yr	1.2	1.3	16	1.3	400	2.4	5*	30*	550*	5*	1000*	700	420	3.8*	90	15	55
51-70 yr	1.2	1.3	16	1.7	400	2.4[d]	5*	30*	550*	10*	1200*	700	420	3.8*	90	15	55
>70 yr	1.2	1.3	16	1.7	400	2.4[d]	5*	30*	550*	15*	1200*	700	420	3.8*	90	15	55
Females																	
14-18 yr	1.0	1.0	14	1.2	400[e]	2.4	5*	25*	400*	5*	1300*	1250	360	2.9*	65	15	55
19-30 yr	1.1	1.1	14	1.3	400[e]	2.4	5*	30*	425*	5*	1000*	700	310	3.1*	75	15	55
31-50 yr	1.1	1.1	14	1.3	400[e]	2.4	5*	30*	425*	5*	1000*	700	320	3.1*	75	15	55
51-70 yr	1.1	1.1	14	1.5	400	2.4[d]	5*	30*	425*	10*	1200*	700	320	3.1*	75	15	55
>70 yr	1.1	1.1	14	1.5	400	2.4[d]	5*	30*	425*	15*	1200*	700	320	3.1*	75	15	55

Pregnancy																
<19 yr	1.4	18	1.9	600f	2.6	6*	30*	450*	5*	1300*	1250	400	2.9*	80	15	60
19-50 yr	1.4	18	1.9	600f	2.6	6*	30*	450*	5*	1000*	700	350h	3.1*	85	15	60
Lactation																
<19 yr	1.6	17	2.0	500	2.8	7*	35*	550*	5*	1300*	1250	360	2.9*	115	19	70
19-50 yr	1.6	17	2.0	500	2.8	7*	35*	550*	5*	1000*	700	310h	3.1*	120	19	70

Reprinted with permission from *Dietary reference intakes: calcium, phosphorus, magnesium, vitamin D, and fluoride*, National Academy Press, Washington, DC; *Dietary reference intakes for thiamin, riboflavin, niacin, vitamin B6, folate, vitamin B12, pantothenic acid, biotin, and choline*, National Academy Press, 1998. Courtesy of the National Academy Press, Washington, DC; and *Dietary reference intakes for vitamin C, vitamin E, selenium, and carotenoids*, National Academy Press, 2000. Courtesy of the National Academy Press, Washington, DC.

Note: This table presents Recommended Dietary Allowances (RDAs) in **bold** type and Adequate Intakes (AIs) in ordinary type followed by an asterisk (*). RDAs and AIs may both be used as goals for individual intake. RDAs are set to meet the needs of almost all (97 to 98%) of the individuals in a group. For healthy, breastfed infants, the AI is the mean intake. The AI for other life-stage groups is believed to cover their needs, but lack of data or uncertainty in the data prevent clear specification of this coverage.

[a] As niacin equivalents. 1 mg of niacin = 60 mg of tryptophan.

[b] As dietary folate equivalents (DFE). 1 DFE = 1 μg food folate = 0.6 μg of folic acid (from fortified food or supplement) consumed with food = 0.5 μg of synthetic (supplemental) folic acid taken on an empty stomach.

[c] Although AIs have been set for choline, few data are available to assess whether a dietary supply of choline is needed at all stages of the life cycle, and it may be that the choline requirement can be met by endogenous synthesis at some of these stages.

[d] Because 10 to 30 percent of older people may malabsorb food-bound B12, it is advisable for those older than 50 years to meet their RDA mainly by taking foods fortified with B12 or a B12-containing supplement.

[e] In view of evidence linking folate intake with neural tube defects in the fetus, it is recommended that all women capable of becoming pregnant consume 400 μg of synthetic folic acid from fortified foods and/or supplements in addition to intake of food folate from a varied diet.

[f] It is assumed that women will continue taking 400 μg of folic acid until their pregnancy is confirmed and they enter prenatal care, which ordinarily occurs after the end of the periconceptional period—the critical time for formation of the neural tube.

[g] As cholecalciferol. 1 μg cholecalciferol = 40 IU vitamin D. Needed in the absence of adequate exposure to sunlight.

[h] RDA for women 19-30 years. Add 10 mg for those 31-50.

Table 1-1B   Tolerable upper intake levels (UL)

Life-Stage Group	Niacin (mg/dl)*	Vitamin B_6 (mg/dl)	Synthetic Folic Acid* (µg/dl)	Choline (mg/dl)	Vitamin D† (µg/dl)	Calcium (g/dl)	Phosphorus (g/dl)	Magnesium (mg/dl)*	Fluoride (mg/dl)
0-6 mo	ND	ND	ND	ND	25	ND	ND	ND	0.7
6-12 mo	ND	ND	ND	ND	25	ND	ND	ND	0.9
1-3 yr	10	30	300	1000	50	2.5	3	65	1.3
4-8 yr	15	40	400	1000	50	2.5	3	110	2.2
9-13 yr	20	60	600	2000	50	2.5	4	350	10
14-18 yr	30	80	800	3000	50	2.5	4	350	10
19-70 yr	35	100	1000	3500	50	2.5	4	350	10
>70 yr	35	100	1000	3500	50	2.5	4	350	10
Pregnancy	35	100	1000	3500	50	2.5	3.5	350	10
Lactation	35	100	1000	3500	50	2.5	4	350	10

Reprinted with permission from *Dietary reference intakes: calcium, phosphorus, magnesium, vitamin D, and fluoride.* National Academy Press, 1997. Courtesy of the National Academy Press, Washington, DC; and *Dietary reference intakes for thiamin, riboflavin, niacin, vitamin B_6, folate, vitamin B_{12}, pantothenic acid, biotin, and choline.* National Academy Press, 1998. Courtesy of the National Academy Press, Washington, DC.

*The ULs for synthetic folic acid, niacin, and magnesium apply only to intakes from supplements, fortified foods, or pharmacologic agents, and not to intakes from food and water.

†As cholecalciferol. 1 µg cholecalciferol = 40 IU vitamin D.

The ULs have been established only for life-stage groups and not for separate genders.

ND = not determinable because of lack of data in this age group. Intake should be from food only to prevent high levels of intake.

climb the stairs rather than taking an elevator or use a bicycle rather than a car to run errands).

Build a healthy base

Let the pyramid guide your food choices

No single food provides all of the necessary nutrients in the amounts needed. By using many different foods, the person has the best chance of obtaining the different nutrients needed. Most food choices should be made from the five primary groups in the Food Guide Pyramid (discussed later in this chapter)—grains (breads, cereals, rice, pasta); vegetables; fruits; milk (milk, yogurt, and cheese); and meat and beans (meat, poultry, fish, dry beans, eggs, and nuts). Fats and sweets can be used occasionally to add variety to the diet. Food choices are determined by many factors, including culture, family background, religion and beliefs, life experiences, food intolerances and allergies, and cost and availability of food. It is possible to obtain a healthful diet with many different eating patterns. For example, milk is a good source of calcium, but adults in many cultures do not drink milk. By making wise food choices (e.g., using cheese, tofu or other soy products fortified with calcium, and fruit juices with added calcium), adequate calcium can be obtained without milk. In general, however, avoiding a whole group places the person at risk for deficiencies of one or more nutrients. For example, people who do not include vegetables and fruits in their diets regularly may not consume enough of the vitamins A and C. Dietary supplements may be needed by some individuals. Women who could become pregnant need a folic acid supplement or regular intake of folic acid-fortified foods. Older adults and people with little sun exposure may need a vitamin D supplement. Individuals who eat no animal products (and many older adults) need a supplement of vitamin B_{12}.

Choose a variety of grains daily, especially whole grains

Whole grains, fruits, and vegetables are an excellent source of fiber. Enriched grains are a good source of folic acid and other B vitamins. Folic acid taken during pregnancy reduces the risk of serious congenital disorders known as neural tube defects and may reduce the risk of coronary artery disease and certain cancers.

Choose a variety of fruits and vegetables daily

Vegetables and fruits are good sources of vitamins, minerals, complex carbohydrates (starch and dietary fiber), and other nutrients and **phytochemicals** (nonnutrients in plant foods that have health-protective effects). Most plant foods are also naturally low in fat. Fiber intake is likely to be low among individuals in many industrialized countries, which can contribute to constipation and an increased risk of cardiovascular disease, diverticulosis, colon cancer, and diabetes. The fiber recommendation for adults in the United States is 25 to 30 g per day, but the average intake is only about half that. Fiber intake can be increased with a diet that includes whole grains, dry beans, and fiber-rich vegetables and fruits daily (see Appendix B). Dark green leafy and yellow vegetables are good sources of β-carotene and other vitamin A precursors and should be chosen frequently.

Phytochemicals include a variety of diverse compounds that act in many ways to prevent or delay chronic illnesses. For example, polyphenols found in tea (especially green tea), cereal grains, and many fruits and vegetables have antioxidant properties and may help reduce the risk of both heart disease and cancer. Flavonoids in citrus and other fruits, vegetables, grains, wine, and tea apparently act by several mechanisms to reduce tumor initiation and growth. Genistein from soy inhibits the growth of human breast and prostate cancer cells, and soy has cholesterol- and triglyceride-lowering effects. Because the identities of all the phytochemicals, their optimal intakes, and their potential interactions with other phytochemicals and nutrients remain unclear, a varied diet with ample servings of plant foods appears the best way to obtain them.

Keep food safe to eat

Foodborne illness results from eating food that contains harmful bacteria, toxins, parasites, viruses, or chemical contaminants. Appendix K summarizes approaches to maintaining food safety.

Choose sensibly

Choose a diet that is low in saturated fat and cholesterol and moderate in total fat

A diet high in saturated fat and cholesterol is linked to elevated blood cholesterol levels and to heart disease. A diet high in total fat is linked to obesity and increased risk of some cancers (e.g., colon, breast). Fat is higher in calories than either protein or carbohydrate, and a high-fat diet (more than 30% of calories from fat) may make it difficult to get the variety of nutrients needed without consuming excessive calories.

The *Dietary Guidelines* recommend that fat supply no more than 30% of calories in the diet, saturated fat account for no more than 10% of calories, and cholesterol intake total no more than 300 mg/day. (These guidelines do not apply to children under the age of 2.) Most of the fat in the diet should be monounsaturated and polyunsaturated fatty acids (Figure 1-1), which are found in olive, canola, sunflower, safflower, soybean, and corn oils, nuts, and high-fat fish. *Trans* fatty acids, found in hydrogenated fats (in most shortenings and stick margarines and many processed foods), raise low-density-lipoprotein (LDL) cholesterol levels, and elevated LDL cholesterol is a risk factor for heart disease. A safe level of trans fatty acid intake has not been established, but the best current advice is to check the ingredient listings on food products and to consume those products containing hydrogenated fats only occasionally. Also, use margarines sold in squeeze bottles and tubs; these products generally contain less hydrogenated fat than stick margarines.

Eating fish regularly appears to reduce the risk of heart disease. Many fish from cold waters are rich in *omega-3* fats, which are used in synthesis of eicosanoids (vital compounds regulating many body processes); omega-3 fatty acids may help to reduce blood pressure and to prevent clumping of platelets, which can block cardiac blood vessels and contribute to myocardial infarction.

In order to control the intake of fat and saturated fat, individuals should use fats and oils sparingly. The Nutrition Facts Label (described later in this chapter) helps consumers choose foods lower in fat, saturated fat, and cholesterol. Fruits, vegetables, and grain products (without added fat) are good choices. Other ways to reduce fat intake include using low-fat milk products, lean meats, fish, and poultry and replacing animal proteins with dried beans (navy, pinto, kidney, garbanzo, etc.) and peas often.

Choose beverages and foods to moderate your intake of sugars

Sugars are one form of carbohydrates. During digestion, all carbohydrates except fiber break down into sugars, and many foods are either natural sources of sugars or have sugar added during preparation. Frequent eating of foods high in sugars and starches between meals and failure to brush the teeth after eating carbohydrates increase the risk of tooth decay. Sugar should be used only in moderation and should be used sparingly if calorie needs are low. The nutrition label lists the amount of sugars in foods.

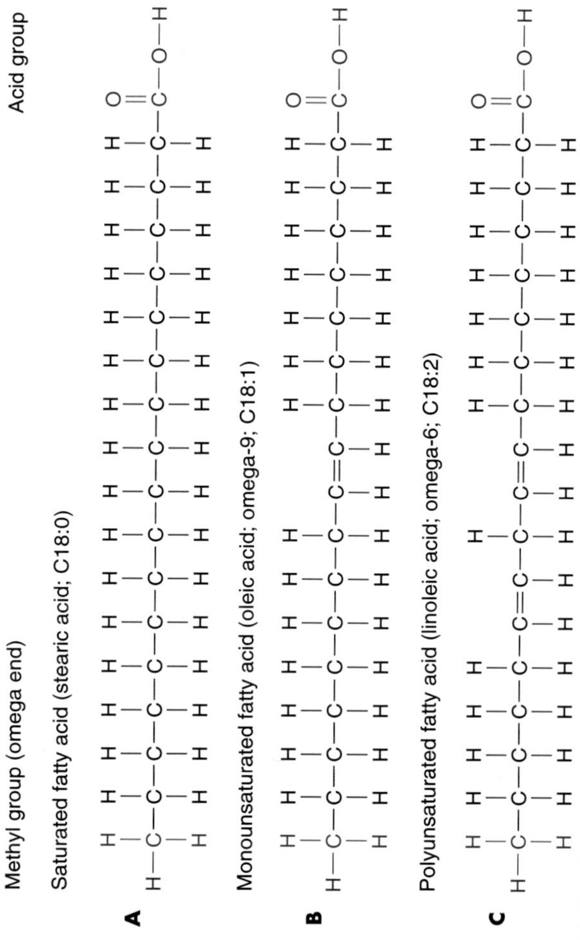

Methyl group (omega end)

Acid group

A   Saturated fatty acid (stearic acid; C18:0)

B   Monounsaturated fatty acid (oleic acid; omega-9; C18:1)

C   Polyunsaturated fatty acid (linoleic acid; omega-6; C18:2)

Polyunsaturated fatty acid (alpha-linolenic acid; omega-3; C18:3)

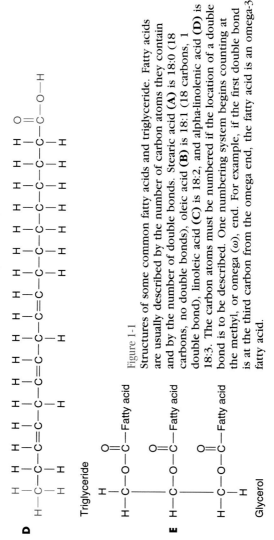

D

Triglyceride

E

Glycerol

Figure 1-1

Structures of some common fatty acids and triglyceride. Fatty acids are usually described by the number of carbon atoms they contain and by the number of double bonds. Stearic acid (**A**) is 18:0 (18 carbons, no double bonds), oleic acid (**B**) is 18:1 (18 carbons, 1 double bond), linoleic acid (**C**) is 18:2, and alpha-linolenic acid (**D**) is 18:3. The carbon atoms must be numbered if the location of a double bond is to be described. One numbering system begins counting at the methyl, or omega (ω), end. For example, if the first double bond is at the third carbon from the omega end, the fatty acid is an omega-3 fatty acid.

Choose and prepare foods with less salt

Most sodium and sodium chloride (salt) in the diet is added during processing and preparation of foods. The suggested **Daily Value (DV)** for sodium on the Nutrition Facts Label is no more than 2400 mg, but most Americans consume at least 1.5 to 2 times this amount. The DV is a reference value based on the RDA and used on food labels to provide a guide to the amount of a particular nutrient that the daily diet should contain. Many people at risk for hypertension reduce their chances of developing this condition by reducing their sodium intake. To help reduce sodium intake, choose fresh fruits and vegetables, most of which are naturally low in sodium; read nutrition labels to help identify foods lower in sodium within each group; and flavor foods with herbs and spices rather than salt or seasoning salts.

If you drink alcoholic beverages, do so in moderation

Alcoholic beverages provide calories but few nutrients. Current evidence suggests that moderate drinking is associated with a lower risk for coronary heart disease in some individuals and that red wine, in particular, may be beneficial. Moderate consumption is defined as no more than one drink per day for women or two drinks per day for men. A drink equals 12 oz of regular beer, 1 glass (5 oz) of wine, or 1.5 oz (1 jigger) of distilled spirits. Higher levels of alcohol intake raise the risk for hypertension, stroke, heart disease, certain cancers, accidents, violence, suicides, birth defects, and overall mortality. Excessive alcohol intake may cause cirrhosis of the liver, pancreatitis, and damage to the brain and heart. Heavy drinkers also are at risk of malnutrition because alcohol contains calories that may substitute for those in more nutritious foods.

Some people should not drink alcoholic beverages at all. These include children and adolescents, individuals of any age who cannot restrict their drinking to moderate levels, women who are trying to conceive or who are pregnant, individuals who plan to drive or take part in activities that require attention or skill, and individuals using many prescription and over-the-counter medications. These individuals can obtain the health benefits of wine by consuming purple grape juice instead.

Food Guide Pyramid

The Food Guide Pyramid (Figure 1-2) is a simple tool for helping individuals to ensure a varied diet. The grain group is at the base and is the largest to demonstrate that it should provide the basis for

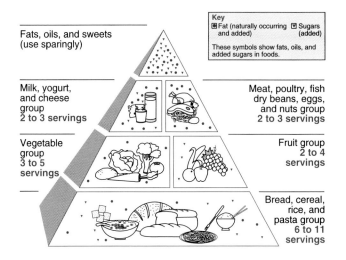

Food group*	Serving size
Grain products	1 slice bread, 1 roll or muffin, 1/2 bagel or hamburger bun
	1 oz ready-to-eat cereal
	1/2 cup rice, pasta, cooked cereal
Vegetable	1 cup raw leafy greens
	1/2 cup of all others, cooked or raw
	1/4 cup vegetable juice
Fruit	1 medium apple, orange, pear, banana
	1/2 cup chopped, cooked, or canned fruit
	1/4 cup juice
Milk	1 cup milk or yogurt
	1 1/2 oz natural cheese or 2 oz processed cheese
Meat and beans	2 to 3 oz cooked lean meat, poultry, or fish
	(1/2 cup cooked dried beans or peas or 1 egg = 1 oz lean meat; 2 tbsp peanut butter or 1/3 cup nuts = 1 oz meat)

* Some foods fit into more than one group. Dry beans, peas, and lentils can be counted as servings in either the meat and beans group or vegetable group, but not in both groups.

Figure 1-2

Food Guide Pyramid: a guide to daily food choices.
(From U.S. Department of Agriculture and U.S. Department of Health and Human Services.)

a healthful diet. The vegetable and fruit groups are next in size to emphasize their importance in nutrition. At the next level are milk products and the group containing meats and plant sources of protein. These groups provide valuable nutrients such as calcium, protein, and iron, but some of the foods in these groups are also rich in fat. Thus, excessive servings from these groups are undesirable. The narrow apex of the pyramid is assigned to fats, oils, and sweets, to illustrate that they should be used in only limited amounts. Many combination foods such as soups, stews, pizza, and casseroles contain servings from more than one food group.

Nutrition Labeling

Nutrition labeling is required on almost all processed foods, meat, and poultry (Figure 1-3). Similar information also appears near fresh produce in many markets. This labeling is a valuable source of information for the consumer who is trying to choose a healthful diet or modify his or her diet (e.g., reduce fat or sodium intake) and is a useful tool for health care professionals engaged in educating their patients about nutrition. The total kilocalorie (kcal) content and kcal from fat must appear on the label to help consumers meet the dietary guidelines recommending no more than 30% of kcal from fat. Also included on the label are the amounts of total fat, saturated fat, cholesterol, sodium, total carbohydrate, dietary fiber, sugars, and protein. Polyunsaturated and monounsaturated fat and potassium are optional. Various vitamins and minerals appear on the label, depending on the food's nutritional composition. Information about most nutrients is expressed in both units of weight (g or mg) and %DV. Labels must express DV in relation to a 2000 kcal diet, a caloric level that meets the energy needs of many adults. For example, fat should provide no more than 30% of the total kcal intake (600 kcal or approximately 65 g per day for the person consuming 2000 kcal). A food that provides 13 g of fat in one serving (see Figure 1-3) provides at least 20% of the fat included in a 2000 kcal diet. Food labels may contain information about DVs for other caloric intakes, if there is room. A shortened form of the food label may be found on small food packages.

The Food and Drug Administration (FDA) has created guidelines to make food labels more informative for consumers who want to choose a healthful diet. These guidelines include definitions for the use of specific terms, such as *low fat* and *light* in food labeling (Box 1-1), as well as a description of 10 types of health claims

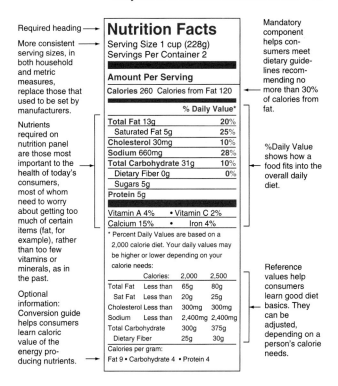

Required heading →

More consistent serving sizes, in both household and metric measures, replace those that used to be set by manufacturers.

Nutrients required on nutrition panel are those most important to the health of today's consumers, most of whom need to worry about getting too much of certain items (fat, for example), rather than too few vitamins or minerals, as in the past.

Optional information: Conversion guide helps consumers learn caloric value of the energy pro- ducing nutrients.

Mandatory component helps con- sumers meet dietary guide- lines recom- mending no more than 30% of calories from fat.

%Daily Value shows how a food fits into the overall daily diet.

Reference values help consumers learn good diet basics. They can be adjusted, depending on a person's calorie needs.

Nutrition Facts

Serving Size 1 cup (228g)
Servings Per Container 2

Amount Per Serving

Calories 260 Calories from Fat 120

	% Daily Value*
Total Fat 13g	20%
Saturated Fat 5g	25%
Cholesterol 30mg	10%
Sodium 660mg	28%
Total Carbohydrate 31g	10%
Dietary Fiber 0g	0%
Sugars 5g	
Protein 5g	

Vitamin A 4%	•	Vitamin C 2%
Calcium 15%	•	Iron 4%

* Percent Daily Values are based on a 2,000 calorie diet. Your daily values may be higher or lower depending on your calorie needs:

		Calories:	2,000	2,500
Total Fat	Less than		65g	80g
Sat Fat	Less than		20g	25g
Cholesterol	Less than		300mg	300mg
Sodium	Less than		2,400mg	2,400mg
Total Carbohydrate			300g	375g
Dietary Fiber			25g	30g

Calories per gram:
Fat 9 • Carbohydrate 4 • Protein 4

Figure 1-3
Nutrition label.
(From *FDA Consumer* 27(4):23, 1993.)

(relationships between diet and specific diseases) that can be included on food labels (Box 1-2).

Cultural Influences on Nutrition

Not all food choices are made because of nutritional considerations, of course. Economic constraints, peer pressure, persuasive adver- tising, and convenience are just a few of the factors influencing food choices. Cultural practices, including those shaped by national, ethnic, or religious background, can exert strong influences on eating patterns.

Box 1-1   Some Terms Used on Food Labels and Their Definitions

Free

Contains none, or an insignificant amount, of a particular component (fat, saturated fat, cholesterol, sodium, sugars, or calories). Per serving a fat-free food contains <0.5 g fat, a sugar-free food contains <0.5 g sugar, and a sodium-free food contains <5 mg sodium.

Good Source or High

Good source: contains 10-19% of the Daily Value for a particular nutrient. High (or "rich in" or "excellent source of"): contains 20% or more of the Daily Value for a particular nutrient. Usually applied to fiber or a vitamin or mineral

Lean or Extra Lean

Lean: contains <10 g fat, <4 g saturated fat, and <95 mg cholesterol per serving and per 100 g. Extra lean: contains <5 g fat, <2 g saturated fat, and <95 mg cholesterol per serving and per 100 g. Used in describing the fat content of meat, poultry, seafood, and game.

Light or Lite

Contains one third fewer calories or one half the fat of the reference food.* A low-calorie, low-fat food can also be referred to as "light in sodium" if it contains 50% or less sodium than the reference food.

Reduced or Less

Contains at least 25% less of a particular component (sugar, fat, cholesterol, saturated fat, or sodium) per serving than the reference food.

Adapted from Stehlin D: A little 'lite' reading, *FDA Consumer* 27(4):29, 1993.
*A reference food is a non-nutritionally altered version of the same food product, e.g., a regular chocolate cake mix would be the reference food for a chocolate cake mix labeled "low-fat."

Box 1-1   Some Terms Used on Food Labels
and Their Definitions—cont'd

Low

Contains only a small amount of a particular food component, e.g., per serving (or per 50 g, if the normal serving size is 30 g or 2 tablespoons or less); low calorie means 40 calories or less, low fat means 3 g fat or less, low cholesterol means 20 mg or less, and low sodium means 140 mg or less. "Very low," applied only to sodium, means 35 mg or less per serving.

More or Added Fiber

Contains at least 2.5 g more fiber per serving than the reference food.

Immigrants and their families gradually adopt the typical American diet, especially as new generations are born in North America. This transition occurs both because it may be difficult or expensive to obtain particular foods and because of a desire to fit in with the dominant society. Nevertheless, it is helpful to be aware of some characteristic cultural food practices. Appreciation of distinct cultural food habits helps the health care professional to demonstrate respect for both the individual and the culture and to be aware of food habits that may need modification. It may be possible to use cultural pride to reinforce or promote healthier eating habits. For instance, obesity is extremely prevalent among native Hawaiians. One program encourages weight loss among native Hawaiians by emphasizing use of native foods, which are lower in fat than the foods chosen by most Americans.

Some cultural food practices that are prevalent in the United States are summarized in Table 1-2. Native Americans are not included in the table because the eating patterns of such a diverse group are not easily categorized. Alcoholism is a serious problem among most Native American groups, however, and diabetes is increasingly common among many tribal groups, particularly those in the Southwest.

Box 1-2 Health Claims Permitted on Food Labels*

Calcium and reduction in the risk of osteoporosis

Foods or supplements must be "high" in calcium and must not contain more phosphorus than calcium.

Sodium and reduction in the risk of hypertension (high blood pressure)

Foods must meet the criteria for "low sodium."

Dietary fat and reduction in cancer risk

Foods must meet the definition of "low fat," and the claim must refer to total fat rather than any specific type of fat. Fish and game must meet the definition for "extra lean."

Dietary saturated fat and cholesterol and reduction in risk of coronary heart disease

Foods must meet the definition of "low saturated fat," "low cholesterol," and "low fat." Fish and game must meet the definition for "extra lean."

Fiber-containing grain products, fruits, and vegetables and reduction of cancer risk

Foods must meet the definition for "low fat" and, without fortification, be a "good source" of dietary fiber. The claim must not mention particular types of fiber.

Fruits, vegetables, and grain products that contain fiber, particularly soluble fiber, and reduction in the risk of coronary heart disease

Food must meet the definition of "low saturated fat," "low cholesterol," and "low fat." It must contain, without fortification, at least 0.6 g soluble fiber per reference amount, and the soluble fiber amount must be listed.

Fruits and vegetables and reduction of cancer risk

Foods must meet the criteria for "low fat" and, without fortification, be a "good source" of fiber, vitamin A, or vitamin C.

Adapted from *FDA Consumer* 32(6):22, 1998.

*The claims cannot state that a particular food or nutrient will prevent disease; "may" and "might" are the preferred terms. The claims must state that disease risk depends on factors other than a particular food or nutrient. For example, regular exercise, in addition to calcium intake, reduces the risk of osteoporosis.

Box 1-2 Health Claims Permitted on Food Labels—cont'd

Folate and reduction in the risk of neural tube defects

Foods must meet the criteria for "good source" of folate and must not provide more than 100% of the Daily Value for vitamins A and D because of their potential risk to fetuses.

Dietary sugar alcohol and reduction in the risk of dental caries (cavities)

Foods or sugarless gums must meet the criteria for "sugar-free" and must contain a sugar alcohol that does not promote tooth decay.

Dietary soluble fiber, such as that found in whole oats and psyllium seed husk, and reduction in the risk of coronary heart disease

Foods must meet the definition of "low saturated fat," "low cholesterol," and "low fat." Foods that contain whole oats or psyllium must provide at least 0.75 or 1.7 g soluble fiber per serving, respectively.

Two types of vegetarian diets are described in the table, but many others exist, including pescovegetarians, who avoid animal products except fish, and individuals who avoid red meats but eat all other animal products. Thus, the term *vegetarian* tells little about food intake, and the health care provider will need to get more information in order to assess the diet and determine whether intervention and teaching are needed.

Physiologic Influences on Nutrition: Digestion and Absorption

During digestion, foods are broken down mechanically by chewing and by mixing motions in the stomach and small intestine. Most carbohydrates, proteins, and fats in the diet are too large to be absorbed even after this mechanical breakdown and must be further digested by enzymes (proteins that produce chemical changes in

Text continued on p. 25

Table 1-2   Cultural Food Practices

Characteristic Food Practices	Health Implications
African-American*	
Cooking methods: Frying common; vegetables often boiled for prolonged periods and seasoned with salt pork (fat-back); gravy often served	*Positives:* Many different vegetables consumed
Foods enjoyed: Chicken, barbecue pork, ham, chitterlings (boiled or fried pig intestines), grits (coarsely ground corn that is boiled and usually served with butter or margarine), greens (especially collards, mustard), okra (boiled or fried), tomatoes, sweet and white potatoes, biscuits, cornbread, melons, peaches, pecans, and peanuts	*Concerns:* Fat and sodium intake often high; many adults have little milk intake (lactose intolerance common); pica (eating nonfood items such as soil or clay) occurs especially among women and may inhibit iron absorption. *Prevalent nutrition-related problems:* Obesity, hypertension, and heart disease; iron deficiency anemia among women
Mexican-American (also applies to some Central Americans)	
Cooking methods: Boiling, stewing; vegetables often cooked for a long time	*Positives:* Wide variety of fruits and vegetables liked
Foods enjoyed: Dry beans (pinto, garbanzo, black beans; beans often mashed and cooked with lard), beef, pork, chicken, fish, goat, eggs, hot sausage, tripe (beef stomach), rice, corn or flour tortillas, sweet pastries, cookies, candies (often candied fruits), chilies, pumpkin, chayote squash, corn, prickly pear cactus leaves (nopales), avocado, tomatoes, citrus, papaya, cilantro	*Concerns:* High fat intake; lard used in Mexico and by recent immigrants; margarine, oils, and mayonnaise widely used in the U.S.; little milk used by adults; sugar intake high *Prevalent nutrition-related problems:* Diabetes and obesity

*This diet is often referred to as African-American "soul food," but many African-Americans have Southern roots. These foods and cooking methods are also typical "home cooking" of Southern whites.

Table 1-2   Cultural Food Practices—cont'd

Characteristic Food Practices	Health Implications
Puerto Rican	
Cooking methods: Frying, boiling, or simmering for prolonged periods with lard or salt pork for seasoning	*Positives:* Many fruits and vegetables used in Puerto Rico
Foods enjoyed: Cafe con leche (coffee with 2 to 5 oz milk), beans (esp. red or white), rice, pork, chicken, eggs, viandas (mixture of plantains, sweet potatoes, and green bananas), breadfruit, mango, avocado, corn, okra, chayote, safrito (relish of tomatoes, green peppers, chilies, onions, spices, and oil or lard)	*Concerns:* High fat intake; adults have little milk intake unless coffee intake is also high; foods used in Puerto Rico are often expensive on the North American mainland, so diets there may have little variety
Food beliefs: Diseases are categorized as hot or cold, and foods are divided into hot, cold, and cool; suitability of a food in sickness or postpartum depends on its category; malt beer believed to be nutritious, often given to children and lactating women	*Prevalent nutrition-related problems:* Obesity; megaloblastic anemia among women in the mainland because of poor folic acid intake

Continued

Table 1-2   Cultural Food Practices—cont'd

Characteristic Food Practices	Health Implications
Southeast Asian (Vietnamese, Cambodian)	
Cooking methods: Stir-frying, steaming *Foods enjoyed:* Fish, duck, chicken, eggs, pork, tofu (soybean curd), chicken—rice noodle soup, green leafy vegetables, white rice, "cellophane" (bean starch) noodles, French bread and pastries, tea	*Positives:* Low-fat cooking methods; limited intake of high-fat animal products; high complex carbohydrates and low sugar intakes *Concerns:* Little milk product use among adults *Prevalent nutrition-related problems:* Osteoporosis among women, anemia, dental caries
Japanese	
Cooking methods: Stir-frying, steaming, broiling, simmering *Foods enjoyed:* Rice, noodles, many vegetables, fish, tofu and other soy products, pickles, green tea	*Positives:* Traditional diet low in fat, high in complex carbohydrates, rich in vegetables *Concerns:* Japanese diet ~4 times as high in sodium as American; gastric cancer rate high in Japan, probably related to use of dried, smoked fish high in nitrates; little milk intake among adults; raw fish (sashimi) consumed by Japanese, potential for food poisoning and tapeworms

Table 1-2   Cultural Food Practices—cont'd

Characteristic Food Practices	Health Implications
Chinese	
Cooking methods: Broiling, steaming, frying, or simmering	*Positives:* Usually a low-fat diet; vegetables used often
Foods enjoyed: Rice, noodles, tofu and other soybean products, pork, chicken, many vegetables, tea	*Concerns:* Sodium intake can be high; lactose intolerance common among adults
Former Soviet Union	
Cooking methods: Boiling, steaming, stewing, pickling of vegetables	*Positives:* Frequent use of grain products (encourage whole-grain breads and flours); use of vegetables in soups, stuffed pastries, salads
Foods enjoyed: Breads, rice, pasta, dumplings, pancake-like breads (blini, oladi), cabbage, potatoes, beets, cucumbers, mushrooms, carrots, berries, pears, cherries, grapes, apples, goose, fresh or smoked salted fish, ground beef, cold cuts, eggs, oil, butter, salad dressings, sour cream or soured milk, whole milk, tea, jams	*Concerns:* Very high-fat diet; sodium intake can be high (pickled vegetables, salted fish) *Prevalent nutrition-related problems:* Heart disease

Continued

specific nutrients) in the lumen or brush border of the intestine (Figure 1-4).

Energy-Providing Nutrients and the Products of Their Digestion
Carbohydrates

Carbohydrates can be large, small, or intermediate in size. *Polysaccharides* such as the starches are the largest carbohydrates. They are found in grains, legumes, potatoes, and other vegetables. Polysaccharides are formed from many *monosaccharide* (glucose,

Table 1-2   Cultural Food Practices—cont'd

Characteristic Food Practices	Health Implications
Jewish	
Cooking methods: Boiling, stewing, many meats salted; "Kashruth," or Jewish food laws, are followed; milk products and meat are not combined in food preparation; utensils used to prepare or serve meat not used for milk products and vice versa; milk consumption must occur at least 3 to 6 hours after meat; "pareve" foods (e.g., fish, eggs, some margarines, and breads) contain neither meat nor dairy products and may be used with either	*Positives:* A wide variety of foods from all groups are included in the kashruth
Foods enjoyed: Milk, cheese, eggs, fish with scales and fins, wide variety of vegetables, fruits, and breads; beef, lamb, poultry must be slaughtered and prepared in kosher manner; packaged foods are marked with a K, ⓚ, U, or other symbol to indicate that they are kosher	*Concerns:* Many meats salted; fasting is practiced on Yom Kippur, but pregnant women and sick individuals are not required to fast; wine is a necessary part of the Passover seder, but grape juice may be substituted or very small amounts of wine consumed
Foods not used: Pork, horsemeat, or meat of any other animal without cloven hooves; fish without fins or scales; shellfish; during Passover (8 days in spring), certain foods (e.g., bread products) must be "kosher for Passover" and no leavenings are used	

Table 1-2   Cultural Food Practices—cont'd

Characteristic Food Practices	Health Implications
Ovolactovegetarian (e.g., Seventh-Day Adventist)	
Cooking methods: All	*Positives:* Lower rates
Foods enjoyed: Milk and milk products, eggs, all fruits, vegetables, soy, and grain products; Seventh-Day Adventists use cereal-based beverages (Postum) and meat analogues made from soy or other vegetable proteins	of certain cancers than general population; diet tends to be lower fat; provides all known nutrients
Foods not used: Meat, poultry, fish; Seventh-Day Adventists avoid caffeinated beverages	*Concerns:* Absorption of iron and zinc may be poor
Strict vegetarian (e.g., vegan)	
Cooking methods: All, steaming and stir-frying popular	*Positives:* Tends to be low in fat and high in fiber, reducing risk of heart disease, obesity, and some cancers; combining grains, legumes, nuts, and seeds yields adequate protein
Foods enjoyed: Grains (esp. whole grains), fruits, vegetables, soy and fermented soy products, oils, nuts and seeds	
Foods not used: Any animal products (milk, eggs, cheese, yogurt, meat, fish, poultry); some avoid fortified foods and nutritional supplements	*Concerns:* Vitamin B_{12} is found only in foods of animal origin, supplements, and fortified foods; fermented soy products (miso and tempeh) are not reliable sources of vitamin B_{12}; calcium intake often low; absorption of iron and zinc often poor; inadequate caloric density for optimal growth in children

Continued

Table 1-2   Cultural Food Practices—cont'd

Characteristic Food Practices	Health Implications
Middle Eastern (Syria, Lebanon, Turkey, Jordan, Iraq, Iran, Greece, Israel, Egypt)	
Cooking methods: Meats cooked in a large amount of animal fat (butter or ghee, a clarified butter from sheep, goat, or camel milk) or oil (olive, sesame) *Foods enjoyed:* Breads (have almost sacred status), rice, pilaf, beans, lentils, yogurt, cheese, lamb, goat, olives, cucumbers, citrus, onions, tomatoes, eggplant, dates, figs, pomegranates, baklava (layered pastry with honey and nuts), seasonings of cinnamon, mint, and oregano *Foods not used:* Muslims avoid alcohol and pork	*Positives:* Fruit served for dessert except on special occasions; breads usually whole-grain and rich in fiber; yogurt used in many foods; avoidance of alcohol-related health problems by Muslims *Concerns:* High-fat cooking methods; females assigned lower status by some Middle Easterners, so may have to eat after males; quantity and variety of available food less for females; fasting during daylight hours required of Muslims for the month of Ramadan; pregnant and lactating women, travelers, or the sick may delay the fast until later in the year

fructose, mannose, or galactose) units, and they must be broken down into these units so that they can be absorbed. *Dextrins* and *oligosaccharides* are compounds made up of chains of glucose molecules (usually 3 to 20 glucose units). They are formed during digestion of starch and must be further digested to allow absorption. Dextrins and oligosaccharides are used commercially in the manufacturing of medical foods for enteral tube feedings and nutritional supplements. *Disaccharides* are sugars composed of two monosaccharides. Sucrose is a disaccharide composed of glucose and fructose. It is found in table sugar, brown sugar, maple syrup,

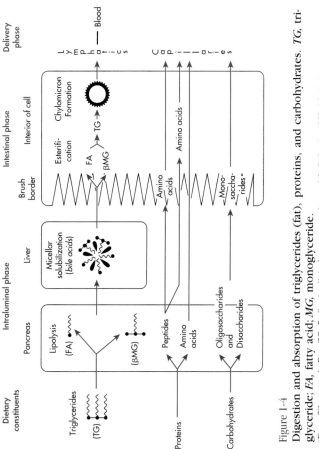

Figure 1-4

Digestion and absorption of triglycerides (fat), proteins, and carbohydrates. *TG,* triglyceride; *FA,* fatty acid; *MG,* monoglyceride.
(From Silverman A, Roy CC: *Pediatric clinical gastroenterology,* ed 3, St Louis, 1983, Mosby.)

and molasses. Lactose is a disaccharide found in milk and consisting of glucose and galactose. Maltose is a disaccharide consisting of two glucose molecules; maltose is not common in the diet, but it is produced during digestion of starch. In addition to being building blocks for larger carbohydrates, the monosaccharides glucose and fructose are found by themselves in foods such as honey and fruits. Dietary monosaccharides and disaccharides are often called *simple sugars.*

Proteins

Dietary *proteins* are compounds made up of hundreds of *amino acids,* or nitrogen-containing molecules. During the digestion of a protein, *polypeptides,* or compounds containing fewer than 100 amino acids, and *peptides* (shorter chains of amino acids), are formed from the protein. These intermediate products must be further digested into amino acids or di- and tripeptides (compounds containing two or three amino acids) to be absorbed. After absorption, the di- and tripeptides are further digested to amino acids, which can be used for synthesis of body proteins.

Fats or lipids

Most dietary fat, and most fat stored in the body, is in the form of *triglycerides* (see Figure 1-1). A triglyceride is a molecule formed from glycerol (a 3-carbon alcohol) bonded or esterified with 3 fatty acids. A *fatty acid* is a chain of carbon atoms (usually 2 to 22 atoms long) with hydrogen attached; the chain contains a methyl group (CH_3) on one end and an acid group (COOH) on the other end. Fatty acids can be saturated (with no carbon-carbon double bonds) or unsaturated (with one or more carbon-carbon double bonds). Triglycerides must be digested into smaller forms to be absorbed. A *diglyceride* is a molecule composed of glycerol bonded to 2 fatty acids; it is produced during triglyceride digestion. A diglyceride is broken down further, into a *monoglyceride* (a molecule composed of glycerol bonded to 1 fatty acid) or to glycerol and fatty acids, and these products can be absorbed.

Process of Digestion and Absorption

Table 1-3 summarizes the major enzymes involved in digestion, the sites where they are released, and the products of their action. Most nutrients are absorbed in the duodenum, jejunum, and ileum (Figure 1-5); therefore, damage to or surgical removal of a significant

Table 1-3   Summary of the Major Digestive Enzymes

Enzyme	Site of Production	Process of Digestion
Carbohydrate Digestion		
Salivary amylase	Mouth	Starch → Oligosaccharides, dextrins, and maltose
Pancreatic amylase	Pancreas (released into intestine)	Starch → Oligosaccharides, dextrins, and maltose
"Brush border" enzymes	Small intestine (inside mucosal cells)	Oligosaccharides and dextrins → Maltose and glucose
Isomaltase and glucoamylase		
Lactase		Lactose → Glucose and galactose
Maltase		Maltose → Glucose
Sucrase		Sucrose → Glucose and fructose
Protein Digestion		
Pepsin	Stomach	Proteins → Polypeptides
Trypsin, chymotrypsin	Pancreas (released into small intestine)	Proteins, polypeptides → Small polypeptides
Carboxypeptidase	Pancreas (released into small intestine)	Polypeptides → Small peptides, amino acids
Aminopeptidase	Intestine	Polypeptides, small peptides → Smaller peptides, amino acids
Dipeptidase	Intestine	Dipeptides → Amino acids
Fat Digestion		
Lingual lipase (significant only in infants)	Mouth	Triglycerides → Diglycerides (glycerol linked to 2 fatty acids), monoglycerides (glycerol linked to 1 fatty acid), glycerol, fatty acids
Lipase	Pancreas (released into small intestine)	Fat → Diglycerides, monoglycerides, glycerol, fatty acids

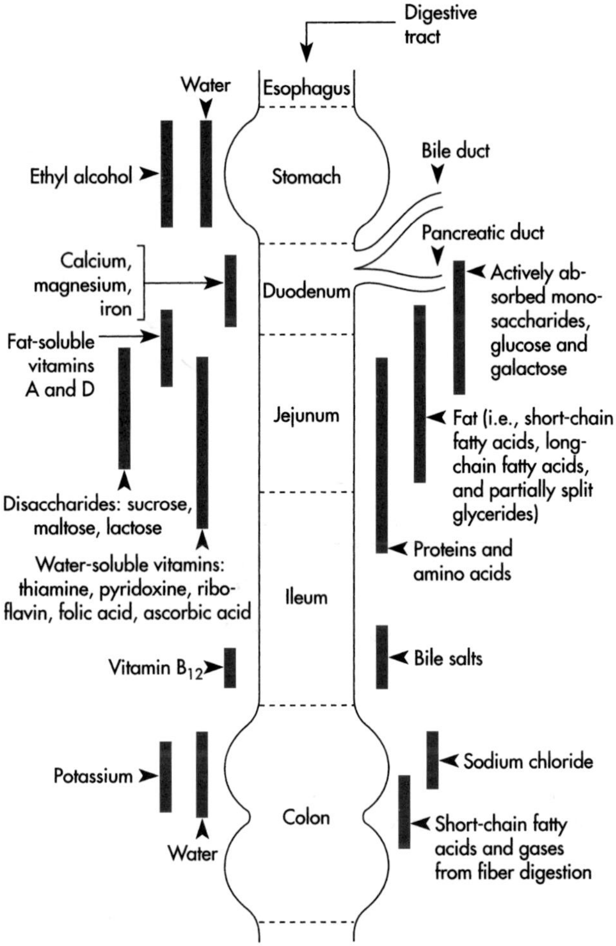

Figure 1-5
Sites of nutrient absorption.
(From Heimburger DC, Weinsier RL: *Handbook of clinical nutrition,* ed 3, St Louis, 1997, Mosby.)

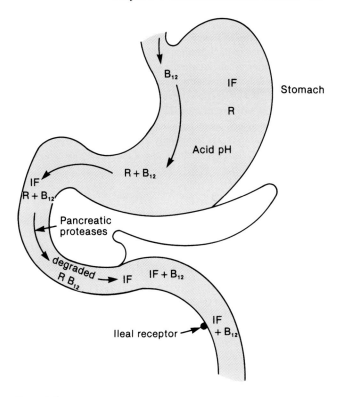

Figure 1-6
Absorption of vitamin B$_{12}$. *IF,* Intrinsic factor; *R,* R protein.
(Reprinted from *Nutrition Research,* 9, Sauberlich HE, Bioavailability of vitamins, 1, Copyright 1985, with permission from Elsevier Science.)

portion of the small intestine often leads to malabsorption of a nutrient or nutrients.

Fat and fat-soluble vitamin absorption is a complicated process (see Chapter 9). Vitamin B$_{12}$ absorption differs from that of other nutrients (Figure 1-6). Vitamin B$_{12}$ is released from foods by hydrochloric acid in the stomach. The free vitamin B$_{12}$ then binds to *R protein,* which is produced by the salivary glands in the mouth. This vitamin-protein complex moves to the small intestine, where trypsin (an enzyme produced by the pancreas) cleaves the vitamin-protein bond, releasing vitamin B$_{12}$. Then vitamin B$_{12}$

binds with intrinsic factor (IF), a protein produced in the stomach. The IF-B_{12} complex travels to the ileum, where the complex binds to specific sites in the intestinal wall and vitamin B_{12} is absorbed. Any condition that interferes with hydrochloric acid or IF production (e.g., gastrectomy, aging) or the absorptive sites in the ileum (e.g., ileal resection, inflammatory bowel disease or other inflammatory process, or mucosal damage during radiation therapy or chemotherapy of cancer) can result in vitamin B_{12} deficiency. In addition, vitamin B_{12} is found only in foods derived from animals (meat, poultry, fish, eggs, milk), and thus vegetarians who avoid these foods may become deficient.

SELECTED BIBLIOGRAPHY

Douglas KC, Fujimoto D: Asian Pacific elders: implications for health care providers, *Clin Geriatr Med* 11:69, 1995.

Dwyer J: Is there a need to change the American diet? *Adv Exp Med Biol* 401:189, 1996.

Eliades DC, Suitor CW: *Celebrating diversity: approaching families through their food,* Arlington, VA, 1994, National Center for Education in Maternal and Child Health.

Food and Nutrition Board, National Academy of Sciences, Institute of Medicine: *Dietary reference intakes: calcium, phosphorus, magnesium, vitamin D, and fluoride,* Washington, DC, 1997, National Academy Press. Available online at www.nas.edu

Food and Nutrition Board, National Academy of Sciences, Institute of Medicine: *Dietary reference intakes for thiamin, riboflavin, niacin, vitamin B_6, folate, vitamin B_{12}, pantothenic acid, biotin, and choline,* Washington, DC, 1998, National Academy Press. Available online at www.nas.edu

Haddad EH: Development of a vegetarian food guide, *Am J Clin Nutr* 59:1248S, 1994.

Healthy People 2010, Washington, DC, 2000, U.S. Department of Health and Human Services.

Kuczmarski MF, Kuczmarski RJ, Najjar M: Food usage among Mexican-American, Cuban, and Puerto Rican adults, *Nutr Today* 30:30, 1995.

National Academy of Sciences: *Recommended dietary allowances,* ed 10, Washington, DC, 1989, National Academy Press.

Nutrition and your health: dietary guidelines for Americans, ed 5, Washington, DC, 2000, USDA and USDHHS.

Romero-Gwynn E, Nicholson Y, Gwynn D et al: Dietary practices of refugees from the former Soviet Union, *Nutr Today* 32:153, 1997.

Truswell AS: Practical and realistic approaches to healthier diet modifications, *Am J Clin Nutr* 67(suppl 3):583S, 1998.

Nutrition Assessment

2

An individual's nutritional status affects performance, well-being, growth and development, and resistance to illness. **Nutrition assessment** is the process used to evaluate nutritional status, identify malnutrition, and determine which individuals need aggressive nutritional support.

Types of Malnutrition

Malnutrition includes both undernutrition and overnutrition. It can result from inadequate intake, disorders of digestion or absorption, or excessive intake of nutrients.

Undernutrition

Protein-calorie malnutrition

Protein-calorie malnutrition (PCM) is undernutrition resulting from inadequate intake, digestion, or absorption of protein or calories. There are two types of PCM: kwashiorkor and marasmus (Figure 2-1); both can occur in infants, children, and adults. **Marasmus** most often results from an inadequate intake of energy nutrients—carbohydrate, fat, and protein—over a period of months or even years. This condition occurs in patients with certain cancers or in individuals in areas with a poor food supply, for example. The individual loses weight, subcutaneous fat, and muscle and appears thin and wasted. Levels of *visceral* proteins such as serum albumin, transferrin, or prealbumin are often normal. This is because the gradual wasting process allows physiological adjustments that are relatively sparing of the visceral organs (e.g., the liver) and the proteins produced in those organs; instead, fat and skeletal muscle are used to meet energy needs. **Kwashiorkor,** on the other hand, can develop rapidly in the patient experiencing trauma, surgery, or infection and receiving inadequate protein or calories. During these acute stresses, it is often impossible to spare the visceral tissues.

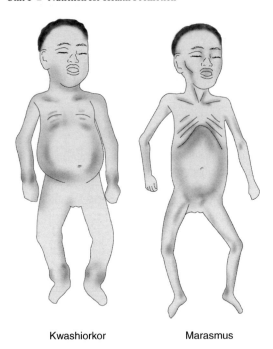

Kwashiorkor   Marasmus

Figure 2-1
Types of malnutrition. Kwashiorkor is characterized by edema,
poor wound healing, and impaired immune function. In marasmus, there is wasting of the subcutaneous fat and the muscle.

Edema accumulates as visceral protein levels fall, causing a decline
in osmotic pressure within the vascular bed. Edema may offset any
change in body mass and prevent weight loss, making the
individual seem deceptively well-nourished. Wound healing and
immune function are compromised, however, and the risk of
complications and death is high. Marasmus and kwashiorkor often
occur together in sick individuals.

Vitamin and mineral deficiencies

Except for iron deficiency anemia, vitamin and mineral deficiencies
rarely occur in isolation. They occur most commonly in groups
or in conjunction with PCM. For example, the individual who
consumes no animal products is at risk of deficiency of vitamin B_{12},
calcium, iron, and zinc.

Overnutrition

The most common forms of overnutrition, present in about half of American adults, are overweight and obesity. Overweight and obesity refer to an excess of body fat, but for simplicity they are often defined as being 10% and 20%, respectively, greater than the ideal body weight. These conditions are associated with numerous health risks, including hypertension, heart disease, type 2 diabetes, stroke, gallbladder disease, osteoarthritis, sleep apnea and respiratory disorders, and certain cancers.

Overnutrition can also occur with excessive intakes of fat-soluble vitamins and some minerals. For instance, excessive intake of vitamin A, especially an intake of 50,000 IU (approximately 10 mg) or more daily over a period of several months, can cause increased intracranial pressure, liver damage, bone and joint pain, and scaly skin. Water-soluble vitamins are usually excreted in the urine without ill effects, but very large amounts of these vitamins may also result in side effects. Megadoses of vitamin C (usually more than 1 g/day), for example, can cause diarrhea, false-negative results on tests for occult blood in the stool, and interference with anticoagulant therapy.

Assessment Procedures

Assessment of nutritional status has four components:

- *A,* anthropometric measurements
- *B,* biochemical or laboratory analyses
- *C,* clinical (physical) assessment
- *D,* diet or nutritional history

Anthropometric Measurements

Anthropometric measurements are measurements of the human body. Essential measurements include height (or length for children less than 2 to 3 years) and weight. Head circumference is included for children less than 2 years of age. Anthropometric measurements are sometimes compared with standard measurements. Appendix C lists healthy weight-for-height for adults. An estimate of the ideal body weight (IBW) for adults may also be obtained with these rules of thumb:

Women: IBW = 100 lb for the first 5 ft of height + 5 lb for every inch over 5 ft

Men: IBW = 106 lb for the first 5 ft of height + 6 lb for every inch over 5 ft

Using these equations, the desirable body weight is within ±10% of the estimated IBW. It should be stressed that these simple equations yield only rough estimates of IBW. Because of variations in body build and other factors, the values determined by these equations may not be very accurate for a particular individual.

Appendix D contains the standardized growth charts for children, showing appropriate height and weight for age and appropriate weight for height. In long-term undernutrition, children exhibit growth retardation, with height low in relation to expected height for age. (Length or height will be below the 5th percentile). Short stature is also found in endocrine and other disorders in children. When short-term undernutrition has occurred, height may be normal for age but weight will be low for height. (Weight-for-height will be less than the 5th percentile; see Appendix D.) Overweight is defined as a weight for height that is above the 90th percentile.

Adjustments to ideal or desirable body weights

Certain physical body changes require adjustments to the ideal or desirable body weights. For amputees, reduce IBW by the following percentages, depending on the extremity lost: hand and forearm, 2.3%; total arm, 5%; foot and lower leg, 6%; and total leg, 16%. These percentages are derived largely from white individuals and may require some adjustment for other racial and ethnic groups. Blacks have proportionally longer lower extremities, and Chinese have shorter extremities than whites. For paraplegic individuals, IBW is approximately 5% to 10% less than the calculated value, and for quadriplegic individuals, IBW is 10% to 15% less than calculated.

Total height may be estimated from knee height for bedridden individuals and those with severe spinal curvature. To measure knee height, bend the knee 90 degrees and measure from the heel to the anterior surface of the thigh.

Men: height in cm $= 71.85 + (1.88 \times K)$

Women: height in cm $= 70.25 - (0.06 \times A) + (1.87 \times K)$

A = age in years, K = knee height in cm

Body composition

Height and weight are useful measurements, but they give little information about body composition. Several methods are available for measuring body composition, including fat content, lean body mass, and bone density. Magnetic resonance imaging (MRI), computerized tomography (CT), ultrasonography, bioelectrical impedance, dual-energy x-ray absorptiometry (DEXA), and densitometry (e.g., underwater weighing) are some of the techniques that can be used. Some of these techniques are quite expensive, however, and they are not available in all settings. Also, CT and DEXA require exposure to radiation. Skinfold measurements are easy and inexpensive to obtain, and they provide an estimate of body fat. The triceps skinfold (TSF) is the most commonly measured (Figure 2-2). It is often used to derive the arm muscle circumference (AMC), which reflects muscle mass. AMC is determined by measuring arm circumference (AC) and TSF at the midpoint of the upper arm and using this equation:

$$AMC \text{ (cm)} = AC \text{ (cm)} - [0.314 \times TSF \text{ (mm)}]$$

Standards for TSF and AMC are found in Appendix E. Generally, TSF and AMC are considered low if less than the 5th percentile and excessive if greater than the 95th. Exceptions exist, however, such as a manual laborer with an AMC greater than the 95th percentile because of increased muscle bulk. Both TSF and AMC are altered by edema of the arm, and a relatively high variability occurs in measurements taken by different examiners. This technique has a

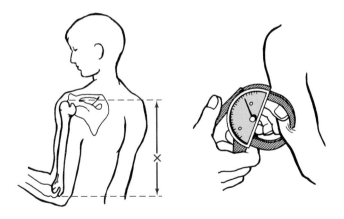

Figure 2-2
TSF and AMC measurements are performed at the midpoint of the upper arm.
(From Heimburger DC, Weinsier RL: *Handbook of clinical nutrition*, ed 3, St Louis, 1997, Mosby.)

great potential for error if the person performing the measurements is not well-trained.

Another anthropometric measurement, waist circumference, is recommended by the National Heart, Lung, and Blood Institute (NHLBI; 1998) for assessing abdominal fat content, a risk factor for cardiovascular disease. Men with waist circumferences >102 cm (40 in) and women with waist circumferences >88 cm (35 in) are at increased risk. The NHLBI has suggested that the waist circumference measurement replace the older technique of calculating the waist/hip ratio (circumference of the waist at its narrowest point divided by the circumference of the hips at their widest point). Ratios greater than 0.95 in men or 0.8 in women are considered evidence of high risk of cardiac disease.

The body mass index (BMI) is a simple tool for evaluating the appropriateness of weight for height (Box 2-1). It does not involve measurement of body composition, and thus it is not an accurate method for assessing the percentage of lean body mass or fat; however, the BMI correlates well with many measures of body fat content, as well as with risk of morbidity. In addition, it is quickly and easily performed in virtually any setting, if accurate measure-

---

Box 2-1   **Body Mass Index (BMI)***

Calculating BMI

$$BMI = \frac{Weight\ (kg)}{Height^2(m)} \quad OR \quad BMI = \frac{Weight\ (lb)}{Height^2\ (in)} \times 704.5$$

Example: An individual weighs 65 kg (143 lb)
and is 1.7 m (5'7") tall.
$$BMI = 65/(1.7)^2 = 22.5\ kg/m^2$$

Classification of BMI
Underweight: <18.5
Normal: 18.5-24.9
Overweight: 25.0-29.9
Obese: ≥30.0
Extreme obesity: ≥40.0

Classification is from the *Clinical guidelines on the identification, evaluation, and treatment of overweight and obesity in adults,* Washington, DC, 1998, NHLCI and NIDDR.

*A nomogram for determining BMI without making any calculations can be found inside the back cover.

ments of height and weight are available. A nomogram for determining BMI without making any calculations can be found inside the back cover of this book.

Biochemical or Laboratory Analyses

Analysis of blood, urine, and other body tissues provides useful information about nutritional status. Table 2-1 lists some tests used in routine nutritional assessment. Specific tests used for evaluation of vitamin and mineral nutrition are listed in Appendix F, along with reference values for nutrition-related laboratory tests.

Laboratory tests are not infallible, and most are affected by factors other than nutrition (see Table 2-1). Circulating proteins are especially problematic. They provide the simplest index of protein nutrition, but their serum or plasma concentrations rise and fall for many reasons that have little to do with nutrition. *Acute phase reactants,* such as C reactive protein, fibrinogen, and α_1-acid glycoprotein usually rise in response to injury, trauma, and infection, while the same conditions can suppress circulating levels of albumin, transferrin, and prealbumin. Good clinical judgment must be used in selecting tests to be performed and interpreting test results. A thorough physical assessment and nutritional history can be as effective in identifying many cases of malnutrition as a battery of laboratory analyses; however, when used appropriately, as in differentiating between types of nutritional anemias, laboratory tests are useful tools.

Using nutrition-related laboratory findings: Nutritional anemias

Nutritional anemias are characterized by low hematocrit (Hct) and hemoglobin (Hgb) concentrations, but several other laboratory findings help to differentiate them (see Table 2-1).

Iron deficiency anemia

Iron deficiency anemia is probably the most prevalent nutritional deficiency in the world and can occur for many reasons, including dietary deficiency, blood loss, and intestinal parasites. Characteristic laboratory findings are:

- Low mean cell volume (MCV) and mean cell hemoglobin concentration (MCHC); microcytic (small), hypochromic (pale) red blood cells
- Elevated serum transferrin (iron transport protein) and total iron binding capacity (TIBC)

Table 2-1   Laboratory Analyses Used in Routine Nutritional Assessment

Area of Concern	Possible Deficiency	Comments
Serum Proteins (one or more are usually evaluated in nutritional assessment)		
↓ Albumin	Protein	Slow to change during malnutrition and nutritional repletion because of long half-life (14-20 days); ↓ in liver disease and nephrosis; good prognostic indicator (e.g., if low, prognosis is poorer than if normal)
↓ Transferrin (iron transport protein)	Protein	Shorter half-life than albumin (7-8 days), so it responds more quickly to undernutrition; ↑ in iron deficiency (a common disorder and one that often occurs in people with PCM) and thus may not be a sensitive indicator of PCM
↓ Prealbumin	Protein	Changes rapidly in malnutrition and during nutritional repletion because of short half-life (2-3 days); ↓ in trauma, inflammation
Hematologic Values		
Anemia (↓ Hct, Hgb)		
Normocytic, or normal-sized RBC (normal MCV, MCHC)	Protein	
Microcytic, or small RBC (↓ MCV, MCH, MCHC)	Fe, Cu	

Parameter	Nutrient	Comments
Macrocytic, or abnormally large RBC (↑ MCV)	Folic acid, vitamin B$_{12}$	
Total lymphocyte count (TLC) (WBC × % lymphocytes) ↓ TLC	Protein	↓ In severe debilitating disease (e.g., cancer, renal disease)
Urinary Values		
↓ Creatinine-height index (CHI)	Protein (reflects lean body mass)	Expected creatinine excretion is 20 mg/kg body weight for children, 17 mg/kg for women, and 23 mg/kg for men; CHI is expressed as percent of the expected value; *Problems:* difficult to collect accurate 24-hr urine; wide variation in day-to-day creatinine excretion
Nitrogen balance*	Protein	Used in evaluation of nutrition therapy; negative values occur when more nitrogen is lost than is consumed (inadequate intake or physiologic stress); positive values occur when more is consumed than lost (e.g., during nutritional repletion); *Problems:* difficult to collect accurate 24-hr urine; retention of nitrogen does not necessarily mean that it is being used for anabolism (tissue building)

MCV, Mean cell volume; *MCH,* mean cell hemoglobin; *MCHC,* mean cell hemoglobin concentration; *Fe,* iron; *Cu,* copper. Reference values for biochemical parameters are given in Appendix F.

*The equation for the calculation of nitrogen balance is: [24-hour protein intake (g) ÷ 6.25] − [24-hour urine urea nitrogen (g) + 4g]

- Low serum iron and ferritin concentrations
- Increased free erythrocyte protoporphyrins (FEP; precursors of heme)

Vitamin B₁₂ or folic acid deficiency anemias

Vitamin B_{12} deficiency occurs when a dietary lack is present (strict vegetarianism) and in conditions that interfere with the process of absorption, such as gastrectomy, disease or resection of the ileum, or aging. Folic acid deficiency is most common in alcoholic individuals with poor diets and in malabsorptive disorders, but many women of childbearing age have borderline folic acid intakes.

The hematologic findings are similar in these anemias, but it is important not to treat vitamin B_{12} deficiency with folic acid because the anemia can be corrected but progressive neurologic damage caused by vitamin B_{12} deficiency will continue. Laboratory tests in these anemias show the following:

- Increased mean cell volume (MCV) in both anemias because red blood cells are large (macrocytic) and immature. (This helps to differentiate these anemias from iron deficiency anemia.)
- Serum transferrin, ferritin, and total iron binding capacity (TIBC) normal or high in most cases. (These findings also differ from those in iron deficiency.)
- Low plasma vitamin B_{12} or serum or red blood cell folic acid concentration. (These tests determine whether the deficiency is in B_{12} or folic acid.)
- Increased urinary levels of methylmalonic acid.
- Abnormal Schilling test (which compares absorption of vitamin B_{12} bound to intrinsic factor to unbound vitamin B_{12}). This result is found only if the person has pernicious anemia (failure to form adequate intrinsic factor); see Figure 1-6.

Clinical or Physical Assessment

Many nutrient deficiencies and excesses become apparent during careful physical assessment of the individual. Table 2-2 describes findings that may indicate malnutrition.

Diet or Nutritional History

Several methods can be used to obtain information about nutrient intake. With all methods, the interviewer should determine whether there have been changes in food intake over the past few months.

Table 2-2   Signs that Suggest Nutrient Imbalance

Area of Concern	Possible Deficiency	Possible Excess
Hair		
Dull, dry, brittle	Pro	
Easily plucked (with no pain)	Pro	
Hair loss	Pro, Zn, biotin	Vit A
Flag sign (loss of hair pigment in strips around the head)	Pro, Cu	
Head and Neck		
Bulging fontanel (infants)		Vit A
Headache		Vit A, D
Epistaxis (nosebleed)	Vit K	
Thyroid enlargement	Iodine	
Eyes		
Conjunctival and corneal xerosis (dryness)	Vit A	
Pale conjunctiva	Fe	
Blue sclerae	Fe	
Corneal vascularization	Vit B_2	
Mouth		
Cheilosis or angular stomatitis (lesions at corners of mouth)	Vit B_2	
Glossitis (red, sore tongue)	Niacin, folate, vit B_{12}, other B vit	
Gingivitis (inflamed gums)	Vit C	
Hypogeusia, dysgeusia (poor sense of taste, bad taste)	Zn	
Dental caries	Fluoride	
Mottling of teeth		Fluoride
Atrophy of papillae on tongue	Fe, B vit	

Pro, Protein; *Vit,* vitamin(s); *Cu,* copper; *Fe,* iron; *K,* potassium; *Zn,* zinc.

Continued

Table 2-2   Signs that Suggest Nutrient Imbalance—cont'd

Area of Concern	Possible Deficiency	Possible Excess
Skin		
Dry, scaly	Vit A, Zn, EFA	Vit A
Follicular hyperkeratosis (resembles goose-flesh)	Vit A, EFA, B vit	
Eczematous lesions	Zn	
Petechiae, ecchymoses	Vit C, K	
Nasolabial seborrhea (greasy, scaly areas between nose and upper lip)	Niacin, vit B_2, B_6	
Darkening and peeling of skin in areas exposed to sun	Niacin	
Poor wound healing	Pro, Zn, vit C	
Nails		
Koilonychia (spoon-shaped nails)	Fe	
Brittle, fragile	Pro	
Heart		
Enlargement, tachycardia, failure	Vit B_1	
Small heart	kcal	
Sudden failure, death	Se	
Arrhythmia	Mg, K, Se	
Hypertension	Ca, K	Na
Abdomen		
Hepatomegaly	Pro	Vit A
Ascites	Pro	
Musculoskeletal, Extremities		
Muscle wasting (especially temporal area)	kcal	
Edema	Pro, vit B_1	
Calf tenderness	Vit B_1 or C, biotin, Se	

EFA, Essential fatty acids; *Ca,* calcium; *Mg,* magnesium; *Na,* sodium; *Se,* selenium.

Table 2-2   Signs that Suggest Nutrient Imbalance—cont'd

Area of Concern	Possible Deficiency	Possible Excess
Beading of ribs, or "rachitic rosary" (child)	Vit C, D	
Bone and joint tenderness	Vit C, D, Ca, P	Vit A
Knock knees, bowed legs, fragile bones	Vit D, Ca, P, Cu	
Neurologic		
Paresthesias (pain and tingling or altered sensation in the extremities)	Vit B_1, B_6, B_{12}, biotin	
Weakness	Vit C, B_1, B_6, B_{12}, kcal	
Ataxia, decreased position and vibratory senses	Vit B_1, B_{12}	
Tremor	Mg	
Decreased tendon reflexes	Vit B_1	
Confabulation, disorientation	Vit B_1	
Drowsiness, lethargy	Vit B_1	Vit A, D
Depression	Vit B_1, biotin	

P, Phosphorus.

24-hour recall

The individual is asked to recall everything he or she consumed the previous day. A sample tool for collection of a 24-hour recall is shown in Box 2-2. The advantage of this method is that it is easily and quickly done; however, the person being interviewed may not be able to recall his or her intake accurately, and snacks and beverages tend to be omitted. The interviewer must be trained in prompting and questioning the individual to obtain complete and accurate information. Serving sizes, in particular, may be reported incorrectly. Having available measuring cups, spoons, and dishes of different sizes may help the interviewee to describe serving sizes more accurately. In addition, the previous day's intake may be atypical for the person.

Box 2-2   24-Hour Recall

The following questions may be used to elicit a 24-hour recall.

1. What time did you get up yesterday? _____
   Was this the usual time? _____
2. When was the first time you had anything to eat or drink?
   _____
   (Avoid mentioning specific meals, e.g., "What did you have for breakfast?")
   What did you have? How much? (For each food, ask for details if type or preparation method is unclear, e.g., was chicken fried or baked?; was milk whole, low-fat, or skim?)
3. When did you eat or drink something again?
   What did you have and how much?
   (Repeat question 3 until the individual has described the entire day.)
4. Did you eat or drink anything else? (Review the day with the individual to see if any snacks have been omitted.)
5. Was this day's intake different from usual?
   If so, in what way? _____
6. Do you eat differently on weekends than on weekdays?
   _____ If so, in what way?

Food frequency questionnaire

The health professional collects information regarding the number of times per day, week, or month the individual eats particular foods. A sample tool, focusing on cholesterol and saturated fat intake, is shown in Box 2-3. When used with a 24-hour recall, the questionnaire can help validate the accuracy of the recall and provide a more complete picture of the individual's intake; it can also save interviewer and patient time. If the goal of the nutritional history is to find out about intake of particular food components or nutrients (e.g., cholesterol and saturated fat), then the questionnaire can be designed to focus on those items. This method provides very limited information, however. Other methods of determining dietary intake can reveal time and circumstances of food intake, which may be of help in identifying and changing poor eating habits (e.g., nighttime snacking during television viewing).

Box 2-3   Food Frequency List for Cholesterol and Fat Intake

How often do you consume each of the following?

	Times/wk	Times/mo	<Once/mo	Never
Eggs	____	____	____	____
Liver	____	____	____	____
Shellfish	____	____	____	____
Other fish	____	____	____	____
Beef or pork	____	____	____	____
Poultry	____	____	____	____
Cheese	____	____	____	____
Butter	____	____	____	____
Whole milk	____	____	____	____
Cream	____	____	____	____
Pastries	____	____	____	____
Gravies	____	____	____	____
Ice Cream	____	____	____	____
Stick margarine	____	____	____	____
Soft margarine	____	____	____	____
Corn, sunflower, or safflower oils	____	____	____	____

Food record

In keeping a food record, the individual records all the foods he or she consumes, with portions weighed, measured, or estimated. Usually this is done for 3 days—a weekend day and 2 weekdays. The food record provides more information than the 24-hour recall, particularly in quantifying the amounts eaten. Nevertheless, a food record relies heavily on the individual's cooperation. Also, food intake may be atypical during the recording period. In some cases, the act of recording one's intake results in a change in eating patterns.

Diet history

The individual is extensively interviewed to elicit detailed information about nutritional status, as well as general health, socio-

---

Box 2-4 Diet History

I. Socioeconomic data
   A. Income
      1. Adequacy for food purchasing
      2. Eligibility for food stamps or other public assistance
   B. Ethnic or cultural background
      1. Influence of culture or religion on eating habits
      2. Educational level
II. Food preparation
   A. Problems in shopping for or preparing food
      1. Skill of person who shops and cooks
      2. Availability of market(s)
      3. Adequacy of facilities for cooking, food storage, and refrigeration
   B. Use of convenience foods
III. Physical activity
   A. Occupation—type, number of hours per week, activity level
   B. Exercise—type and frequency
   C. Handicaps
IV. Appetite and perception of taste and smell—quality, any changes over the last 12 months
V. Allergies, intolerances, food avoidances, and special diets
   A. Foods avoided and reason
   B. Special diet—what kind, why followed, and who recommended it

---

economic status, and cultural impact on nutrition. The diet history usually includes information similar to that collected by the 24-hour recall and food frequency questionnaire, as well as other information listed in Box 2-4. An accurate diet history requires an experienced interviewer, and it can be very time-consuming. This method provides more information than either the 24-hour recall or the 3-day food record, however, and it can give an indication of food habits over several months or years. Table 2-3 illustrates diet history findings that may indicate nutritional deficits.

Box 2-4   Diet History—cont'd

   VI. Oral health/swallowing
       A. Dentures; completeness of dentition
       B. Problems with chewing, swallowing, and saliva-
          tion
  VII. Gastrointestinal problems
       A. Heartburn, bloating, gas, diarrhea, vomiting,
          constipation—frequency of problems, any associ-
          ation with food intake or other occurrences
       B. Remedies used—laxatives, antacids
 VIII. Medical or psychiatric illnesses
       A. Type of disease
       B. Type and duration of treatment
   IX. Medications
       A. Vitamins, minerals, or other nutritional sup-
          plements—frequency, type, amount, and recom-
          mended or prescribed by whom
       B. Other medications—frequency, type, amount, and
          duration of use
    X. Recent weight change
       A. Amount of loss or gain and over what period of
          time (most significant if during past year)
       B. Intentional or unintentional; if intentional, what
          method was used
   XI. Usual food intake—description of a "typical" day's
       intake, or 24-hour recall with use of food frequency
       questionnaire

Evaluating nutrient intake
Food composition method

Tables of food composition or computer databases can be used to
calculate the amount of each nutrient in the diet. Nutrient intake is
then compared with some standard, usually the Dietary Reference
Intakes (DRIs) (see Chapter 1). The DRIs can serve as goals, but
because they are set so that they cover the needs of practically all
healthy people in the population, a particular individual may not
require the full DRI of a nutrient to maintain good nutritional status.
For this reason, an intake equivalent to two thirds of the DRI

Table 2-3   Evaluation of Nutritional History

Area of Concern	History	Possible Deficiency
Inadequate intake	Alcohol abuse	kcal, pro, vit B_1, niacin, folate
	Avoidance of food groups:	
	Fruits and vegetables	Vit A, C
	Breads and cereals	Vit B_1 and B_2, fiber
	Meat, eggs, dairy products	Vit B_{12}, protein, Fe, Zn
	Dairy products	Ca, vit B_2
	Constipation, hemorrhoids, diverticulosis	Fiber
	Poverty, disadvantaged environment	Various nutrients, especially pro and Fe
	Multiple food allergies	Depends on specific allergies
	Weight loss	kcal, other nutrients
Inadequate absorption	Drugs (especially antacids, cimetidine, anticonvulsants, cholestyramine, neomycin, antineoplastics, laxatives)	Various nutrients (see Appendix H)
	Malabsorption (diarrhea, weight loss, steatorrhea)	kcal; vit A, D, E, K; pro; Ca; Mg; Zn
	Parasites	Fe
	Surgery	
	Gastrectomy	Vit B_{12}, Fe, folate
	Intestinal resection	kcal; vit A, D, E, K; Ca; Mg; Zn; vit B_{12} if distal ileum

Modified from Heimburger DC, Weinsier RL: *Handbook of clinical nutrition*, ed 3, St Louis, 1997, Mosby.
Pro, Protein; *Vit*, vitamin(s); *Fe*, iron; *Ca*, calcium; *Mg*, magnesium; *Zn*, zinc.

Table 2-3   Evaluation of Nutritional History—cont'd

Area of Concern	History	Possible Deficiency
Impaired utilization	Drugs (especially antineoplastics, oral contraceptives, isoniazid, colchicine, corticosteroids)	Various nutrients (see Appendix H)
	Inborn errors of metabolism (by family history)	Depends on disorder
Increased losses	Diabetes	Zn, Cr
	Alcohol abuse, cirrhosis of the liver	Mg, Zn
	Blood loss	Fe
	Diarrhea, fistula	Pro, Zn, fluid, electrolytes
	Draining abscesses or wounds	Pro, Zn
	Nephrotic syndrome	Pro, Zn
	Peritoneal dialysis or hemodialysis	Pro, water-soluble vit, Zn
	Vomiting (persistent)	Fluid, electrolytes, kcal, other nutrients
Increased requirements	Fever	kcal, vit B_1
	Hyperthyroidism	kcal
	Physiologic demands (infancy, adolescence, pregnancy, lactation)	Fe, Ca, other nutrients
	Surgery, trauma, burns, infection	kcal, pro, vit C, Zn
	Neoplasms (some types)	kcal, pro, other nutrients

Cr, Chromium.

is often assumed to be adequate for healthy people. On the other hand, sick individuals may need more of some nutrients than specified by the DRI.

The food composition method can provide specific information about a wide group of nutrients and food components. Computer databases make the process rapid and easy. A free computer database at www.ag.uiuc.edu is available to anyone, and the simple instructions make it possible for laypeople to use this nutrition analysis tool. Some caveats should be noted, however, in the use of any nutrient database. Foods consumed may not have exactly the same nutrient composition as those in the database because of variations in growing and storage conditions, food processing, and cooking procedures. Moreover, gaps exist in the food composition data in published tables and databases. Many foods have not been analyzed for all trace elements, for example. Despite these caveats, the databases are among the most useful and widespread methods for nutrition analysis.

The healthy eating index

The Healthy Eating Index (1995) is a scoring system with 10 categories based upon the Food Guide Pyramid and the *Dietary Guidelines for Americans* (Table 2-4). Each category is scored from 0 to 10 (perfect score), so that the best possible score is 100. A score of 0 is given for a food group if no servings are included from that group, and a score of 10 is given if the recommended number of servings is consumed (see footnote to Table 2-4). A score between 0 and 10 is given if some foods from the group are eaten, but not the recommended number of servings (e.g., a score of 3 is given if the recommendation is for 9 servings of grains and only 3 are consumed). Combination foods are categorized according to their major components. The Index gives a simple summary of diet quality, showing not only nutrient intake but also progress toward achieving the *Dietary Guidelines*. Evaluation of the diet in this manner is a useful tool for nutrition education of lay individuals because they can readily see the shortcomings in their diets.

Nutrition Screening

Health care providers rarely have the time to perform a complete nutrition assessment on every patient. It is most important that

Table 2-4 Scoring the Healthy Eating Index

	Criteria for Score of 0*	Criteria for Score of 10*
Food Group		
1. Grains	0 servings	6-11 servings†
2. Vegetables	0 servings	3-5 servings†
3. Fruits	0 servings	2-4 servings†
4. Milk	0 servings	2-3 servings†
5. Meat/beans	0 servings	2-3 servings†
Dietary Guidelines		
6. Total fat	45% or more of kcal from fat	30% or less of kcal from fat
7. Saturated fat	Less than 10% of kcal from saturated fat	15% or more of kcal from saturated fat
8. Cholesterol	450 mg or more	Less than 300 mg
9. Sodium	4800 mg or more	Less than 2400 mg
10. Variety	6 or fewer different foods over a 3-day period	16 or more different foods over a 3-day period

From the Center for Nutrition Policy and Promotion, United States Department of Agriculture: *Healthy Eating Index,* Washington, DC, 1995, USDA.
*All scores except variety are for a 1-day period.
†The recommended number of servings per day depend on kcal needs. For diets of 1600 kcal or less, the number of servings required to score a 10 in each group would be: grains, 6; vegetables, 3; fruits, 2; milk, 2; meat, 2. For 2200 kcal diets, the number of servings required to score a 10 in each group would be: grains, 9; vegetables, 4; fruits, 3; milk, 2; meat, 2.4. For diets of 2800 kcal and greater, the number of servings required to score a 10 in each group would be: grains, 11; vegetables, 5; fruits, 4; milk, 2; meat, 2.8. No matter what their kcal level, pregnant or breastfeeding women and teenagers and young adults up to age 24 must consume 3 milk servings to score a 10 for that group.

individuals who are nutritionally at risk or those who are malnourished be identified quickly; thorough assessment can then be performed on these individuals and intervention can be planned as necessary. Nutrition screening of individuals consists of gathering some readily available subjective and objective information.

Any of the following findings may indicate the presence of mal-nutrition or nutritional risk:

- Unplanned loss of ≥10% of usual body weight within 6 months or ≥5% of usual body weight in 1 month; in infants (after the first week of life) and children, any weight loss (or failure to gain adequate weight) that causes deviation from the child's usual percentile (see Appendix D)
- Body mass index (see Box 2-1) >25 or <18.5, or weight 10% greater than or less than ideal body weight; in infants and children, weight or length less than the 10th percentile or greater than the 90th percentile
- Presence of chronic disease
- Increased metabolic requirements (e.g., trauma, burns, systemic infection)
- Altered diet or diet schedules (e.g., recent surgery, serious illness, receiving total parenteral nutrition or tube feedings)
- Inadequate food intake (for adults, risk is greater if inadequate intake continues or is expected to continue for 7 days or more; infants and children are considered at risk with a shorter period of inadequate intake)

Estimating Nutrient Needs
Energy (Calorie) Needs

Energy expenditure can be divided into three components: (1) **basal energy expenditure,** or energy required for basic life processes such as respiration, cardiac function, and maintenance of body temperature; (2) the thermic effect of food, or the energy required for ingestion, digestion, absorption, and metabolism of nutrients from food; and (3) physical activity. Basal (or resting) energy expenditure (BEE) is determined largely by the amount of lean body mass (also known as the fat-free mass). It can be measured by indirect calorimetry. This technique, which requires a metabolic cart, is not available in all settings, and therefore established formulas are often used to estimate caloric needs.

Daily energy needs for adults are often estimated as shown in Table 2-5. These estimates are useful for a quick assessment of the adequacy of energy intake and for teaching lay individuals about energy needs. The estimates may not reflect accurately the energy

Table 2-5   Estimates of Daily Energy Needs for Adults

Status/Activity Level	Kcal/kg	Kcal/lb
Obese	21	9.5
Sedentary or hospitalized	25-30	11-13.5
Moderately active (regular aerobic exercise plus routine activities)	30-35	13.5-16
Very active (manual laborer, athlete) or patient with major burns or trauma	40	18

expenditure of a particular person. Several more detailed formulas are often used in clinical practice in an effort to derive more individualized estimates of energy expenditure. Two of these formulas are shown in Box 2-5.

The lean body mass (LBM, or fat-free mass) is responsible for most of the energy expenditure. Obese people contain more of both fat and LBM than do normal-weight individuals, but LBM accounts for only about 25% of the excess weight in the obese. That is why the aforementioned guidelines suggest a reduced energy allowance for the obese. Elderly people have less LBM and a higher fat content, on average, than their younger counterparts. LBM decreases approximately 10% between the ages of 25 and 60 years, another 10% between 60 and 75, and then declines more rapidly (as much as 20% to 25% more by age 90). For this reason, estimates of caloric needs for elderly persons should usually fall at the bottom end of the suggested range. Rather than drastically limiting their caloric intake to maintain a desirable body weight, elderly people should be encouraged to exercise at a moderate intensity on a regular basis (e.g., walk as briskly as can be tolerated for 30 to 60 minutes almost every day). Regular exercise has two advantages: maintenance of LBM and increase in energy expenditure. With increased energy expenditure, and thus an increase in energy needs, it is easier for the elderly to obtain a diet adequate in vitamins, minerals, and other nutrients.

Protein Needs

Protein needs vary with the degree of malnutrition and stress. For healthy adults or those undergoing elective surgery, 0.8 to

Box 2-5 Selected Equations Used in Estimating Energy Expenditure

Harris-Benedict Equations

Developed in healthy individuals; used for calculating energy needs of both well and sick individuals

1. *First calculate the BEE*

   For women, BEE (kcal/day) =
   655 + 9.6(W) + 1.7(H) − 4.7(A)

   For men, BEE (kcal/day) =
   66 + 13.7(W) + 5(H) − 6.8(A)

   W = weight in kg (1 lb = 0.45 kg); H = height in cm
   (1 in = 2.54 cm); A = age in years

2. *Multiply by an activity factor to obtain an estimate of total energy expenditure*

   Sedentary, obese,* or hospitalized individual: 1.2 to 1.3

   Active nonhospitalized normal weight individual: 1.4 to 1.6

Example: A woman who has a sedentary job is 26 years old, 162.5 cm (5'4") tall, and 84 kg (185 lb).

   BEE = 655 + 9.6(84) + 1.7(162.5) − 4.7(26) = 1615 kcal/day

   Estimated total energy expenditure = 1615 × 1.2 = 1938 kcal/day

Ireton-Jones Equations

Developed in and used for sick hospitalized patients†

   EEE(v) = 1784 − 11(A) + 5(W) + 244(S) + 239(T) + 804(B)

   EEE(s) = 629 − 11(A) + 25(W) − 609(O)

   EEE = estimated total energy expenditure in kcal/day, v = ventilator-dependent, s = spontaneously breathing, A = age in years, W = actual weight in kg, S = sex (m = 1, f = 0). Diagnosis: T = trauma, B = burn, O = obesity (if present = 1, absent = 0).

Example: If the woman in the example above suffered respiratory failure and needed ventilatory support following a near-drowning incident, her EEE would be as follows.

   EEE(v) = 1784 − 11(26) + 5(84) + 244(0) + 239(0) + 804(0) = 1918 kcal/day

*Because the obese need less energy per kg than normal-weight people, use of an activity factor of 1.2 has been found to correlate best with measured energy expenditure (Ireton-Jones 1999).

†Both of the Ireton-Jones equations can be applied to obese individuals, although obesity appears as a factor only in the equation for spontaneously breathing patients.

1 g/kg body weight is usually adequate. Athletes and individuals in catabolic states (sepsis, major trauma, and burns) may need as much as 1.2 to 2.0 g/kg daily. Individuals with liver or kidney failure may require lower protein intakes (see Chapters 12 and 17).

Assessing State of Hydration

The state of hydration is an important part of nutritional assessment. On one hand, fluid overload is a hazardous state that may compromise cardiorespiratory function. It is usually reflected in rapid weight gain (more than approximately 0.1 to 0.2 kg [1/4 to 1/2 lb]/day in an adult over a period of several days). On the other hand, fluid deficits (**dehydration**) can become severe enough to cause shock and coma.

There are three types of dehydration, which can be distinguished by the serum sodium level:

1. *Hypertonic or hypernatremic:* Serum sodium >150 mEq/L. This occurs because loss of water is greater than loss of sodium. Causes include inadequate water intake (e.g., hospitalized elderly individuals who may not feel or be able to express thirst, infants given improperly diluted powdered or concentrated formula, individuals with diarrhea and inadequate fluid intake) and osmotic diuresis (e.g., excessive urination in hyperglycemia).
2. *Isotonic:* Serum sodium 130 to 150 mEq/L. This is the most common form of dehydration; it occurs because of loss of balanced amounts of sodium and water. Causes include diarrhea, vomiting, and nasogastric suction with inadequate replacement of fluid and electrolytes.
3. *Hypotonic or hyponatremic:* Serum sodium <130 mEq/L. Sodium is lost in excess of water. Causes include viral gastroenteritis with rehydration with plain water, tea, or other low-sodium fluids; excessive sweating without fluid and electrolyte replacement; cystic fibrosis; diuretic therapy.

Dehydration can be graded as mild, moderate, or severe. The amount of weight loss, along with clinical signs (Table 2-6), can be used to determine the severity of the fluid deficit.

Table 2-6   **Judging Severity of Fluid Deficit**

	Mild, 3%-5%	Moderate, 6%-9%	Severe, ≥10%
Blood pressure	↔	↔	↔ to ↓
Pulses	↔	↔ to ↓	↓↓
Heart rate	↔	↑	↑*
Skin turgor	↔	↓ to ↓↓	↓↓ to ↓↓↓
Fontanelle (infants)	↔	Sunken	Sunken
Mucous membranes	Slightly dry	Dry	Dry
Eyes	↔	Sunken	Deeply sunken
Capillary refill	↔	Delayed	Delayed†
Mental status	↔	↔ to ↓	↔ to ↓↓↓
Urine output	↓	↓↓‡	↓↓↓‡
Thirst	↑	↑↑	↑↑↑

Key: ↔, normal; ↓, slightly decreased; ↓↓, moderately decreased; ↓↓↓, severely decreased; ↑, slightly increased; ↑↑, moderately increased; ↑↑↑, severely increased.
*May become bradycardic in very severe dehydration.
†Skin cool and mottled.
‡<1 ml/kg/h

Selected Bibliography

Center for Nutrition Policy and Promotion, United States Department of Agriculture: *Healthy Eating Index,* Washington, DC, 1995, USDA.

Clinical guidelines on the identification, evaluation, and treatment of overweight and obesity in adults, Washington, DC, 1998, National Heart, Lung, and Blood Institute and National Institute of Diabetes, Digestive, and Kidney Diseases.

Forbes GF: Body composition: overview, *J Nutr* 129 (1S):270S, 1999.

Haymond MW: Nutritional and metabolic endpoints, *J Nutr* 129(1S): 273S, 1999.

Ireton-Jones CS: Strategies for feeding obese patients. Presented at the American Society for Parenteral and Enteral Nutrition 23rd Clinical Congress, San Diego, CA, February 1, 1999.

Klein S, Kinney J, Jeejeebhoy K, et al.: Nutrition support in clinical practice: review of published data and recommendations for future research directions, *JPEN* 21:133, 1997.

Osterkamp LK: Current perspective on assessment of human body proportions of relevance to amputees, *J Am Dietet Assoc* 95:215, 1995.

Weinsier RL, Heimburger DC: Distinguishing malnutrition from disease: the search goes on, *Am J Clin Nutr* 66:1063, 1997.

Pregnancy and Lactation

3

Pregnancy

The idea that the pregnant woman is "eating for two" has been discredited, at least in terms of quantity; however, the quality of food intake during pregnancy deserves special attention to promote optimal health for both the mother and the child.

Special Concerns

Nutritional needs

Nutritional deficiencies during pregnancy can have adverse effects on both the mother and her infant. Maternal diets are most likely to be low in iron, zinc, calcium, and folic acid. Some of the more serious effects of deficiencies are summarized in Table 3-1. Requirements for some important nutrients are described later in this chapter. Food sources of these nutrients are listed in Appendix A.

Preconceptual weight, weight gain, and energy needs

Enlargement of maternal breasts, uterine tissue, blood volume, and energy (fat) stores, as well as development of the placenta, amniotic fluid, and fetus, contribute to maternal weight gain during pregnancy (Figure 3-1). Appropriate weight gain does not necessarily equal good nutritional status, of course, but the amount of weight gain during pregnancy is closely related to pregnancy outcome. The mother's weight before pregnancy is another factor involved in pregnancy outcome. Maternal and fetal risks are increased in the following cases:

1. *Underweight:* Women who are underweight before pregnancy are more likely to experience preterm labor and to deliver **low birth weight (LBW;** less than 2500 g or 5.5 lb) infants. LBW is the single greatest risk factor for the survival of the newborn.

Table 3-1   Nutritional Deficiencies During Pregnancy

| | Potential Effects of Deficiency | |
Nutrient	Maternal	Fetal
Kcal*	Anemia Endometritis	Prematurity Low birth weight (LBW)
Protein	Hypoproteinemia with edema ? Increased incidence of preeclampsia	? LBW (difficult to separate from effects of kcal deprivation)
Iron	Microcytic, hypochromic anemia	Fetal death; LBW; premature birth
Zinc	Amnionitis	Fetal malformations, including neural tube defects
Folic acid	Megaloblastic or macrocytic anemia	Neural tube defects

*Especially if underweight before pregnancy.

2. *Overweight:* Women who are overweight before pregnancy are more likely to have hypertension and diabetes. Fetal death rates are highest in pregnancies where the mother weighs more than 77.3 kg (170 lb).

3. *Inadequate weight gain:* For normal-weight and underweight women, maternal weight gain is directly related to infant birth weight, and the risk of delivering an LBW infant is increased by inadequate gain.

4. *Excessive weight gain:* Overeating, multiple gestation, edema, and pregnancy-induced hypertension are some of the causes of greater-than-expected weight gain. Very high total weight gain, especially in short women (less than 157 cm or 62 in) is associated with increased risk of fetopelvic disproportion, operative delivery, birth trauma, and infant mortality. Moreover, excessive fat stores tend to be retained after pregnancy, increasing the woman's likelihood of being overweight or obese.

The optimum amount of weight gain during pregnancy is determined largely by the mother's weight before pregnancy. Recommendations have been developed for desirable ranges for total weight gain and rate of weight gain based on body mass index

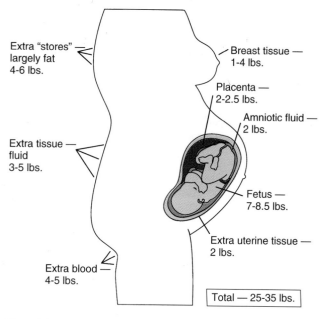

Extra "stores" largely fat 4-6 lbs.

Breast tissue — 1-4 lbs.

Placenta — 2-2.5 lbs.

Amniotic fluid — 2 lbs.

Extra tissue — fluid 3-5 lbs.

Fetus — 7-8.5 lbs.

Extra uterine tissue — 2 lbs.

Extra blood — 4-5 lbs.

Total — 25-35 lbs.

Figure 3-1
Components of maternal weight gain at 40 weeks of gestation.
(From Worthington-Roberts BS, Williams SR: *Nutrition in pregnancy and lactation,* ed 5, New York, 1997, McGraw-Hill. Used with permission of The McGraw-Hill Companies.)

(BMI), an indicator of the appropriateness of weight for height. BMI = weight in kg/(height in m)^2. For example, a woman weighing 51 kg (112 lb), 1.57 m (5'2") in height, would have a BMI = $51/(1.57)^2 = 20.7$. A nomogram for determining the BMI is shown inside the back cover of this book.

Recommended total weight gain during pregnancy is as follows: underweight women (BMI <19.8), 12.5 to 18 kg (28 to 40 lb); normal-weight women (BMI 19.8 to 26), 11.5 to 16 kg (25 to 35 lb); overweight women (BMI 26 to 29), 7 to 11.5 kg (15 to 25 lb); and obese women (BMI >29), ≥6.8 kg (15 lb) (Figure 3-2). Young adolescents (less than 2 years past menarche) should be encouraged to make their weight gain goal the upper end of the recommended range for their BMI because their infants are smaller than those of

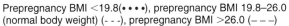

Prepregnancy BMI <19.8(• • • •), prepregnancy BMI 19.8–26.0 (normal body weight) (- - -), prepregnancy BMI >26.0 (– – –)

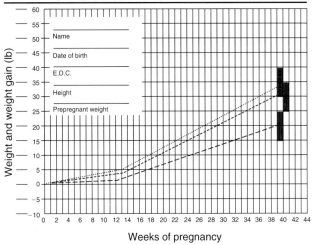

Figure 3-2

Prenatal weight gain chart. The dotted and dashed lines show desirable weight gain based on prepregnancy BMI. To use, write the woman's prepregnant weight on the left axis, on the line to the left of 0. Fill in the horizontal blanks above her prepregnant weight (e.g., if her prepregnant weight was 123 lb, the line just above 0, indicating a gain of 5 lb, should be filled in with 128 lb; the second line, corresponding to a 10-lb gain, should read 133 lb). At each prenatal visit, the woman can plot her current weight against her weeks of gestation and evaluate her weight gain in relation to the desirable gain.

(Reprinted with permission from *Nutrition during pregnancy and lactation.* Copyright 1992 by the National Academy of Sciences. Courtesy of the National Academy Press, Washington, DC.)

adult women for any given amount of maternal gain. Outcome of a twin pregnancy appears to be best if weight gain is approximately 16 to 20.5 kg (35 to 45 lb).

The pattern of weight gain is important in evaluating weight changes during pregnancy. Most women gain approximately 1.5 to

2 kg (3 to 5 lb) during the first trimester of pregnancy, when the fetus and the changes in maternal tissues are relatively small. Recommended weekly weight gains during the second and third trimesters are 0.5 kg (1.1 lb) for underweight women, 0.4 kg (1 lb) for normal-weight women, and 0.3 kg (0.66 lb) for overweight women. Gain of 1 kg (2.2 lb) or less per month in the second or third trimester by normal-weight women and 0.5 kg or less (1 lb) by obese women should be investigated, as should a gain of 3 kg (6.6 lb) or more per month. The Recommended Dietary Allowances (RDA; 1989) suggest that during the second and third trimesters the woman should consume 300 kcal/day more than her nonpregnant intake to promote an adequate gain. (See Chapter 1 for discussion of RDA.) In twin gestations, a gain of 0.75 kg (1.65 lb) per week during the second and third trimesters appears appropriate.

Protein

A total of 60 g of protein per day is recommended. This amount, which is easily provided by the average diet in the United States, is necessary for normal growth of the fetus, enlargement of the uterus and breasts, formation of blood cells and proteins as the blood volume expands, and production of amniotic fluid.

Iron

The red blood cell mass expands by about 15% during pregnancy, which requires a substantial increase in the maternal content of iron. Iron is also needed for deposition of fetal stores. **Pica,** the consumption of substances usually considered nonfoods, can interfere with iron nutriture in two ways: (1) displacing nutritious foods in the diet (both calcium and iron intakes have been found to be lower in women with pica than those without pica by some investigators), and (2) interfering with absorption of iron and other nutrients from foods and nutritional supplements. Women who practice pica have been found to have significantly lower levels of hemoglobin, mean cell hemoglobin, and ferritin (a storage form of iron) than women who do not practice pica (Rainville, 1998). Ice or freezer frost, soil or clay, chalk, glue, cornstarch, and laundry starch are common pica substances. As many as 20% of women at high risk for pica may practice it. Women at highest risk for pica are most likely to be African-Americans, live in rural areas, to have practiced pica during childhood, and to have family members who practice pica. The pica substances preferred are usually items that their family members have consumed or that they themselves consumed before pregnancy.

Zinc

Absorption of zinc is inhibited by large intakes of iron and folic acid. Women taking iron and folic acid supplements need to consume rich sources of zinc (e.g., shellfish, meats, and tofu and other soy products) daily. Whole grains, milk, cheese, and eggs contain smaller but important amounts of zinc. Vegetarians are especially apt to have marginal zinc status, both because meats and shellfish are some of the best sources of zinc and because phytates and oxalates found in whole grains and green leafy vegetables inhibit zinc absorption.

Calcium

Pregnant women are encouraged to consume at least 1000 mg of calcium per day, and pregnant adolescents are advised to consume 1300 mg. This can be achieved with a daily intake of 3 cups of milk or yogurt plus additional foods such as green leafy vegetables or bread products made with milk. The requirement for calcium in the fetal skeleton is a major reason for the increase in maternal needs.

Folic acid (folate)

The recommended intake of folic acid increases from 400 μg in the nonpregnant state to 600 μg in pregnancy. It is needed for both maternal red blood cell production and the DNA synthesis entailed in fetal and placental growth. Data indicate that women with folic acid deficiency are more likely to give birth to infants with neural tube defects.

Vitamin C

An extra 10 mg of vitamin C in addition to the adult RDA of 60 mg is recommended during pregnancy. In addition to its role in development of connective tissue, vitamin C improves iron absorption and facilitates activation of folic acid.

Potentially harmful substances

Caffeine

The effect of caffeine intake on the fetus is not fully known. Some investigators have reported that heavy caffeine use is associated with spontaneous abortions, decrease in birth weight, and decrease in maternal and fetal hemoglobin and hematocrit levels. Pregnant women should consume no more than 300 mg caffeine daily (see Appendix G).

Alcohol

There is no known safe level of alcohol intake during pregnancy, and thus alcohol is best avoided altogether by pregnant women. Heavy drinking (2 or more drinks/day; see Chapter 1) during pregnancy can result in **fetal alcohol syndrome (FAS),** which may include some or all of the following features: microcephaly, prenatal and postnatal growth failure, mental retardation, facial abnormalities (Figure 3-3), cleft palate, skeletal-joint abnormalities, abnormal palmar creases, cardiac defects, and behavioral abnormalities. Even women who consumed less than two drinks per day have delivered infants with some features of FAS. Avoiding alcohol altogether is the only known way to prevent FAS.

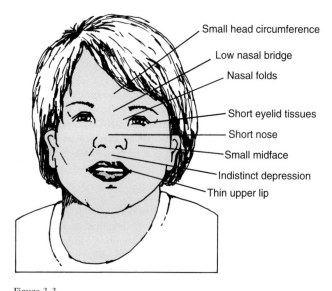

Figure 3-3
Abnormal findings of the head in fetal alcohol syndrome.
(From Wardlaw GM, Insel PM, Seyler MF: *Contemporary nutrition: issues and insights,* ed 2, New York, 1994, McGraw-Hill. Used with permission of The McGraw-Hill Companies.)

Cigarette smoking

Infants of women who smoke during pregnancy have lower birth weights than infants of nonsmoking mothers. In addition, women who smoke have an increased risk of preterm delivery, perinatal mortality, placenta previa, and possibly spontaneous abortion. The mechanism by which smoking affects the fetus is not completely understood, but it is likely that it causes intrauterine hypoxia, perhaps through reduced placental blood flow. Also, smoking increases the metabolic rate and thus caloric needs. Weight gain and prepregnant weight tend to be lower in smokers than in nonsmokers, and the diets of smokers are reported to be poorer than those of nonsmokers. Women who smoke have decreased levels or increased needs for several nutrients, including vitamin C, folic acid, zinc, and iron. Women who stop smoking during pregnancy have been successful in increasing the birth weights of their infants. Vitamin and mineral supplementation of the woman who continues to smoke is advisable, but supplementation does not counteract the detrimental effects of smoking on the fetus. Smoking cessation should be the goal for all women who smoke.

Illicit drugs

Increased risk of intrauterine growth retardation (IUGR) and preterm labor is associated with both marijuana and cocaine abuse. The risk of abruptio placentae is also increased by cocaine. Moreover, infants of mothers who abuse crack cocaine often display persistent learning and behavioral abnormalities. It is difficult to determine exactly what impact illicit drugs have on the nutritional status of the pregnant woman because drug abuse is often accompanied by abuse of other substances, such as alcohol or cigarettes, poverty, and poor education, all of which have detrimental influences on nutritional status. Vitamin and mineral supplements are recommended for women who abuse drugs, but supplements cannot be expected to correct the problems associated with drug use during pregnancy. Every effort should be made to convince the pregnant woman to stop using drugs.

Pregnancy Complications with Nutritional Implications

Nausea and vomiting

Nausea and vomiting, or "morning sickness," are common during the first trimester of pregnancy. "Morning sickness" is a misnomer because the symptoms can occur at any time of the day. Although annoying, nausea and vomiting are rarely severe and prolonged enough to impair nutritional status. Severe nausea and vomiting that may continue throughout pregnancy occurs in about 3.5/1000 births. Known as **hyperemesis gravidarum,** this condition results in loss of fluids and electrolytes and limits intake of all other nutrients.

Constipation

Constipation is most common during the last half of pregnancy. Contributing factors include decreased gastrointestinal (GI) motility resulting from increased progesterone levels, increased pressure on the GI tract by the bulky uterus, effects of iron supplementation, and decreased physical activity.

Pregnancy-induced hypertension

Pregnancy-induced hypertension (PIH), also called *preeclampsia* or *toxemia,* is characterized by hypertension, albuminuria, and excessive edema. It generally occurs in the third trimester. The cause is unknown, but diets adequate in protein, kcal, calcium, and sodium are associated with the lowest incidence of PIH. Obesity increases the risk of PIH. Bedrest and antihypertensive medications are used in the treatment of PIH. A severe sodium restriction (1 to 1.5 g daily), which was historically used in prevention and treatment of PIH, is not normally part of the current prenatal regimen.

Diabetes

For the diabetic woman who becomes pregnant or the woman who develops **gestational diabetes mellitus** (diabetes that is first evident during pregnancy), the goal is to maintain normoglycemia during pregnancy. Insulin requirements usually decline during early pregnancy but increase during the second trimester and remain high until delivery. Gestational diabetes often can be managed by dietary modification alone, but some women with type 2 diabetes who become pregnant may require insulin during pregnancy.

Poor control of blood glucose levels during pregnancy is associated with an increased number of congenital malformations and fetal deaths. In fact, it is important for diabetic women to achieve good control before conception; an increased risk of preeclampsia and of producing infants with malformations is present for those who do not.

Nutritional Care

Assessment

Assessment is summarized in Table 3-2.

Intervention and teaching

Objectives of intervention and teaching during pregnancy are for the woman to do the following:

1. Recognize and alter any practices or findings that could interfere with optimal nutritional status and pregnancy outcome.
2. Establish with the health care provider a goal for weight gain within the recommended range and achieve this goal with an appropriate rate of gain.
3. Cope with physiologic changes during pregnancy that interfere with optimal nutritional intake or comfort.

Selecting a balanced diet

Nutritional needs for healthy pregnant women, except perhaps those for iron, can be met through a varied diet of normal foods. The Food Guide Pyramid (see Chapter 1), with an increase to 3 or 4 servings of milk, yogurt, or cheese daily, can be used as a guideline for teaching the pregnant woman to plan an adequate diet.

The Special Supplemental Food Program for Women, Infants, and Children (WIC) provides vouchers for selected food items rich in protein, iron, and vitamin C to women who need this assistance. Low-income women may also be eligible for the Food Stamp program.

When the woman's diet is found to be poor and there is little likelihood of its improving, or when other risk factors (adolescent pregnancy, maternal smoking, use of illicit drugs or alcohol, or multiple gestation) exist, vitamin-mineral supplementation may be required (see the discussion that follows).

Adequate energy and weight gain

The extra 300 kcal needed daily are easily obtained by increasing intake of milk products by one or two servings per day and making small increases in intake of protein foods, fruits, or vegetables. There is little room in the diet for high-kcal foods that are low in nutrients.

Women may be surprised to learn how large the desirable weight gain in pregnancy is, and women who have always worked to keep

Text continued on p. 77

Table 3-2 Assessment of Nutrition in Pregnancy and Lactation

Areas of Concern	Significant Findings
Inadequate Kcal Intake and Weight Gain	*History* Limited income; body image concerns; nausea and vomiting; lack of knowledge about optimal gain during pregnancy, nutritional needs during pregnancy and lactation; stress or fatigue; prepregnant weight <90% of ideal or BMI <19.8; poor obstetric history during previous pregnancies (e.g., spontaneous abortion, delivery of an LBW infant); heavy smoking; illicit drug use; unmarried; adolescent pregnancy *Physical Examination* Pregnancy: failure to demonstrate adequate weight gain (see Figure 3-2); lactation: poor milk production, inadequate gain by infant
Excessive Kcal Intake	*History* Emotional stress, indulgence, and boredom from interruption of job routine; decrease in activity because of awkwardness during pregnancy or interruption of job routine; prepregnant weight >120% of ideal or BMI >26 *Physical Examination* Pregnancy: weight gain > recommended range (see Figure 3-2); lactation: weight gain or maintenance of weight >120% of ideal body weight or BMI >26
Inadequate Protein Intake	*History* Limited income; strict vegetarianism*; nausea and vomiting during pregnancy; lack of knowledge about

*Strict vegetarians consume no milk products, eggs, meat, poultry, or fish. Lacto-vegetarians use milk products, and ovolactovegetarians use both milk products and eggs.

Table 3-2 Assessment of Nutrition in Pregnancy
and Lactation—cont'd

Areas of Concern	Significant Findings
Inadequate Protein Intake—cont'd	*History—cont'd* needs; fatigue (especially during lactation); frequent pregnancies (>3 within 2 years) or high parity; poor obstetric history during previous pregnancies (e.g., spontaneous abortion, delivery of an LBW infant); alcohol or illicit drug use; multiple gestation *Physical Examination* Edema (some lower extremity edema is normal during pregnancy; look for edema in hands and periorbital area); changes in hair color and texture; hair loss *Laboratory Analysis* Serum albumin <3.2 g/dl; ↓ lymphocyte count
Inadequate Vitamin Intake	
Vitamin C	*History* Failure to consume vitamin C–containing foods daily because of poverty, alcohol or drug abuse, or dislike of these foods; increased needs because of smoking, long-term oral contraceptive or salicylate use, multiple gestation *Physical Examination* Bruising, petechiae, bleeding gums *Laboratory Analysis* ↓ serum vitamin C

Continued

Table 3-2 Assessment of Nutrition in Pregnancy and Lactation—cont'd

Areas of Concern	Significant Findings
Inadequate Vitamin Intake—cont'd	
Folic acid	*History*
	Failure to use a daily supplement or foods rich in folic acid; delivery of a previous infant with a neural tube defect; increased needs because of alcohol or drug abuse, smoking, or multiple gestation
	Physical Examination
	Pallor; glossitis
	Laboratory Analysis
	Hct <33%; ↑ MCV; ↓ serum folate
Vitamin B_{12}	*History*
	Strict vegetarian with failure to use a supplement or foods fortified with vitamin B_{12}
	Physical Examination
	Maternal findings: glossitis, pallor, ataxia; infant breastfed by strict vegetarian: delayed growth, pallor, glossitis, developmental delay
	Laboratory Analysis
	↓ Hct; ↑ MCV (in mother or infant); ↓ serum vitamin B_{12} (in mother or infant)
Vitamin D	*History*
	Failure to consume vitamin D–fortified milk because of strict vegetarianism, lactose intolerance, dislike of milk, or cultural practices; little exposure of skin to sunlight because of residence in northern latitudes in winter or cultural prohibitions against exposing the body

Table 3-2   Assessment of Nutrition in Pregnancy and Lactation—cont'd

Areas of Concern	Significant Findings
Inadequate Mineral Intake	
Iron (Fe)	*History*
	Failure to consume a daily supplement and foods rich in Fe because of vegetarianism, limited income, or dislike of these foods; frequent pregnancies or high parity with depletion of stores; adolescent with increased needs for her growth as well as that of the fetus; anemia during a previous pregnancy; pica; menorrhagia; multiple gestation
	Physical Examination
	Pallor, especially of conjunctiva; blue sclerae; koilonychia (spoon-shaped nails)
	Laboratory Analysis
	Hct <33%; Hgb <11 g/dl; ↓ MCV, MCH, MCHC, serum ferritin, serum Fe; ↑ free erythrocyte protoporphyrin (FEP)
Zinc (Zn)	*History*
	Use of supplement containing >30 mg Fe (competition between Zn and Fe for absorption); use of folate or calcium supplement; avoidance of animal protein foods; frequent pregnancies or high parity with depletion of stores; adolescent with increased needs for her growth as well as that of the fetus; pica; alcoholism with increased excretion
	Physical Examination
	Seborrheic dermatitis; alopecia; diarrhea

Continued

Table 3-2   Assessment of Nutrition in Pregnancy
and Lactation—cont'd

Areas of Concern	Significant Findings
Inadequate Mineral Intake—cont'd	
Zinc—cont'd	*Laboratory Analysis* ↓ Serum Zn
Calcium (Ca)	*History* Lactose intolerance; dislike of milk products; strict vegetarianism or cultural food patterns that avoid milk (e.g., Japanese, Mexican); frequent pregnancies or high parity with depletion of stores; adolescent with increased needs for her growth as well as fetus
Potentially Harmful Substances (During Pregnancy)	
Caffeine	*History* Daily consumption of coffee, tea, and soft drinks (other than caffeine-free); use of over-the-counter cold or analgesic medications (not usually recommended during pregnancy; the woman should consult her physician before using)
Alcohol	*History* Use of alcoholic beverages, especially if >1 oz/day or more than 3 or 4 times/wk
Cocaine/other illicit drugs	*History* Use of drugs, especially on a regular basis, during pregnancy *Laboratory Analysis* Positive urinary drug screen

their weight under control may be resistant to achieving the recommended weight gain. Explanation of the components of that weight gain (see Figure 3-1) may help them to understand the importance of weight gain.

Excessive weight gain is associated with the development of diabetes and hypertension; excessive fat accumulation can be difficult to correct after delivery.

Protein

The extra protein needed in addition to the prepregnant intake can be provided by 1 cup of milk and 1 oz of meat or an equivalent meat substitute per day. Protein intake in excess of the recommendations has not been shown to be beneficial.

Minerals and vitamins

Iron: A supplement of 30 mg of ferrous iron is recommended during the second and third trimesters of pregnancy. Ferrous sulfate, 150 mg, provides 30 mg of elemental iron and is often prescribed because it is inexpensive and relatively well absorbed.

Teaching in relation to iron supplementation and iron nutrition includes the following guidelines:

- Take the supplement between meals or at bedtime because certain food components interfere with iron absorption. These include phytates (in whole grains), oxalates (in deep green leafy vegetables), and tannins in tea and coffee.
- Take the supplement with liquids other than milk, coffee, and tea, which inhibit iron absorption.
- Take the supplement at bedtime if it tends to cause GI distress.
- Even with supplementation, include in the daily diet good sources of iron, such as meats and legumes, and vitamin C sources, which enhance iron absorption.
- Keep the supplement out of the reach of children.

Calcium: Supplements are not routinely recommended for pregnant women. Instead, women are encouraged to consume several good dietary sources of calcium daily:
- Dairy products, particularly milk, buttermilk, yogurt, and cheese, are among the richest calcium sources available (Figure 3-4). Three to four daily servings meet most of the needs of pregnant women.

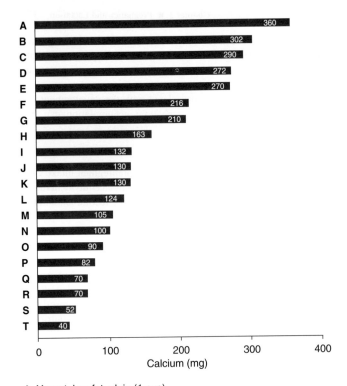

A Yogurt, low-fat, plain (1 cup)
B Milk, skim (1 cup)
C Milk, whole (1 cup)
D Cheese, Swiss (1 oz)
E Yogurt, low-fat, fruit-flavored (1 cup)
F Cheese, cheddar (1 oz)
G Tortilla, corn, "lime" treated (1)
H Cheese food, American (1 oz)
I Orange juice, calcium-fortified ($^1/_2$ cup)
J Turnip greens, cooked ($^1/_2$ cup)
K Tofu (soybean curd), raw ($^1/_2$ cup)
L Sardines, canned, bones eaten (1oz)
M Frozen yogurt ($^1/_2$ cup)
N Pudding, chocolate, ready-to-eat ($^1/_2$ cup)
O Ice cream, vanilla, 10% fat ($^1/_2$ cup)
P Almonds (1 oz or ~25 nuts)
Q Cheese, cottage, 1% fat ($^1/_2$ cup)
R Tortilla, wheat (1)
S Mustard greens, boiled ($^1/_2$ cup)
T Chickpeas (garbanzos), cooked ($^1/_2$ cup)

Figure 3-4
Sources of calcium in the diet.

- Sardines and other canned fish are excellent calcium sources if the bones are eaten.
- Foods made with milk, such as pancakes, waffles, puddings, and cream soups, provide moderate amounts of calcium.
- Most deep green leafy vegetables contain calcium; however, some of these vegetables, such as Swiss chard and spinach, are poor calcium sources because they contain oxalates that prevent absorption of the calcium.
- A commercial enzyme preparation (Lactaid or Lactrase) can be used when consuming milk if the woman has lactose intolerance (cramping, bloating, and diarrhea following milk consumption, resulting from lack of lactase, the enzyme that digests lactose). Lactose-intolerant individuals usually tolerate yogurt and hard cheeses, which contain little lactose. Some individuals with lactose intolerance can tolerate milk as long as they drink only 0.5 to 1 cup at a time.
- Women who do not drink enough milk because they do not like it can use juices and cereal products fortified with calcium.

Other minerals: Good dietary sources of all minerals, especially zinc, should be consumed daily. Sources of zinc include oysters and other shellfish, red meats, poultry, fish, dairy products, legumes, and whole grains (see Appendix A).

Vitamins: Vitamins of greatest concern for the pregnant woman are folic acid, vitamin C, and vitamin D; daily intake of good sources is recommended. Reliable sources of these vitamins include the following:
- Folate: Fruit, juices, green vegetables, and whole grains
- Vitamin C: One to two servings of citrus fruits, broccoli, green peppers, or strawberries
- Vitamin D: Regular exposure of the skin to sunlight using sunscreen or consumption of vitamin D–fortified milk and cereals

Multivitamin-multimineral supplements: The Institute of Medicine (1992) recommends a daily multivitamin and multimineral supplement for women who consume poor diets and those who are at high nutritional risk, such as women carrying more than one fetus, using cigarettes or alcohol heavily, or using illicit drugs. Specifically, this supplement should provide: *iron,* 30 mg; *zinc,* 15 mg; *copper,* 2 mg; *calcium,* 250 mg; *vitamin B_6,* 2 mg; *folic acid,* 300 μg; *vitamin C,* 50 mg; and *vitamin D,* 5 μg.

The supplement should be taken between meals or at bedtime because foods in the GI tract may interfere with its absorption.

A supplement will not remove the risk of potential complications associated with alcohol use, drug abuse, or smoking; abstinence from these practices is the only truly effective measure for preventing their complications.

Single-nutrient supplementation in special circumstances: In a few instances, women may be deficient in or at risk for deficiency of one specific nutrient. The Institute of Medicine (1992) recommends the following for daily supplementation of women at risk:

■ *Vitamin D:* 10 μg or 400 IU is suggested for strict vegetarians or other women with little intake of vitamin D–fortified milk, especially for women with little exposure of the skin to sunlight.
■ *Calcium:* 600 mg is recommended for women under age 25 who consume less than 600 mg of calcium (two 8-oz glasses of milk) a day, because the bones of these women may still be increasing in density. Calcium citrate is a well-absorbed form of calcium that is often used as a supplement. To maximize absorption, it should be taken 1 to 2 hours before or after the iron supplement, and it should not be taken with bran or whole-grain cereals.
■ *Vitamin B$_{12}$:* 2 μg is suggested for strict vegetarians.
■ *Zinc and copper:* 15 mg and 2 mg, respectively, are recommended for women who require therapeutic doses of iron (more than 30 mg daily) to treat anemia, because iron may inhibit absorption and utilization of these minerals.

Avoiding or limiting agents that may harm the fetus

■ *Caffeine:* Insufficient data are available to make a recommendation regarding caffeine use during pregnancy; however, until such data are available, it would be wise to abstain from caffeine use or to limit daily intake to no more than 300 mg (approximately two 6-oz cups of coffee). Sources of caffeine other than coffee may be found in Appendix G.
■ *Alcohol:* Abstinence is the only safe practice. If the mother does not find this possible, she should be urged to limit her intake to small amounts consumed infrequently.
■ *Smoking and drug abuse:* These practices have extremely adverse effects on the fetus, and the woman should be assisted to stop these practices if at all possible.

■ *Artificial sweeteners:* Aspartame (NutraSweet), an artificial sweetener, has not been found to have adverse effects on the normal mother or fetus, but its use should be avoided by pregnant women homozygous for phenylketonuria (PKU). Saccharin, another artificial sweetener, has not been shown to be safe for use during pregnancy.

Using nutritional measures to cope with common discomforts

Nausea and vomiting: Suggestions for coping:

■ Eat small, frequent meals; hunger can worsen nausea.
■ Avoid fluids for 1 to 2 hours before and after meals.
■ Consume plain, starchy foods (crackers, dry toast, Melba toast, rice, pasta or noodles, plain boiled or baked potatoes, unsweetened cooked or ready-to-eat cereals) during times of nausea because they are easily digested and unlikely to cause nausea. Spicy foods can worsen nausea.
■ Decrease intake of fats and fried foods. Fat delays gastric emptying and can increase nausea.
■ Minimize exposure to strong food odors. Avoid cooking foods with strong odors during times of nausea, maintain adequate ventilation in the kitchen, and use lids on pots during cooking.
■ Avoid brushing teeth immediately after eating because this causes some individuals to gag.
■ Try salty foods (e.g., potato chips) or tart foods (e.g., lemonade), which are tolerated well by some women with nausea.

The woman suffering from hyperemesis gravidarum may require hospitalization to receive intravenous fluids for rehydration. Peripheral parenteral nutrition (containing glucose, amino acids, vitamins, and electrolytes) or an enteral tube feeding may be used initially. When vomiting has diminished, small amounts of low-fat, easily digested starches, skinless poultry, and lean meats are reintroduced orally, and the diet is gradually advanced as tolerated. Occasionally, nausea and vomiting will be so severe and prolonged that the woman requires prolonged enteral tube feeding or total parenteral nutrition (see Chapters 9 and 10).

Constipation: To improve bowel evacuation:

■ Increase intake of dietary fiber to at least 25 to 30 g/day (see Appendix B).

- Consume approximately 50 ml fluid/kg body weight daily, to ensure that adequate fluid is available to form soft, bulky stools.
- Exercise (e.g., walk briskly) regularly to improve muscle tone and stimulate bowel motility.

Using nutritional measures to help control PIH and diabetes

PIH: A moderate restriction of sodium to 2 to 3 g/day may be prescribed to help control PIH. Omit the following foods and seasonings from the diet: salt, seasoning salts, and obviously salty foods, such as potato chips and pretzels; smoked or canned meats, fish, and poultry; condiments and seasonings, such as prepared mustard, catsup, Worcestershire or soy sauce; canned soups and vegetables (unless they are low-sodium); bouillon; prepared mixes for cakes, casseroles, breads and muffins, gravies or sauces, and puddings (especially instant); frozen entrees; commercially prepared pies and pastries; and salted butter, margarine, peanut butter, and cheese.

Good choices for a low-sodium diet include fresh, canned, or frozen fruits; fresh vegetables and those canned or frozen without salt (check label); and unprocessed meats, poultry, and fish.

Diabetes: The diet for diabetes in pregnancy is discussed in Chapter 18. Strict control of blood glucose is currently advocated in many diabetes treatment centers, with insulin-dependent women receiving several daily injections or continuous infusions with an insulin pump.

Lactation

Human milk is an ideal food for the infant, and any mother who is interested in breastfeeding should be encouraged to do so. The advantages of breastfeeding are summarized in Box 3-1.

Special Concerns

Nutritional requirements

Kilocalories

The RDA (1989) suggests that the lactating woman consume about 500 kcal per day more than her nonpregnant intake. Because this level is inadequate to meet the energy cost of producing milk, maternal stores deposited during pregnancy are used to provide the extra kcal required. Thus, return to prepregnant weight is often more rapid in women who breastfeed.

Box 3-1   Advantages of Breastfeeding

Infant Benefits

Reduced risk of diarrheal diseases, respiratory diseases, bacterial meningitis, and otitis media. Human milk contains a variety of antiinfective factors and immune cells, such as IgA, IgM, IgG, B- and T-lymphocytes, neutrophils, macrophages, complement, and lactoferrin, that are not found in infant formula. In addition, human milk appears to contain immunomodulating factors that stimulate the infant to produce interferon and other agents of immunity.

Reduced risk of overfeeding.

Ease of digestion. Lactalbumin protein in human milk forms a soft, easily digested curd in the infant's stomach. Lipase enzyme in human milk improves the digestion of milk fat.

Improved absorption of zinc and iron, compared with absorption from formula.

Potential for reduced risk of allergic diseases, type 1 diabetes mellitus, Crohn's disease and ulcerative colitis, sudden infant death syndrome, and lymphoma

Potential for enhanced cognitive development. Infants fed human milk have been found to have higher scores on intelligence tests at school age than those fed formula. These findings may be related to the fact that human milk is rich in certain long-chain polyunsaturated fatty acids believed to be needed for neurologic development. These fatty acids are especially important for preterm infants, who are more immature neurologically than term infants.

Maternal Benefits

Less postpartum bleeding and more rapid uterine involution. Oxytocin levels are increased in the breastfeeding mother.

Convenience (once lactation is established).

Economy.

More rapid postpartum weight loss.

Increased child spacing because of delayed resumption of ovulation. Note that this does not mean that breastfeeding is a reliable method of contraception.

Reduced risk of ovarian and premenopausal breast cancer.

Improved bone mineralization in the postpartum period, with a reduced risk of postmenopausal hip fractures.

Mutual Benefit

Promotion of maternal-infant bonding.

Protein

Recommendations for protein are 65 g during the first 6 months of lactation and 62 g during the second 6 months. This amount is easily obtained in the U.S. diet; women often consume this much protein or more even before becoming pregnant.

Vitamins and minerals

Vitamin B_{12} and calcium are of special concern during lactation. Vitamin B_{12} deficiency has been found to affect approximately two thirds of lactating women who have followed strict vegetarian diets for several years; deficient women often produce milk with very low vitamin B_{12} levels. Megaloblastic (macrocytic) anemia, poor growth, and neurologic abnormalities have occurred in infants breastfed by such mothers.

The RDA for calcium during lactation remains the same as during pregnancy (1000 mg/day for adult women, and 1300 mg/day for teens; Food and Nutrition Board, 1997). For women who do not drink milk, other good sources of calcium are listed in Figure 3-4 or Appendix A. The use of milk in cooking (e.g., in mashed potatoes, grain products, and soups) can greatly increase milk intake. If the woman's diet appears likely to be inadequate, a daily calcium supplement is advisable.

Foods and other substances to avoid

Lactating women are sometimes told to avoid "gas-forming" foods such as onions, cabbage, legumes, chocolate, and spicy foods. There is little basis for these prohibitions. Very rarely a mother will note that some food she consumes causes a rash, diarrhea, or irritability in her infant on a consistent basis. Elimination of this food from her diet readily corrects this problem.

Excessive maternal alcohol intake during lactation appears to have a detrimental effect on infant motor development and can impair the mother's milk ejection reflex. If a woman chooses to drink alcohol during lactation, it would be best for her to limit her intake to no more than one drink per day. Drugs of abuse, including amphetamines, cocaine, heroin, marijuana, and phencyclidine hydrochloride (angel dust), should be avoided during lactation.

The iron content of milk from mothers drinking three or more cups of coffee per day has been found to be approximately one third lower than in mothers drinking less than three cups. Only 1% of the caffeine consumed by the mother is passed into her milk, but infants are unable to metabolize and excrete caffeine as effectively as adults. Some infants of mothers who consume caffeine have been noted to have irritability and insomnia, and mothers who note these symptoms would be well advised to limit their intake of caffeine from coffee, tea, chocolate, soft drinks, and some over-the-counter drugs.

Diabetes

Breastfeeding may have a positive effect on blood glucose control in type 1 diabetes. Successful breastfeeding is associated with a kcal prescription of at least 31 kcal/kg of maternal weight (14 kcal/lb). Women with diabetes should be carefully monitored for mastitis because it is more common in diabetic than in nondiabetic women.

Nutritional Care

Assessment

Assessment is summarized in Table 3-2.

Intervention and teaching

The objectives of intervention and teaching are for the woman to do the following:

1. Maintain an adequate diet to replenish stores that were diminished during pregnancy and produce sufficient milk for growth of the infant.
2. Lose the weight gained during pregnancy.
3. Avoid nutritional practices that could harm the infant.
4. Establish a successful breastfeeding relationship with her infant.

Eating a balanced diet and achieving prepregnant weight

Food guide: The Food Guide Pyramid (see Chapter 1), with inclusion of approximately 3 to 4 servings of milk, yogurt, or cheese, is appropriate during lactation. A variety of foods from all food groups should be consumed.

Kilocalories: The increased kcal needs should be met by use of additional milk products and small increases in meat and meat substitutes, fruits and vegetables, and whole-grain or enriched breads and cereals. Fatigue and the demands of the infant on the woman's time may interfere with food preparation. Commercially prepared foods such as low-salt and low-fat frozen meals may be helpful during the early postpartum period.

Protein: Most of the extra protein needed is provided by the consumption of 3 to 4 cups of milk or equivalent products per day.

Calcium: Those individuals who do not consume dairy products should follow the suggestions given for pregnant women. Careful selection of high-calcium foods (see examples in Figure 3-4) and use of foods prepared with milk (e.g., pancakes and waffles) will ensure an adequate calcium intake.

Fluid: To produce adequate milk, women need 35 to 50 ml of fluid/kg of body weight per day (16 to 23 ml/lb/day) plus an additional 500 to 1000 ml. This amount should be sufficient for most women. Water, milk, tea, decaffeinated coffee, soft drinks, fruit juices, and ices can be used to meet fluid needs. If energy intake is likely to be excessive, then emphasis should be placed on skim milk and calorie-free beverages. Women may perceive 100% fruit juices as healthful drinks, but these contain about 60 kcal in 120 ml and are a significant source of energy if used to quench thirst.

Vitamin B$_{12}$: Strict vegetarian mothers need a supplement or soy milk fortified with vitamin B$_{12}$.

Exercise: It is important to exercise regularly after the birth of the baby to promote weight control, reshape the figure, and foster a feeling of health and well-being. The lactating woman can participate in any activity she enjoys. It is essential that she have adequate fluid intake during and after exercise to replace losses in perspiration and to avoid interfering with milk production. After very heavy exercise, lactic acid may accumulate in the milk and cause the infant to reject the following feeding. This condition is usually temporary, with the infant feeding well at the next feeding.

Avoiding practices that could harm the infant

In a few circumstances, mothers should not be encouraged to breastfeed. These include the following:

- Galactosemia (congenital inability to metabolize galactose, a component of lactose) in the newborn.
- Serious maternal infections that pose a threat to the infant, such as sputum-positive tuberculosis. In the United States and other industrialized nations, women positive for the human immuno-deficiency virus (HIV) are advised not to breastfeed because the

virus is present in milk. In developing countries, however, the issue is more complicated. The antiinfective properties of human milk, which protect the infant from many diarrheal and respiratory infections associated with high mortality, may outweigh the risk of transmission of HIV posed by breastfeeding. Human T-lymphotrophic virus infection and active herpes simplex on the breast may also be contraindications to breastfeeding.

■ Maternal need for certain drugs that are secreted in milk (Box 3-2).
■ Maternal disinclination to breastfeed.

Certain medical conditions are compatible with breastfeeding as long as there is careful supervision by the health care provider:

■ Phenylketonuria (PKU) in the infant: Human milk is relatively low in phenylalanine, and many PKU infants can be totally or partially breastfed if their phenylalanine levels are closely monitored.
■ Severe "breast milk jaundice" (serum bilirubin concentration approaching 20 mg/dl): Human milk contains an inhibitor of bilirubin conjugation and excretion, and therefore in some cases of severe hyperbilirubinemia, pediatricians may recommend temporary interruption of breastfeeding. After 12 to 24 hours of formula feeding, bilirubin usually declines, and breastfeeding can continue. The mother should be reassured that her milk is not bad for the infant and assisted in pumping her breasts if necessary during the interruption of breastfeeding.
■ Hepatitis B: Carriers of hepatitis B may breastfeed as long as their infants have received hepatitis B immune globulin at birth and hepatitis B vaccine before hospital discharge.

Certain personal practices are potentially harmful during breastfeeding:

■ Lactating women should be encouraged to avoid regular and heavy drinking, even though there are currently insufficient data available regarding the effects of alcohol intake during lactation.
■ Smoking should be avoided. Nicotine appears in milk, but the major risk to the infant is from "passive smoking"—exposure to tobacco pollutants within the home environment.
■ Heavy use of caffeine (more than 300 mg daily) might increase the infant's risk of iron deficiency. Decaffeinated beverages are preferable to those containing caffeine.

Box 3-2   Drugs and Breastfeeding

Drugs That Are Contraindicated During Breastfeeding

Amphetamine (Biphetamine)
Bromocriptine (Parlodel)
Cocaine
Cyclophosphamide (Cytoxan, Neosar)
Cyclosporine (Sandimmune)
Doxorubicin (Adriamycin)
Ergotamine (Bellergal-S, Cafergot, Ergostat, Wigraine)
Heroin
Lithium (Eskalith, Lithobid, Lithane)
Marijuana
Methotrexate (Folex)
Nicotine
Phencyclidine (PCP)

Drugs That Require Temporary Cessation of Breastfeeding (times to stop breastfeeding are only guidelines; testing milk is the best way to ensure radioactivity is no longer present)

Gallium-67 (72 hr)
Iodine-123 (have milk tested)
Iodine-123 hippuran (24 hr)
Iodine-125 (have milk tested; 2 to 4 wk)
Iodine-131 (36 hr for test dose, 2 wk for therapeutic dose)
Iodine-131 hippuran (24 hr)
Iodine-131 macroaggregate (10-12 days)
Radioactive sodium (1 to 4 days)
Technetium-99m (24 hr)

Modified from Committe on Drugs, American Academy of Pediatrics: *Pediatrics* 93:137, 1994; Lawrence RA: *Breastfeeding: a guide for the medical profession,* ed 4, St Louis, 1994, Mosby; The Lactation Study Center, Rochester, New York; and Logsdon BA: *J Am Pharmaceut Assoc* NS 37:407, 1997. Consult these sources for further information about maternal drug usage and breastfeeding.

Establishing successful breastfeeding

Many actions by health care providers can enhance the likelihood of successful breastfeeding. Early and sustained contact between the infant and mother (e.g., the opportunity to breastfeed within the first hour of life and to room in with the infant in the hospital) is

---

Box 3-2   Drugs and Breastfeeding—cont'd

Drugs Whose Effect on Nursing Infants Is Unknown but May Be of Concern

Amitriptyline (Elavil, Etrafon, Limbitrol, Triavil)
Amoxapine (Asendin)
Chloramphenicol (Chloromycetin)
Chlorpromazine (Thorazine)
Chlorprothixene (Taractan)
Desipramine (Norpramin)
Diazepam (Valium)
Dothiepin
Doxepin (Adapin, Sinequan)
Fluoxetine (Prozac)
Fluvoxamine maleate
Haloperidol (Haldol)
Imipramine (Tofranil)
Lorazepam (Ativan)
Mesoridazine (Serentil)
Metoclopramide (Reglan)
Metronidazole (Flagyl, MetroGel, Protostat)
Perphenazine (Etrafon, Triavil, Trilafon)
Prazepam (Centrax)
Quazepam (Doral)
Temazepam (Restoril)
Tinidazole
Trazodone (Desyrel)

Drugs That Should Be Used Only with Caution

Aspirin
Clemastine (Tavist)
Phenobarbital (Donnatal, Kinesed, Quadrinal, Tedral)
Primidone (Mysoline)
Sulfasalazine (Azulfidine)

---

an important measure. The infant should not be supplemented with water, glucose solutions, or formula unless the infant's medical condition makes supplementation necessary. In general, supplements and pacifiers should be used only after lactation is established, if at all. When juices, formula, and solid foods are introduced, the mother's milk production declines, and these foods and fluids are generally unnecessary until at least 6 months of age. Growth spurts occur during infancy, and the infant may seem continually hungry at these times. The mother can be reassured that this is normal and that her milk is sufficient; more frequent feedings will increase her milk supply so that the infant's needs are met.

For the infant, some signs of successful breastfeeding include a moist tongue and good hydration, weight gain of 15 to 30 g/day after the milk comes in, at least 3 to 4 bowel movements and 4 to 6 urinations daily after day three of life, and rhythmic sucking with audible swallowing during breastfeeding. Some signs of success in the mother include milk "coming in" by 72 hours after delivery (the breasts feel full and warm, and milk may leak), comfortable feedings, and letdown of milk, evidenced by the infant's swallows, leaking of milk, and softening of the breasts after feeding.

SELECTED BIBLIOGRAPHY

American Academy of Pediatrics Work Group on Breastfeeding: Breastfeeding and the use of human milk, *Pediatrics* 100:1035-1039, 1997.

American Diabetes Association: Gestational diabetes mellitus, *Diabetes Care* 22 (suppl 1):S74-S75, 1999.

Butterworth CE Jr, Bendich A: Folic acid and the prevention of birth defects, *Ann Rev Nutr* 16:73, 1996.

Dallongeville J, Marecaux N, Fruchart JC, Amouyel P: Cigarette smoking is associated with unhealthy patterns of nutrient intake: a meta-analysis, *J Nutr* 128:1450, 1998.

Ellings JM, Newman RB, Bowers NA: Prenatal care and multiple pregnancy, *J Obstet Gynecol Neonatal Nurs* 27:457, 1998.

Food and Nutrition Board, National Academy of Sciences, Institute of Medicine: *Dietary reference intakes: calcium, phosphorus, magnesium, vitamin D, and fluoride,* Washington, DC, 1997, National Academy Press.

Institute of Medicine, National Academy of Sciences: *Nutrition during pregnancy and lactation: an implementation guide,* Washington, DC, 1992, National Academy Press.

National Academy of Sciences: *Recommended dietary allowances,* ed 10, Washington, DC, 1989, National Academy Press.

Nehlig A, Debry G: Consequences on the newborn of chronic maternal consumption of coffee during gestation and lactation: a review, *J Am Coll Nutr* 13:6, 1994.

Newman V, Fullerton JT, Anderson PO: Clinical advances in the management of severe nausea and vomiting during pregnancy, *J Obstet Gynecol Neonatal Nurs* 22:483, 1993.

Position of the American Dietetic Association: use of nutritive and nonnutritive sweeteners, *J Am Dietet Assoc* 93:816, 1993.

Prentice A: Calcium requirements of breast feeding mothers, *Nutr Rev* 56:124-130, 1998.

Rainville AJ: Pica practices of pregnant women are associated with lower maternal hemoglobin level at delivery, *J Am Dietet Assoc* 98:293, 1998.

Rees JM: Nutrition for pregnant and childbearing adolescents: demographics, developmental needs, behavior, and outcome, *Ann NY Acad Sci* 817:246, 1997.

Schieve LA, Cogswell ME, Scanlon KS: An empiric evaluation of the Institute of Medicine's pregnancy weight gain guidelines by race, *Obstet Gynecol* 91:878, 1998.

Slusser W, Powers NG: Breastfeeding update 1: immunology, nutrition, and advocacy, *Pediatrics in Review* 18:111-119, 1997.

Infancy, Childhood, and Adolescence

During infancy, childhood, and adolescence, adequate nutrition is essential for the promotion of growth and the establishment of a framework for lasting health. Growth is the simplest and most basic parameter for evaluation of nutritional status in children.

Evaluating Growth

Adequate nutrition is reflected in a child's progress on standardized growth charts depicting height/length for age, weight for age, weight for stature, head circumference for age (up to 36 months of age), and body mass index for age. Sex- and age-specific charts are available for children from birth through 20 years (see Appendix D).

Each child establishes an individual growth pattern and should follow this pattern consistently. Children should be evaluated for nutritional or medical disorders when one of the following occurs:

- They are consistently below the 5th or above the 95th percentile for any growth parameter. Some normal children fall outside the boundaries of the 5th and 95th percentile markings, but all children outside these boundaries should be evaluated to be sure that their growth patterns are reasonable for them (e.g., consistent with the size of their parents and other family members).
- They fail to stay within one percentile marking of their previous growth parameter (e.g., weight has been at 75th percentile marking, and it then declines below the 50th percentile).
- Weight and height (or length) are inconsistent with each other (e.g., weight is at the 90th percentile but height is at the 25th percentile).

Infancy

Special Concerns

Human milk and infant formula

Human milk is ideally suited to meet the needs of the term infant (see Box 3-1). The composition of human milk changes over the first few weeks of lactation. **Colostrum,** the milk produced for about the first 3 to 5 days, is yellowish, rich in immunoglobulins and lymphocytes, and higher in protein than mature human milk. Mature human milk is produced after about 10 to 14 days. It appears watery and may be bluish; it has more lactose and lipid than does colostrum. Transitional milk, produced in the period between colostrum and mature milk production, has some features of each type of milk.

Either human milk or iron-fortified infant formula meets the nutritional needs of term infants for the first 4 to 6 months of life. Commercial formulas closely resemble human milk. Standard formulas and human milk contain about 20 kcal/oz (66 kcal/100 ml). Absorption and utilization of nutrients from human milk are generally very good. Commercial formulas contain higher levels of protein and most minerals than human milk to compensate for less complete absorption and utilization. The formula-fed infant may grow more rapidly than the breastfed one, but more rapid growth has not been shown to be an advantage for a healthy term infant.

Commercial formulas are manufactured with or without added iron. The low-iron formulas are virtually iron free, as is cow's milk. Anemia is common in infants receiving low-iron formulas. For infants who are not breastfed, use of iron-fortified formulas for the first year of life provides a reliable source of dietary iron. Commercial formulas are available in three forms: ready-to-feed, concentrate (to be diluted with an equal volume of water), and powder. The three forms are the same in nutritional value (except for fluoride), and the concentrate or powdered forms are almost always less expensive than ready-to-feed.

Frequency and amount of feedings

Infants vary considerably in their feeding patterns, but after the first few weeks of life most breastfed infants feed at approximately 3-hour intervals and formula-fed infants feed at 4-hour intervals. Overfeeding is more likely than underfeeding, but parents frequently worry about whether they are feeding their infants enough, especially if the infants are breastfed. Infants who are gaining weight steadily and are wetting at least six to eight diapers per day are usually taking in enough milk or formula.

Nutritional Problems in Infancy

Acute gastroenteritis

Acute episodes of diarrhea and vomiting, usually associated with viral illness, are common during infancy and early childhood. These illnesses damage the intestinal mucosa and diminish the absorptive surface. In addition, the increased motility of the GI tract during gastroenteritis may not allow sufficient time for fat absorption. Fatty foods often worsen diarrhea and delay gastric emptying, which may increase vomiting.

Much of the intestine's maltase (an enzyme that is involved in digestion of maltose, glucose oligosaccharides [corn syrup solids] and starch) is retained during gastroenteritis. Salivary and pancreatic amylases (enzymes active in starch digestion) are also adequate. Therefore, it is best to choose foods low in fat and high in glucose oligosaccharides or starch during and immediately after a bout of gastroenteritis.

Diarrhea can result from malabsorption of sorbitol and fructose in fruit juices. If diarrhea is chronic, rather than acute, then the child's intake of fruit juices should be evaluated. Intakes of juice should be restricted to no more than 12 fluid oz (360 ml) daily.

Food hypersensitivity

In infants and small children, symptoms of **food hypersensitivity** or allergy (an immunologic reaction to ingestion of a food or food additive) can include anaphylaxis, failure to thrive, vomiting, abdominal pain, diarrhea, rhinitis, sinusitis, otitis media, cough, wheezing, rash, urticaria, and atopic dermatitis. Egg white, cow's milk, peanuts, nuts from trees, wheat, and fish are among the most allergenic foods for children. A significant proportion of infants allergic to cow's milk are also allergic to soy and thus cannot tolerate soy formulas. Protein hydrolysate formulas (in which the protein is hydrolyzed so that no large protein molecules are present to stimulate an allergic response) such as Nutramigen are often used for infants with allergic symptoms. Eighty-five percent of children with milk allergy outgrow it by their third year of life. Reintroduction of milk or any other suspected allergen into the diet should be done in a setting where epinephrine, intravenous fluids, and respiratory support are available.

Failure to thrive

Failure to thrive describes the infant who does not regain his or her birth weight by 3 weeks of age or the infant who exhibits continuous weight loss or failure to gain weight at the appropriate rate (see Appendix D). This condition results from an inadequate food supply or illness in the infant. *Organic* failure to thrive is a condition in which a physiologic reason for the infant's failure to thrive is apparent. Insufficient milk production by the breast-feeding mother and cystic fibrosis in the infant are two examples of this condition. When no physical cause is apparent, the infant has *inorganic* failure to thrive. Impairments in the parent-child relationship, knowledge deficits in the parent or caregiver, and poor parenting skills are some reasons for inorganic failure to thrive.

Nutritional Care

Assessment

Assessment is summarized in Table 4-1.

Intervention and parent teaching

Goals of intervention and teaching are to assist the infant to consume an adequate diet for optimal growth and development; to avoid practices that may contribute to obesity, poor dentition, or other health problems; and to eat a wide variety of foods.

Human milk feedings

The following information should be included when instructing the breastfeeding mother:

- Make sure that the infant "latches on" well. The infant's mouth should cover as much of the areola (the dark area around the nipple) as possible and never cover just the nipple (Figure 4-1). If the infant is grasping only the nipple or nursing is painful to the mother, then she should insert her finger between the breast and the infant's mouth to break the seal and then reposition the infant's mouth before beginning again. Improper grasp of the nipple makes nipples sore and may lead to cracking.
- Feed the infant from both breasts at each feeding. Begin each feeding with the breast the infant ended with at the last feeding, to ensure that the breast is drained at least every other feeding. Emptying the breasts encourages milk production. If twins are being breastfed, feed each baby on alternate breasts every other

Table 4-1   Assessment in Growth and Development

Areas of Concern	Significant Findings
Inadequate Kcal or Protein Intake	*History* Poverty; chronic illness or frequent acute illnesses; altered parent-infant relationship manifested by failure to feed infant adequately; fear of becoming obese; obsession with thinness (older children and adolescents); poorly planned vegetarian diet *Physical Examination* Length, height, or weight <5th percentile, or decrease in these parameters by >one percentile marking; edema, ascites; hair changes: alopecia, loss of pigmentation (flag sign), altered texture; muscle wasting; TSF <5th percentile for age; tooth erosion, gastric bleeding, weak and flabby muscles, poor skin turgor (signs of self-induced vomiting) *Laboratory Analysis* ↓ Serum albumin, transferrin, and prealbumin, lymphocyte count, serum K^+ (self-induced vomiting)
Excessive Kcal Intake	*History* Overfeeding; sedentary lifestyle: frequent and prolonged television viewing, lack of regular physical activity; one or both parents overweight or obese *Physical Examination* Weight >95th percentile for length/height; TSF >95th percentile for age

Table 4-1   Assessment in Growth and Development—cont'd

Areas of Concern	Significant Findings
Inadequate Mineral Intake	
Iron (Fe)	*History*
	Poverty; dislike of iron-containing foods; vegetarianism; increased needs (especially adolescent females); excessive milk consumption by toddlers; infant receiving cow's milk before 12 months of age
	Physical Examination
	Pallor; blue sclerae; koilonychia (spoon-shaped nails); short attention span; diminished learning ability
	Laboratory Analysis
	↓ Hgb, Hct, MCV, MCH, MCHC, serum Fe, serum ferritin; ↑ free erythrocyte protoporphyrin (FEP), serum transferrin
Zinc (Zn)	*History*
	Poverty; dislike of zinc-containing foods; vegetarianism (large intake of grains and vegetables containing phytates and oxalates that impede absorption); abnormal losses (severe or prolonged diarrhea)
	Physical Examination
	Seborrheic dermatitis; anorexia; weight or length <5th percentile for age, or decline in these parameters by >1 percentile marking; diarrhea
	Laboratory Analysis
	↓ Serum Zn
Calcium (Ca)	*History*
	Failure to consume milk products, calcium-fortified soy milk or formula, or a calcium supplement daily because of food preferences, vegetarianism, dieting, or frequent reliance on fast foods

Continued

Table 4-1   Assessment in Growth and Development—cont'd

Areas of Concern	Significant Findings
Inadequate Vitamin Intake	
A	*History*
	Failure to consume vitamin A (liver, deep green, leafy, or deep yellow vegetables) at least every other day; frequent reliance on fast foods
	Physical Examination
	Dry skin, mucous membranes, or cornea; follicular hyperkeratosis (resembles gooseflesh); poor growth, susceptibility to infection
	Laboratory Analysis
	↓ Serum retinol
B_{12}	*History*
	Child or adolescent following strict vegetarian diet without a supplement or use of fortified soy milk*; infant breastfed by strict vegetarian mother
	Physical Examination
	Pallor; glossitis; neurologic abnormalities (altered sensation, altered sense of balance)
	Laboratory Analysis
	↓ Serum vitamin B_{12}, Hct; ↑ MCV

*Young children should not follow strict vegetarian regimens because of the difficulty of ensuring that the diet contains adequate kcal and protein for growth. Lactovegetarian diets and ovolactovegetarian diets can be adequate for children.

feeding. One baby is likely to be a more vigorous feeder than the other.
■ Exposing the nipple to the air helps to heal it if it becomes sore or cracked (e.g., leave flaps of nursing bra down for 20 minutes after feedings). Massaging a drop of colostrum or milk into the

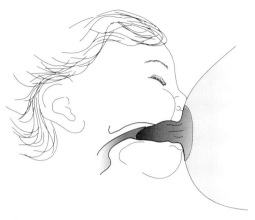

Figure 4-1
Infant properly latched on at the breast. Note that most of
the areola is in the infant's mouth.

nipple is also helpful. Begin with brief feedings (< 5 minutes per
breast) to avoid nipple soreness, but progress to 15 to 20 minutes
per breast. Milk fat is usually released only after 10 to 20 minutes
of suckling, and the infant needs the fat to grow properly and to
be satisfied between feedings.

■ Avoid offering bottle feedings (expressed human milk or
formula) until the mother's milk supply is established, usually 4
to 6 weeks after birth. The artificial nipple is different and may
confuse the infant, causing him or her to refuse the breast. After
that time, it may be possible to give a bottle so that the mother
can be away from the infant. Many mothers who return to work
outside the home continue to breastfeed for months, either by
pumping their breasts during breaks at work or by adjusting their
breastfeeding schedule to only two to three feedings per day.

■ Use different infant positions (e.g., cradle hold across the
mother's body, lying beside the mother, and football hold with
the infant's head in the mother's hand, nursing from the breast on
the same side of the body as that hand) to drain different portions
of the breast and decrease the risk of clogging the milk ducts.
Clogging causes discomfort and may lead to mastitis or breast
infection. If signs of clogging or mastitis (redness, enlargement,
and pain in a portion of the breast) occur, then the mother should

nurse more frequently, beginning on the affected side. The baby is hungrier at the beginning of the feeding and will nurse more effectively, helping to relieve the clogging.

Formula feeding

When teaching the parents of a formula-fed infant, include the following information:

- Hold the infant closely during feedings. Never prop a bottle or leave an infant unattended during feeding, both for safety reasons and because feedings are an important time for nurturing.
- Be attuned to the infant's degree of hunger. Never encourage him or her to take more at a feeding than he or she seems to want. Table 4-2 gives general guidelines as to the amount of formula to feed, but the individual infant may have different needs.
- Burp the infant regularly during feeding, every 0.5 to 1 oz initially and less often as the infant grows.
- Positioning the infant on the right side or sitting up after feedings encourages gastric emptying.

Introducing solid foods

There is no need to introduce solid foods before 4 to 6 months of age. Reasons for delaying consumption of solid food include the following:

- The tongue extrusion reflex, which tends to push solid foods out of the mouth, does not fade until the infant is about 4 months of age.
- Production of pancreatic amylase, an important enzyme for digestion of starches in infant foods, is low before 4 months.
- Infants can maintain good head control at 4 months of age and can sit fairly well by 6 months of age. Thus, they are better prepared than younger infants to participate in the feeding process; for example, an infant can turn his or her head away from the spoon to indicate that he or she is full.
- Eczema and other atopic diseases are more common in infants who have undergone early introduction of solid foods; the greater the diversity of foods introduced, the greater the risk.
- Early introduction of solid food has no effect on sleep patterns. Many parents introduce solid foods early, erroneously believing that this will cause the infant to sleep through the night.

Table 4-2   Approximate Daily Amount of 20 kcal/oz Formula
Needed by Infants Younger Than 6 Months

Infant Weight			
kg	lb	Caloric Need	Ounces of Formula Needed
3	6.6	324	16.2
4	8.8	432	21.6
5	11.0	540	27.0
6	13.2	648	32.4

- Solid foods can inhibit absorption of iron and other nutrients from human milk.
- Introduction of solid foods before 4 to 6 months of age is associated with a shorter duration of lactation.

Method of introducing solid foods. When introducing solid foods, the parents should follow these guidelines:

- Begin with foods that provide needed nutrients. For breastfed infants, this means good sources of iron, zinc, protein, and kcal. Iron-fortified infant cereals and pureed meats, vegetables, and fruits are usually among the first foods. Within this group of foods, the order of introduction is not of major importance.
- Introduce only one new food every 3 to 5 days, and observe the infant for hypersensitivity reactions after each food. If a reaction is thought to have occurred, then stop that food for several weeks and try again later. If the same thing occurs after the second or third trial, then the infant is probably sensitive to this food. Use single-grain cereals until it is clear that the infant tolerates all grains contained in mixed cereals.
- Wait until late in infancy or after infancy to introduce egg white and shellfish, which are among the foods most likely to cause allergy.
- Begin with about 1 tsp at a time, and advance the amount as the infant seems ready.
- Offer solid foods at the beginning of feedings while the infant is hungry.
- Thin foods with formula or expressed breast milk initially (e.g., 1 spoon of cereal to 6 spoons of formula or milk) to help the

infant make the transition from human milk or formula to foods with thicker consistencies.

■ Feed the infant with a spoon. Adding foods to formula in a bottle deprives the infant of a chance to learn feeding skills. Infants with certain medical disorders are exceptions to this rule. Thickening the formula with infant cereal may help to control gastroesophageal reflux, for example.

■ Never feed the infant from the jar. If any food is left over, amylase enzyme in the saliva will digest starches in the food, making it watery. Also, bacteria from the mouth contaminate the food and might cause spoilage.

■ Avoid serving desserts regularly; these are usually low in nutrients and establish a desire for sweets.

■ Consider the developmental state of the infant in choosing foods. For instance, between 7 and 9 months of age the infant's purposeful grasp improves and he or she picks objects up and moves them to his or her mouth. This is an ideal time to offer finger foods such as toast, zwieback, dry cereals, and cheese slices.

Home preparation of infant foods. Some parents may wish to prepare food at home for the infant. When preparing infant foods at home, the parents should follow certain guidelines:

■ Use fresh or frozen fruits, vegetables, and meats. Canned foods may contain lead, and canned vegetables and meats contain salt unless they are "no salt added" products.

■ Cook foods in as little water as possible, and do not overcook; this preparation preserves the vitamin content.

■ Add no sugar or salt. Infants have a well-developed sense of taste and do not require flavor enhancers. The infant receives enough sodium from unsalted foods, and routine use of sugar and salt causes the infant to develop a taste for these unnecessary food additives.

■ Puree foods in a blender or food grinder initially; chop or mash foods once the infant has more teeth and can chew lumpier foods.

■ Freeze prepared foods in ice trays for later use; one to two cubes can be used each time for an infant-sized serving.

■ Avoid home-prepared spinach, carrots, beets, turnips, or collard greens, which may contain enough nitrates to cause methemoglobinemia, inhibiting the transport of oxygen by the red blood cells.

Minimizing the risk of obesity

To minimize the risk of obesity, parents can:

■ Reduce formula and milk intake as infants consume more solids.
■ Recognize and respond to cues that the infant has reached satiety. Satiety cues from a younger infant include withdrawing from the nipple, falling asleep, closing the lips tightly, and turning the head away. Cues from an older infant include closing the lips tightly, shaking the head "no", playing with or throwing utensils or food, and handing the cup or bottle back to the parent.
■ Never insist that the infant finish a bottle, dish, or jar of food. Before 6 months, an average serving size is about 2 to 5 tablespoons, and after 6 months, it is approximately 1/2 to 1 jar of baby food. Infants' needs vary widely, however, and an individual infant may not need an average serving.

Transition from formula to cow's milk

The American Academy of Pediatrics, Committee on Nutrition (1998) recommends that infants receive human milk or iron-fortified formula for the first year of life. It is especially important that skim milk not be used. The reasons for these recommendations are as follows. Infants given cow's milk before 12 months of age are likely to develop iron deficiency anemia. Cow's milk, whether whole, low-fat (1% or 2% fat), or skim, can cause gastrointestinal blood loss in infants. Also, cow's milk is extremely low in iron and has excessive amounts of protein, calcium, phosphorus, and sodium for infants; excreting the unneeded nitrogen and minerals can place stress on the kidneys by increasing the renal solute load. Finally, skim milk lacks essential fatty acids, which are needed for optimal growth and maintenance of skin integrity.

Recommended supplements

The American Academy of Pediatrics, Committee on Nutrition (1998) has made the following recommendations:

■ *Vitamin D:* 400 IU daily is recommended for breastfed infants who are not exposed to the sun regularly.
■ *Vitamin B_{12}:* approximately 0.3 to 0.5 µg daily is needed for breastfed infants of strict vegetarian mothers.
■ *Iron:* 10 mg daily is recommended for breastfed infants older than 6 months if they do not consume good sources of dietary iron (such as iron-fortified infant cereal) daily.

- *Fluoride:* 0.25 mg fluoride daily is needed for infants over 6 months of age who are fed human milk, ready-to-feed formula, or formula reconstituted with water containing less than 0.3 parts per million (ppm) fluoride. No fluoride supplementation is recommended before 6 months of age.

Promoting dental health

Nursing bottle caries results from prolonged contact of sugar-containing fluids (milk, juice, fruit drinks) with developing teeth. If infants are put to bed with a bottle, then it should contain only water so that exposure of the teeth to sweet fluids is minimized. When infants are put to bed with a bottle, they suck on it periodically and keep the mouth full of fluid. Avoid giving the infant a bottle or breastfeeding whenever he or she cries. Learn to distinguish cries of hunger from cries for other needs, and feed only in response to hunger.

Promoting feeding safety

Infants less than 1 year of age should not consume honey. Clostridium botulinum spores in honey can cause infant botulism. Symptoms range from constipation through progressive weakness and diminished reflexes to sudden death. Botulism in older persons is almost always caused by consuming the toxin released by the bacteria, not by consuming spores.

Coping with gastroenteritis

The Provisional Committee on Quality Improvement of the American Academy of Pediatrics (1996) has made specific recommendations regarding management of acute gastroenteritis in children 1 month to 5 years of age who live in developed countries and who have no other known illnesses. These recommendations are as follows:

Children with diarrhea but no dehydration. These children should continue to receive an age-appropriate diet.

- Infants who are breastfed can continue to nurse. Infants and children who normally drink milk-based formulas or animal milks usually tolerate them during diarrheal episodes; they should be monitored closely for malabsorption and worsening diarrhea.
- Complex carbohydrates (rice, wheat, potatoes, bread or toast, and

cereals), lean meats and poultry, yogurt, fruits, and vegetables appear to be best tolerated. The classic, very restricted BRAT diet (bananas, rice, applesauce, and toast) is low in energy, protein, and fat and is not recommended.

■ Fatty foods and foods high in simple sugars (including fruit juices, fruit drinks, and soft drinks) are to be avoided.

Children with dehydration. Oral rehydration therapy (ORT) is the preferred method for correcting fluid and electrolyte losses in children with mild to moderate dehydration. The degree of dehydration can be determined using the criteria in Table 2-5. ORT is less expensive than intravenous treatment and can be administered at home in many instances. A variety of solutions designed for ORT are commercially available (Table 4-3).

■ Children with mild dehydration should have dehydration corrected with ORT, 50 ml/kg. To replace continuing losses, give 10 ml/kg of ORT for every stool and estimate the amount of any emesis and replace it. As soon as dehydration is corrected, feedings can be given as for the child without dehydration.

■ Children with moderate dehydration can be treated with 100 ml/kg of ORT over 4 hours, along with replacement of ongoing losses as for mild dehydration. The state of hydration should be

Table 4-3   Appropriate and Inappropriate Solutions for Oral Rehydration

Composition	Rehydration Solutions*	Solutions Inappropriate for Oral Rehydration			
		Cola	Apple Juice	Chicken Broth	Sports Drink
CHO	70-140	700	690	0	255
Na	45-90	2	3	250	20
K	20-25	0	32	8	3
Base	30-48	13	0	0	3
Osm	250-310	750	730	500	330

*Carbohydrate-electrolyte solutions that are commercially available (e.g., Pedialyte [Ross], Infalyte [Mead Johnson], Rehydralyte [Ross], WHO/UNICEF oral rehydration salts).
CHO, carbohydrate; *Na,* sodium; *K,* potassium.; *Osm,* osmolality.
All concentrations are mmol/l, except osmolality, which is mOsm/kg water.

assessed every hour until rehydration is accomplished; this usually requires that treatment be given in a supervised setting such as a physician's office or emergency room. Once the child is rehydrated, feedings can resume as described previously.

■ Severe dehydration leads to shock. Bolus administration of intravenous fluids such as normal saline or Ringer's lactate is the usual treatment.

Vomiting is common with acute gastroenteritis, and ORT is possible even with vomiting occurring. The parent or other caregiver should administer 5 ml aliquots every 1 to 5 minutes. As fluid and electrolyte imbalances are corrected, vomiting often decreases. At this point, the caregiver can gradually increase the volume of ORT and the interval between doses. Some children object to the salty taste of the ORT solutions. The solutions may be better accepted if frozen into ice pops. Some of the commercial solutions are flavored to improve their acceptance.

Toddlers and Preschoolers

Special Concerns

Caloric intake

As the growth rate slows during the toddler and preschool years, caloric needs (per kg) are not as high as they were during infancy, and the appetite declines. Caloric needs in early childhood are approximately 1000 kcal plus 100 kcal per year of life. That is, a 3-year-old needs about 1300 kcal/day. Needs for protein, vitamins, and minerals remain high, however. Thus, there is little room for "empty calories" from high-fat or high-sugar foods.

Mineral intake

The highest incidence of iron deficiency in the United States is found in children under age 5. Children at special risk include Mexican-Americans, Native Americans, the poor, and those who consume one quart or more of milk per day. Milk, which is low in iron, may take the place of iron-rich foods in the diet. Iron deficiency is associated with decreased attentiveness, narrow attention span, and impaired problem-solving ability.

The recommended calcium intake for toddlers is 500 mg/day, and for preschoolers it is 800 mg/day. Development of bones and teeth depends on adequate calcium intake. Furthermore, the habit of consuming a diet rich in calcium is important for the prevention of osteoporosis in later life. Milk and cheese are the richest calcium sources in the diets of most young children. Juices, fruit drinks, and other beverages should not be allowed to replace milk in the diet.

Nutritional Care

Assessment

Assessment is summarized in Table 4-1.

Parent teaching

The goals of teaching are to foster development of good eating habits that will ensure adequate nutrient intake and minimize the risk of obesity and other health problems.

Developing good eating habits

Children need to consume a variety of foods from all food groups. The Food Guide Pyramid can be used to plan children's diets; the recommended number of daily servings from each food group is shown in Figure 4-2. Parental food habits strongly influence those of children, so parents may need to make an effort to eat a balanced and varied diet and avoid voicing distaste for any foods. Both adults who smoke and their children are likely to have poorer diets than those of nonsmoking families. In families in which the parents have not been able to stop smoking, children's diets need to be carefully assessed and parents should be instructed in the principles of a healthful diet if necessary.

Young children begin to develop food likes and dislikes (Box 4-1). Parents should continue to encourage their children to eat a variety of foods, while respecting children's preferences as much as possible. Children sometimes refuse foods simply because they are unfamiliar with them, but parents should not take this refusal to be permanent. Children's opinions of particular foods improve after they are served those foods repeatedly.

The American Heart Association and American Pediatric Association (1998) do not recommend restricting dietary fat and cholesterol routinely before age 2. After that time, a diet with no more than 30% of the kcal in the form of fat is healthful. Fried foods, peanut butter, regular luncheon meats and cheeses, and butter or margarine should be used only in moderation.

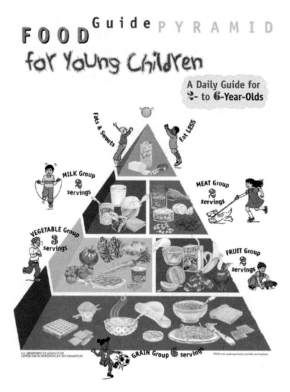

Figure 4-2
Food Guide Pyramid for Young Children.
(From U.S.D.A. Center for Nutrition Policy and Promotion.)

The "age + 5" guideline encourages a daily fiber intake equal to the child's age plus 5 grams (e.g., intake for a 4-year-old should be approximately 9 g daily). This recommendation continues throughout childhood and adolescence. Fiber helps to reduce the risk of heart disease and improves bowel function. Appendix B lists good fiber sources.

Food jags

Food jags, during which children consume only one or two foods for several days, are common. Parents should avoid making an issue

---

Box 4-1   Food Preferences of Young Children

Likes	Dislikes
Crisp, raw vegetables	Strong-flavored vegetables such as cabbage and brussels sprouts; overcooked vegetables
Foods that can be served and eaten without help, such as finger foods (sandwiches cut into strips or shapes, raw fruit or vegetables cut into small pieces, cheese cubes) and milk and other beverages that can be poured from a child-sized pitcher	Highly spiced foods
	Large servings of beverages or foods
	Foods served at temperature extremes
Foods served lukewarm	Combination foods (e.g., mixed vegetables) where flavors mingle and textures become similar; exceptions: pizza, spaghetti, macaroni and cheese
Single foods that have a characteristic color and texture; preferably, different foods should not even touch each other on the plate	

---

of food jags because this disapproval can put parents into the position of struggling with the child for control of the child's behavior. Parents should provide a variety of nutritious foods at each meal, and they should not allow the child to eat only sweets. Food jags are not usually harmful; intake over a period of several weeks balances out.

Feeding skills

Young children want to feed themselves and need to learn the necessary skills. Although the process is messy, it should be encouraged. Overemphasis on neatness creates stress at mealtimes and could interfere with the development of good eating habits.

Mineral intake

To ensure an adequate intake of iron, the child needs to eat at least two servings of meat, poultry, fish, or legumes and six servings of enriched or whole-grain breads and cereals daily (see Figure 4-2).

Deep green, leafy vegetables can also supply some iron. Consuming good vitamin C sources daily improves iron absorption.

To ensure adequate intake of calcium, children should:

■ Drink milk regularly unless they are lactose intolerant (which is less common in children than in adults). There is no significant difference in the absorption of calcium from chocolate milk and unflavored milk, so chocolate milk can be used if the child prefers it.

■ Eat cheese often. Parents can offer cheese for snacks, use cheese in main dishes such as macaroni and cheese or Welsh rarebit, or use cheese sauce over vegetables. Low-fat or "part skim" versions of some cheeses help to reduce children's fat intake, which is often excessive.

■ Eat yogurt often with meals or as a snack.

■ Avoid excess fruit juice intake. Preferably, juice should be limited to no more than 4 fl oz (120 ml)/day, and whole fruit, a good source of fiber, should make up the remainder of the fruit servings. In no case should juice intake exceed 12 fluid oz (360 ml) per day. Although calcium-fortified juice can be a valuable source of calcium, fruit juice often displaces milk in the diet.

Minimizing the risk of obesity

Parents may be concerned about what they perceive to be poor food intake by toddlers and preschoolers. They need to be reminded that the growth rate is slowing, and children's appetites will reflect this change. Some steps that parents can take to reduce the risk of obesity are:

■ Avoid overwhelming the child with servings that are too large. More can be served if the child is still hungry after the initial serving.

■ Most foods should be chosen from the five food groups nearer the bottom of the Food Guide Pyramid (see Figure 4-2), because caloric needs are too low to allow for consumption of many sweets or high-fat foods.

■ Keep fruits or vegetables available, include them in every meal, and offer them as snacks. Children learn to control their own energy intake when parents provide healthful foods but let the children determine the amount that they will consume. Fresh, frozen, or canned fruits and raw vegetables make better snacks than chips, cookies, or candy.

■ Limit the amount of time that young children watch television, and encourage daily activities that use large muscle groups. Excessive television watching promotes inactivity and exposes children to multiple cues to eat. Food advertisements make up more than half of all advertising during children's programming, and advertisements often promote foods with low nutrient density (those containing few nutrients in proportion to the calories provided). Parents should serve as active role models for children.

■ Limit fruit juice intake to 12 fluid oz (360 ml) or less a day, preferably no more than 4 fl oz (120 ml) daily. Larger intakes are associated with obesity in children. Water is the preferred beverage if children are thirsty.

Promoting dental health

Good dental health is promoted by encouraging the child to consume a diet adequate in calcium and phosphorus. Four servings of milk daily provide the calcium and phosphorus needed. Avoid offering sticky carbohydrates such as chewy candies, cookies, and pastries, which cling to the teeth. Develop the habit of regular brushing as soon as the child has teeth, and begin flossing as soon as teeth touch each other.

Fluoride makes the teeth more caries-resistant; therefore, the American Dental Association and the American Academy of Pediatrics (1995) recommend providing some children with fluoride supplements. If the local water supply contains <0.3 ppm fluoride, then the recommended daily supplement of fluoride is 0.25 mg before age 3, 0.5 mg between ages 3 and 6, and 1 mg from 6 to 16 years. If the water supply provides 0.3 to 0.6 ppm fluoride, then the recommended dosage for fluoride supplementation is 0 to 3 years of age, none; 3 to 6 years, 0.25 mg; 6 to 16 years, 0.5 mg. No supplement is routinely recommended for children of any age whose water supply provides >0.6 ppm fluoride.

Promoting feeding safety

Most deaths resulting from asphyxiation by food occur in children under age 3. To help prevent asphyxiation:

■ For children under age 3, avoid foods such as hot dogs, hard candy, caramels, jelly beans, gum drops, nuts or peanuts, grapes, and raw carrots, which are difficult to chew or swallow and are an appropriate size to block the airway.

- If the parent chooses to give the child foods that are likely to be aspirated, the parent should modify these foods to make them less likely to obstruct the airway. Grapes can be quartered, carrots cooked, and meat cut into very small pieces. Hot dogs can be cut lengthwise into four strips.
- Provide adult supervision for very young children while they eat.
- Insist that children sit down while they eat.
- Keep eating times as calm as possible. A child who is laughing or extremely excited could inhale food.

School-Age Children

Special Concerns

Influences on food consumption

Peers, teachers, and other significant adults begin to influence food choices during the school years, and home influences decline. As children grow older and have more money to spend, they consume more snacks and meals outside the home. Vending machines and fast-food restaurants offer foods that are likely to be high in fat, salt, and sugar and low in vitamins and minerals. Furthermore, a growing number of latchkey children may spend several hours of each day without adult supervision. Among the many issues regarding the welfare of these children is a concern about the quality of their food intake.

Attention deficit/hyperactivity disorders

Attention Deficit/Hyperactivity Disorders (ADHDs) are characterized by focusing on irrelevant stimuli, impulsive behavior, overactivity (not in all children), inconsistency, and lack of persistence. The Feingold diet has been recommended as a treatment for ADHDs. It excludes foods containing salicylates, compounds that cross-react with salicylates, artificial flavors, colors, and preservatives. Controlled studies have not provided clear-cut evidence that this diet is effective. Positive effects from the diet may be a result of the placebo effect or of the fact that it takes pressure off the child (placing the blame for his or her behavior on the diet, rather than on the child). Unfortunately, some of the supposed salicylate-containing foods such as oranges, peaches, grapes, raisins, apples, berries, and cherries are nutritious and are commonly enjoyed by children. A modified Feingold diet, restricting only food additives, allows a more varied diet, even though it, too, increases the difficulty of food purchasing and preparation. There should be no objection if the family wants to follow such a diet, unless they substitute the diet for medication or counseling needed by the child or family or unless emphasis on the diet promotes behavioral problems by forcing the child to be "different" from his or her peers.

Sugar has also been proposed as a cause of ADHDs, but identifying the cause of ADHDs is difficult, largely because most research must depend on subjective reports by parents. Studies done so far indicate that parents expect their children to be hyperactive after consuming large amounts of sugar-containing foods, and this parental expectation may explain why children sometimes have behavioral problems after high sugar intake. Also, sugar intake tends to be high at parties and on holidays, when children are usually excited; the children's excitement over the event itself can confuse parents into thinking that sugar is causing the problem.

Reducing the risk of chronic health problems

Eating habits with long-lasting effects are set during childhood. Dietary intake can influence the incidence of chronic health problems such as obesity, heart disease, cancer, and osteoporosis. A recent survey of U.S. children (Muñoz et al. 1997) found that only 1% received the recommended number of servings from all food groups, and only approximately one third consumed the recommended number of servings from any single food group. Intakes of vitamin B_6, iron, calcium, zinc, and fiber were low in children who failed to consume the recommended number of servings from any food group. Fat intake in the children surveyed exceeded the recommended level.

Over the past 20 years, the prevalence of overweight among U.S. children has more than doubled, to approximately 33%. Thus, prevention of overweight is one of the highest priorities in child health. The ideal diet is low in fat, high in calcium and complex carbohydrate (starch and fiber), and adequate but not excessive in kcal. A sedentary lifestyle, e.g., excessive viewing of the television and electronic games or computers, contributes to overweight and obesity.

Nutritional Care

Assessment

Assessment is summarized in Table 4-1.

Child and family teaching

The goals of teaching are to develop sound eating habits that minimize the risk of obesity and other health problems while providing adequate amounts of all nutrients and fiber. Specifically, teaching should include choosing a balanced diet and encouraging physical activity.

Choosing a balanced diet while minimizing the risk of obesity

Children need to eat foods from all food groups daily. Their diet should be low in fat, high in calcium, and adequate but not excessive in kcal. Parents can encourage children to eat a nutritious diet by involvement and example. Establish a rule that all family members eat at least one meal together daily (if at all possible). The example of parents, as well as exposure to new foods, encourages children to eat a variety of foods. Also, it is easier to control the amount of sodium, sugar, and fat in home-prepared foods than in items obtained outside the home.

Involve children in obtaining or preparing food. Children can be involved in gardening if the family grows some vegetables, in choosing food at the market (with adult guidance), and in age-appropriate cooking and food preparation tasks. This involvement gives children a personal stake in the family meals and is a good way to introduce elementary nutrition.

Make nutritious snacks available at all times, especially for latchkey children, to discourage the consumption of high-kcal, low-nutrient foods. Good choices for snacks include fresh or dried fruits; yogurt; air-popped or other low-fat popcorn; cheese, especially low-fat varieties; cottage cheese with raisins or other fruits; unsalted, dry-roasted seeds or nuts; bran or oat muffins; fruit juice frozen into pops; and peanut butter (in moderation because of the high fat content).

Prepare foods attractively, because meals with "eye appeal" are more likely to be enticing to youngsters. Choose appealing color combinations for foods served in a meal, and be sure that vegetables are not overcooked, to avoid causing their colors and textures to deteriorate. Bread for sandwiches can be cut with cookie cutters into inviting shapes, and pancakes can be poured in the shape of the child's initials or other fun shapes. If vegetable intake is a problem, try incorporating vegetables into other foods (e.g., bake carrot or zucchini muffins, or add finely grated vegetables to meatballs or meatloaf).

Encouraging regular exercise

Children need daily physical activity that involves use of large muscle groups—either team sports or individual aerobic exercises. Parent example and involvement is important. The NIH Consensus Development Panel on Physical Activity and Cardiovascular Health (1996) recommended that both children and adults accumulate at least 30 minutes of moderate-intensity exercise daily. Brisk walking, biking, ball playing, skating, and swimming are good family activities.

Identifying factors in the child's environment that may contribute to excessive weight gain

The child's social, emotional, and family environment may contribute as much as the nutritional and physical environment to the problem of overweight. The mother who has always struggled with maintaining her weight at a stable level may put undue pressure on her child to stay slim, for example. The child's self-esteem and sense of independence can suffer as a result. Ultimately, this attitude may contribute to development of eating disorders. Parents need help from the health care team when they are too rigid in trying to control the child's eating and exercise behaviors or too disorganized to provide children with the structure and support they need to maintain a healthy body weight. Children benefit from counseling and modeling of behaviors that help them to improve their self-esteem and self-reliance.

Adolescence
Special Concerns
Dietary intakes

Caloric needs for adolescent growth are high. Despite these needs, many adolescents do not consume an adequate diet. In a survey of U.S. children, only approximately 4% of teenage boys and 3% of teenage girls consumed the recommended number of servings from at least four of the five food groups (Muñoz et al. 1997). Fruit intake was low among both sexes, and consumption of dairy products was especially low among girls. The average fat intake among adolescents and younger children was approximately 35% of total calories, which is well above the recommended level (< 30% of total calories).

Dieting

About three fourths of girls in high school have dieted at least once, and 40% are on diets at any one time. Fad diets are popular but are more likely to promote transient water loss than lasting changes in eating habits. Magazines aimed at adolescent girls focus on physical appearance, with thinness given extreme importance. The cultural emphasis on a slim figure contributes to the prevalence of anorexia nervosa and bulimia (see Chapter 8), eating disorders that usually develop during the teen years.

Minerals

Lack of calcium and iron is particularly common among teenage girls. Bone growth requires an increase in calcium intake, with a DRI of 1,300 mg/day. Growth and onset of menstruation necessitate an increase in iron needs; the RDA for adolescent girls is 15 mg/day. Fast foods and traditional snack foods tend to be low in calcium and iron. Also, girls concerned about their weight often consider dairy products, rich sources of calcium, too fattening to include in their diets.

Food habits of adolescents

Snacks furnish about 40% of kcal in adolescent diets. Although snacking is not bad in itself, traditional snack foods such as chips, cookies, and soft drinks are low in nutrients. Ice cream, shakes, hamburgers, and pizza provide important nutrients, but they are also high in fat, sodium, and kcal. Adolescents rely heavily on fast-food restaurants, which have limited menus and serve foods that, for the most part, are high in calories, fat, and sodium.

In one survey (Newmark-Sztainer et al. 1999), adolescents identified the top four factors affecting their food choices. These were hunger and the availability of food to meet that hunger, the appeal of the food, time considerations, and convenience. Because the teenage years are usually a time of good health, the teens surveyed indicated that health considerations were of little concern to them. Some of the teens noted that parents need to teach good health and nutrition habits when children are younger because adolescence is not likely to be a time when they are open to such teaching. Teens have such busy schedules that convenience is an overwhelming concern for them. Thus, parents need to ensure that nutritious snacks and convenience foods are readily available at home, and schools need to keep vending machines and snack bars stocked with fruits, yogurt, and other healthful items.

Vegetarianism

The teen years are a time of experimentation, which may take the form of adopting vegetarianism. There are many types of vegetarians (see Chapter 1). Unless carefully planned, vegetarian diets may be nutritionally inadequate.

Plant sources of protein include legumes (soybeans; peanuts; beans such as pinto, navy, northern, or kidney; and peas such as blackeye and Crowder), grains, nuts and seeds, and vegetables other than legumes. Plant sources of protein differ from animal sources such as meat, milk, and eggs, in that most plant sources are not **complete proteins.** A complete protein is one that contains all of the **essential amino acids** in sufficient amounts and in proportion to one another so that it can support growth and maintenance of tissues. Essential amino acids are those that cannot be synthesized in the body in the amounts needed for the building of tissues and therefore must be provided by the diet. Most plant proteins are low in one or more essential amino acids and are therefore **incomplete proteins.** Fortunately, the amino acid patterns of the different plant protein sources vary. For example, most grains are low in the amino acid lysine but contain moderate amounts of methionine, and conversely most legumes are relatively low in methionine but contain moderate amounts of lysine. Consuming proteins from a variety of plant sources on a daily basis is the best way to ensure that the diet includes adequate amounts of all amino acids. Use of milk products also helps to ensure that the diet has high-quality protein sources, and adolescents should be encouraged to include milk, cheese, and yogurt in their diets.

Vegetarians who avoid dairy products often have difficulty consuming enough calcium. Furthermore, plant foods are usually lower in zinc and iron than animal products, and phytate (in whole grains) and oxalate (in chocolate, green leafy vegetables, and rhubarb) form complexes with minerals and inhibit their absorption. Calcium-fortified juice, cereals, tofu, and soy milk can be valuable sources of calcium for vegetarians who do not use dairy products.

Vitamin B_{12} is found naturally only in animal products. Vegetarians who consume no eggs, dairy products, or other animal proteins are unlikely to receive enough vitamin B_{12}.

Nutritional Care

Assessment

Assessment is summarized in Table 4-1.

Teaching

The goal is to help adolescents learn to make wise food choices that provide the necessary nutrients while maintaining a desirable body weight. Following are some specific teaching topics.

Eating a balanced, nutritious diet and maintaining desirable body weight

Adolescents can follow the guidelines of the Food Guide Pyramid for adults (see Chapter 1). It is especially important for them to learn to select diets with a wide variety of foods that are low in fat and cholesterol; high in vitamins, minerals, and fiber; and moderate in kcal. Following are some guidelines that will help them to achieve these diets.

To control fat and cholesterol intake:

- Limit use of fried foods to one serving per day or less.
- Eat only two to three servings of red meat per week; choose poultry, fish, or grain and legume main dishes on the other days.
- Limit meat intake to about 5 oz/day. This is sufficient even for most athletes in training.
- Use dairy products made with skim milk whenever possible. Chapter 15 provides additional information for limiting fat and cholesterol intake.
- Fiber has a cholesterol-lowering effect. Continue to follow the "age + 5" rule (grams of fiber consumed daily should equal the age plus 5) begun in early childhood.

To ensure adequate vitamin and mineral intake:

- Consume three to four servings of milk or milk products daily (especially important for adolescent girls). It is difficult to consume enough calcium in the diet without using milk products. Skim milk and yogurt, cheese, and cottage cheese made of skim milk are low in kcal and may be acceptable to dieting teens. Calcium-fortified juice and cereals are reliable calcium sources, and Figure 3-4 shows other dietary calcium sources.

- Use a daily supplement if the diet is low in milk products or other good sources of calcium (see Appendix A). Calcium citrate is a well-absorbed form of calcium. Calcium carbonate, a common antacid, is 40% calcium. To improve absorption, it should be taken with foods, but preferably not with bran or whole grains.
- Eat meat, poultry, fish, legumes, enriched or whole grains, or deep green, leafy vegetables daily to receive dietary iron (see Appendix A). Even if they use a variety of these foods daily, adolescent girls may still have an inadequate or marginal iron intake. A daily supplement (15 mg) may be needed. Ferrous sulfate, 20% iron, is inexpensive and well-absorbed.
- If both calcium and iron supplements are used, take them at least 1 to 2 hours apart.

To avoid excessive kcal intake:

- Limit fat intake.
- Choose high-fiber foods (see Appendix B), because they are bulky and require more chewing than low-fiber, refined foods. The person feels full after eating fewer kcal. Whole grains, legumes, and crisp salads without excessive additions such as dressing, eggs, meat, and bacon are nutritious, low-kcal foods.
- Obtain approximately 60 minutes of moderate exercise most days of the week. Some teens wish to participate in team sports, which can be encouraged. Others need to choose individual activities that they will continue on a long-term basis. Chapter 6 shows how to calculate the target heart rate for cardiovascular fitness and includes recommendations for becoming and remaining physically fit.
- Make sure that snacks are nutritious and low in kcal, because they are such an important part of the adolescent's diet. Some examples are fresh or dried fruits; fresh vegetables with a dip made of low-fat yogurt and herbs; air-popped popcorn; bagels (plain or with low-fat cream cheese or other low-fat topping); fruit ices; and yogurt, cottage cheese, or cheese made with skim milk.

Avoiding unhealthy weight loss practices

Because teens are so interested in weight-reduction diets, they need to be taught to recognize a safe and effective diet. Fad diets promise and often deliver quick results, but much of the weight loss is fluid and lean body mass, rather than fat. A good diet meets the criteria given in Box 7-6.

Eating disorders often appear during adolescence. Magazines and television programming focused on adolescents place a priority on slimness. Adolescents who are seriously committed to certain sports or recreational activities, such as gymnastics, figure skating, or ballet, may feel compelled to maintain unrealistically low body weights. Primary prevention of eating disorders should be the goal. Some topics to include in a primary prevention program are: (1) normal physiologic, social, and psychologic changes during puberty, the normal increase in fat deposition, and the diversity that occurs among individuals; (2) general nutrition, meal skipping, and other eating habits; (3) physical activity—its importance and appropriate levels; (4) weight control—realistic and safe methods of weight control, realistic goals for weight, myths and fads about dieting, the physiologic and psychologic effects of food restriction and chronic dieting; (5) body image issues and how to determine one's appropriate body weight; (6) autonomy and self-esteem; and (7) information about anorexia and bulimia. If parents observe their children to be dieting and experiencing weight loss, they need to intervene early. The prognosis is much better if intervention occurs early in the course of the illness. See Chapter 8.

Following an adequate vegetarian diet plan

Some individuals may choose a vegetarian diet. Table 4-4 demonstrates that a vegetarian diet can be a healthful one. To ensure that nutritional intake is adequate, the adolescent vegetarian needs to be taught certain guidelines:

■ Consuming a wide variety of grains, legumes, nuts, and seeds allows the vegetarian to obtain adequate levels of amino acids. A diet including eggs and dairy products ensures that the vegetarian has complete protein in the diet, but an adequate diet without animal products is possible with careful planning.
■ Whole grains, legumes, and deep green, leafy vegetables contain iron and zinc. Additional iron can be obtained from dried fruits, molasses, soy sauce, and use of iron cookware.

Table 4-4   Sample Vegetarian Diet Plan

Breakfast	
6 oz calcium-fortified orange juice	1 Fruit
⅔ cup oat bran cereal	1 Grain
1 sliced peach	1 Fruit
1 cup fortified soy milk	1 Milk
Lunch	
2 bean burritos	1 Protein + 2 Grain
½ cup Spanish rice	1 Grain
½ cup tomato wedges	1 Vegetable
Dinner	
1½ cups spaghetti	3 Grain
1 cup sauce (tomato and textured vegetable [soy] protein)	1 Protein + ½ Vegetable
1 cup mixed greens	1 Vegetable
½ cup broccoli flowerets	1 Vegetable
1 cup soy milk	1 Milk
Snack	
1½ cups frozen tofu dessert	1 Milk
TOTAL SERVINGS	7 Grain
	3½ Vegetable
	2 Fruit
	2 Protein
	3 Milk

- Iron from plant sources is better absorbed if it is consumed with a vitamin C–containing food such as citrus fruit.
- Coffee and tea inhibit iron absorption; thus it is best not to consume these beverages with meals.
- Adolescent girls, in particular, benefit from daily use of dairy products or a calcium supplement. Dairy products are among the richest dietary sources of calcium, and lactose in dairy products stimulates calcium absorption. See Figure 3-4 for other sources of calcium.

■ Vegetarians need to consume vitamin B_{12}–containing products several times per week. Eggs, dairy products, and all other animal products contain vitamin B_{12}. Some soy milk and nutritional yeast is fortified with vitamin B_{12} (consult the label). If no dietary vitamin B_{12} sources are used, then the individual will need a vitamin B_{12} supplement.

Using nutritional supplements safely

High doses of vitamin A taken systemically, including synthetic vitamin A products used in treatment of acne (isotretinoin), are teratogenic. Sexually active girls taking vitamin A supplements need instruction in effective methods of contraception, as do all other sexually active teens.

SELECTED BIBLIOGRAPHY

American Academy of Pediatrics Committee on Nutrition: Fluoride supplementation for children: interim policy recommendations, *Pediatrics* 95:777, 1995.

American Academy of Pediatrics Committee on Nutrition: *Pediatric nutrition handbook,* ed 4, Elk Grove Village, IL, 1998, American Academy of Pediatrics.

Baer MT, Harris AB: Pediatric nutrition assessment: identifying children at risk, *J Am Dietet Assoc* 97(suppl 2): S107, 1997.

Conference on Dietary Fiber in Childhood: A summary of conference recommendations on dietary fiber in childhood, *Pediatrics* 96(no. 5, part 2):1023, 1995.

Duggan C, Nurko S: "Feeding the gut": the scientific basis for continued enteral nutrition during acute diarrhea, *J Pediatr* 131:801, 1997.

Johnson RK, Wang M, Smith MJ, Connolly G: The association between parental smoking and the diet quality of low-income children, *Pediatrics* 97:312, 1996.

Muñoz KA, Krebs-Smith SM, Ballard-Barbash R, Cleveland LE: Food intakes of US children and adolescents compared with recommendations, *Pediatrics* 100:323, 1997.

Newmark-Sztainer D, Story M, Perry C, Casey MA: Factors influencing food choices: findings from focus group discussions with adolescents. *J Am Dietet Assoc* 99:929, 1999.

NIH Consensus Development Panel on Physical Activity and Cardiovascular Health: Physical activity and cardiovascular health. *JAMA* 276:241, 1996.

Provisional Committee on Quality Improvement, Subcommittee on Acute Gastroenteritis: Practice parameter: the management of acute gastroenteritis in young children, *Pediatrics* 97:424, 1996.

Rauh-Pfeiffer A, Kelleher D, Duggan C: Obesity and low-fat diets in pediatrics, *Curr Opin Pediatrics* 10:329, 1998.

Sylvester GP, Achterberg C, Williams J: Children's television and nutrition: friends or foes? *Nutr Today* 30:6, 1995.

Wolraich ML, Wilson DB, White JW: The effect of sugar on behavior or cognition in children, *JAMA* 274:1617, 1995.

Aging

5

Physical and psychosocial changes of aging may have a negative impact on nutritional status. On the other hand, optimal nutrition may have positive effects on the physical and emotional health of the elderly.

Special Concerns
Physiologic and Psychosocial Changes

Many physiologic and psychosocial changes that affect nutritional status occur with aging. Some of these are summarized in Table 5-1.

Osteoporosis

Osteoporosis, or loss of skeletal mass, deserves special attention because of the prevalence of the disorder and the morbidity associated with it. About one third of women and one sixth of men who reach age 90 will have a hip fracture related to osteoporosis. Throughout life, bone is constantly being formed and resorbed. After the third decade in women and the fourth decade in men, more bone is lost than is formed. Women generally have smaller, less dense bones than men, and bone loss is accelerated by the decline in estrogen levels at the time of menopause. Women are therefore more likely to develop signs and symptoms related to osteoporosis. About 80% of older individuals with significant osteoporosis are women. The most vulnerable individuals are white or Asian women, women who have had early oophorectomies, and individuals who are immobile for prolonged periods. Inadequate calcium intake over a long period is believed to predispose people to osteoporosis. In addition, the renal activation of vitamin D and the ability of vitamin D to stimulate calcium absorption may be impaired in the elderly, so that absorption of calcium is diminished. Hyperparathyroidism is relatively common in the elderly, as a response to the decrease in calcium absorption. The increase in

Table 5-1   Nutritional Implications of Changes Related to Aging

Change	Nutritional Implications
Physiologic Changes and Impairments of Physical Function	
Decreased muscle mass (sarcopenia) and increased percentage of body fat	Decline in basal metabolic rate of about 2% per decade after age 30; daily kcal need declines; potential for weight gain and obesity
Decreased skin capacity for cholecalciferol (vitamin D) synthesis; decreased renal activation of cholecalciferol and/or resistance of the gut to stimulation of vitamin D	Impaired absorption of calcium, contributing to osteoporosis
Diminished sense of taste and smell	Disinterest in food; anorexia; some individuals salt or sugar their food heavily to compensate for loss of taste
Poor vision, especially in dim light	Difficulty shopping for or preparing food; decreased appeal of food because it cannot be seen well; difficulty feeding self
Periodontal disease (occurs in about 80% of older adults); causes discomfort and tooth loss	Difficulty eating; food choices limited (raw or crisp fruits and vegetables and high-fiber grains often avoided; softer, low-fiber foods, which are frequently higher in kcal, are substituted); can contribute to weight loss, weight gain, or constipation
Decreased secretion of hydrochloric acid (needed for absorption of vitamin B_{12}), pepsin (protein digestive enzyme), and bile (needed for fat absorption)	Potential for impaired absorption of calcium, iron, zinc, protein, fat, fat-soluble vitamins, vitamin B_{12}

Continued

Table 5-1   Nutritional Implications of Changes Related
to Aging—cont'd

Change	Nutritional Implications
Physiologic Changes and Impairments of Physical Function—cont'd	
Increased prevalence of lactose intolerance	Decreased use of milk; poor intake of calcium possible, contributing to osteoporosis
Decreased gastrointestinal motility	Constipation, which can cause anorexia; hemorrhoids; diverticulosis
Decreased sensation of thirst	Potential for dehydration (volume deficit)
Decreased body water	Potential for dehydration (volume deficit)
Increased prevalence of chronic illness	Potential for anorexia; need for modified diets, which may be unappealing and may result in poor intake; need for hospitalizations and diagnostic testing, which interfere with intake
Frequent use of medications; use of multiple medications	Potential for impaired appetite, decreased absorption or utilization of nutrients, increased requirements for nutrients; constipation (see Appendix H for nutritional implications of specific drugs)
Impaired mobility; weakness	Difficulty shopping for or preparing food (fresh fruits and vegetables and milk products are especially bulky and hard to carry and may be omitted from the diet); difficulty feeding self; decreased energy expenditure, which contributes to weight gain

Table 5-1   Nutritional Implications of Changes Related
to Aging—cont'd

Change	Nutritional Implications
Psychosocial Changes	
Fixed income	Potential for difficulty affording food or being unwilling to spend money on food, particularly foods perceived as expensive, e.g., milk, meats, fruits, vegetables, which are important sources of calcium, riboflavin, protein, iron, zinc, vitamins C and A, and fiber
Lack of socialization; loneliness	Apathy about meals; poor intake; potential for alcohol abuse
Vulnerability to advertising and food fads related to alleviation of the effects and discomforts of aging	33%-72% of older Americans use vitamin supplements, although studies indicate that their diets are usually not low in the vitamins they are supplementing; wasting of limited income on diet or health aids with dubious value; potential for toxic intakes of vitamins, particularly A and D
Confusion, memory loss	Potential for forgetting to eat or forgetting what has been eaten (and therefore consuming an unbalanced diet)

release of parathyroid hormone stimulates mobilization of calcium from the bone and worsens osteoporosis. Supplements of vitamin D and calcium are used in cases of hyperparathyroidism. Other factors contributing to osteoporosis are use of corticosteroid or anticonvulsant medications, smoking, gastrointestinal disease causing malabsorption, hypogonadism in men, liver and renal disease, and multiple myeloma.

Changes in the eye

Prolonged exposure to oxidative stresses in the environment affects many tissues, and the lens and the retina of the eye are especially vulnerable. Some evidence suggests that the antioxidant vitamins (A, C, and E) and zinc may play roles in protecting the aging eye. Smokers, in particular, have reduced risk of cataract formation if they take a daily multivitamin supplement. Age-related macular degeneration (ARMD), an irreversible cause of visual loss in middle-aged and elderly individuals, appears to be less common in people with higher circulating levels of **carotenoids** (vitamin A precursors). Carotenoids are concentrated in the macula of the retina. Zeaxanthin and lutein are the two carotenoids believed to be the most important in prevention of ARMD. Many supplements contain β-carotene but not the other carotenoids. Spinach and leafy greens, corn, broccoli, pumpkin, brussels sprouts, and celery are good sources of zeaxanthin and lutein.

Chronic and Acute Illnesses

Malnutrition is, unfortunately, a common finding among the elderly, and acute or chronic disease processes are often contributing factors. Disease processes may interfere with food intake or increase nutritional requirements, require modified diets that are unappealing to the individual, or require drug therapy that influences nutritional status (see Appendix H).

Coronary heart disease and type 2 (non–insulin-dependent) diabetes are two nutrition-related chronic diseases that become increasingly prevalent with aging. Diet modifications used in treatment of these disorders are described in Chapters 15 and 18.

Nutritional Care

The goals of care are to alter nutritional factors that may increase the risk of chronic illness and to help the individual maintain health, well-being, and functional capacity.

Assessment

The Nutrition Screening Initiative has developed a checklist that the elderly can use to screen themselves for nutritional risk (Box 5-1); friends or family members can fill out the checklist for an elderly person who is unable to complete it. Health care providers can use the information from the screening tool to target individuals who

Box 5-1   Determine Your Nutritional Health

The warning signs of poor nutritional health are often overlooked. Use this checklist to find out if you or someone you know is at nutritional risk.

Read the statements below. Circle the number in the yes column for those that apply to you or someone you know. For each yes answer, score the number in the box. Total your nutritional score.

	Yes
I have an illness or condition that made me change the kind and/or amount of food I eat.	2
I eat fewer than 2 meals per day.	3
I eat few fruits or vegetables or milk products.	2
I have 3 or more drinks of beer, liquor, or wine almost every day.	2
I have tooth or mouth problems that make it hard for me to eat.	2
I don't always have enough money to buy the food I need.	4
I eat alone most of the time.	1
I take 3 or more different prescribed or over-the-counter drugs a day.	1
Without wanting to, I have lost or gained 10 pounds in the last 6 months.	2
I am not always physically able to shop, cook, and/or feed myself.	2
TOTAL	

Reprinted with permission by the Nutrition Screening Initiative, a project of the American Academy of Family Physicians, The American Dietetic Association and the National Council on the Aging, Inc. and funded in part by a grant from Ross Products Division, Abbott Laboratories, Inc. *Continued*

Box 5-1   Determine Your Nutritional Health—cont'd

Total Your Nutritional Score. If it's—

0-2	Good! Recheck your nutritional score in 6 months.
3-5	You are at moderate nutritional risk. See what can be done to improve your eating habits and lifestyle. Your office on aging, senior nutrition program, senior citizens center, or health department can help. Recheck your nutritional score in 3 months.
6 or more	You are at high nutritional risk. Bring this checklist the next time you see your doctor, dietitian, or other qualified health or social service professional. Talk with them about any problems you may have. Ask for help to improve your nutritional health.

Reprinted with permission by the Nutrition Screening Initiative, a project of the American Academy of Family Physicians, The American Dietetic Association and the National Council on the Aging, Inc. and funded in part by a grant from Ross Products Division, Abbott Laboratories, Inc.

need in-depth assessment and nutrition intervention. Assessment of nutrition in the aging by the professional is summarized in Table 5-2.

The institutionalized elderly have been reported to be especially vulnerable to weight loss and other nutritional problems. This is probably related to the prevalence of chronic diseases, use of multiple medications with nutritional impacts, and depression or other psychological problems. Thus, thorough assessment and appropriate nutritional intervention are especially important for elderly individuals in long-term care facilities.

Obtaining accurate values for height in the elderly can be problematic, because loss of vertebral mineralization and volume in intervertebral disks results in loss of height. Long bones, however, do not shorten with age. Knee height (length from sole of foot to anterior thigh with both ankle and knee bent at 90-degree angle) can be used to estimate height.

For women: Estimated height in cm = 84.88 + (1.83 × knee height in cm) + (−0.24 × age in years)

For men: Estimated height in cm = 60.65 + (2.04 × knee height in cm)

Table 5-2   Assessment of Nutrition in Aging

Area of Concern	Significant Findings
Underweight and Undernutrition (Protein-Calorie Malnutrition)	*History*
	Loss of 4.5 kg (10 lb) or more in the last 6 months; fixed income, inadequate money for food; usually eats alone, loss of spouse or friends; difficulty chewing or swallowing, pain in mouth, teeth, gums; poor appetite; follows a modified diet; regular use of medications (particularly those that impair appetite, e.g., digoxin), especially if three or more are used; has a chronic disease; avoids one or more food groups or eats inadequate servings; has more than one alcoholic drink per day (woman) or more than 2 drinks per day (man); difficulty getting to market or transporting purchases home; lack of food preparation skills; lack of facilities for food storage or preparation; difficulty feeding self
	Physical Examination
	Weight <90% of standard for height or BMI <18.5; lack of body fat, TSF <5th percentile; muscle wasting; edema; glossitis, angular stomatitis
	Laboratory Analysis
	↓ Serum albumin, transferrin, prealbumin, lymphocyte count

Continued

Table 5-2   Assessment of Nutrition in Aging—cont'd

Area of Concern	Significant Findings
Overweight/Obesity	*History*
	Gain of 4.5 kg (10 lb) or more in the last 6 months; excessive intakes, especially of fat, snack items, and sweets; increase in intake of kcal-dense refined foods because of difficulty chewing high-fiber foods; little physical activity
	Physical Examination
	Weight >120% of of ideal for height or BMI >25; TSF >95th percentile
Inadequate Fluid Balance (Potential for Fluid Deficit)	*History*
	Altered mental status (confusion or coma) with inability to feel or express thirst; decreased thirst sensation with aging; vomiting, diarrhea, febrile illness, or extremely hot weather
	Physical Examination
	Poor skin turgor; dry, sticky mucous membranes; rapid weight loss over 1-2 wk; oliguria; lethargy, hypotension
	Laboratory Analysis
	↑ Hct, BUN, serum Na

Intervention and Teaching

Guidelines for choosing a healthful diet

The elderly can be encouraged to use the Food Guide Pyramid (see Chapter 1) as a tool for diet planning and a reminder to include a variety of foods in their diets. Food is the preferred source of

Table 5-2   Assessment of Nutrition in Aging—cont'd

Area of Concern	Significant Findings
Inadequate Calcium and Vitamin D Intake	*History* Avoids milk because of lactose intolerance, difficulty carrying milk home from the market, inadequate money, etc.; little sun exposure because of chronic illness or residing in a nursing home or other institution; vertebral or hip fractures *Laboratory Analysis* ↓ Bone density on radiographs
Impaired Vitamin B_{12} Status	*History* Achlorhydria (inadequate hydrochloric acid production); meats and milk avoided because of difficulty chewing, lactose intolerance, cost, etc. *Physical Examination* Pallor, weakness, paresthesias (abnormal sensations in feet or legs), difficulty walking *Laboratory Analysis* ↓ Hct, ↑ MCV, ↓ plasma vitamin B_{12}
Inadequate Zinc (Zn) Intake	*History* Decreased animal protein or whole grain intake because of low income or difficulty chewing *Physical Examination* Hypogeusia, dysgeusia (altered sense of taste); dermatitis; poor wound healing *Laboratory Analysis* ↓ Serum Zn

nutrients in the elderly, just as it is in other age groups. Unlike supplements, food provides a variety of phytochemicals and functional components (nutrients or other food components that have functions that are not necessarily nutritional in nature). Soy is an example of a "functional" food. Genistein, a component of soy, apparently reduces the risk of heart disease; soy also provides phytoestrogens (estrogenlike compounds in plants) that are reported to reduce the risk of some cancers and to provide some relief from menopausal symptoms.

The elderly are susceptible to food fads and **nutritional quackery,** similar to other age groups. They may rely on these beliefs to treat chronic illnesses or other health problems. The elderly need instruction in ways of recognizing quackery (e.g., heavy reliance on anecdotal and testimonial evidence, rather than clinical trials; insistence that certain foods or supplements can cure disease; distrust of the food supply as a means of meeting nutritional needs). A multivitamin-multimineral supplement (usually without iron because of the prevalence of hemochromatosis, an iron storage disorder, in the North American population) may be of value to the elderly. Little evidence suggests that most elderly individuals need liquid meal replacements or other nutritional supplements, however.

Achieving and maintaining desirable weight

Impaired physical function is more common among overweight and underweight elderly than among their normal-weight peers. Overweight can impair mobility, whereas underweight is associated with debility and can predispose the individual to infectious illnesses.

Overweight

Teaching elderly patients to facilitate weight control can include the following:

- Explain the need for controlling caloric intake (or increasing physical activity level) to prevent progressive weight gain as metabolic rate declines. Gradual weight loss or maintenance of body weight is usually possible with intakes of approximately 1,200 to 1,500 kcal per day for women and 1,500 to 1,800 calories for men.
- Assist the individual in identifying foods, such as fruits,

vegetables, whole grains, and low-fat dairy products, that are relatively low in kcal but that make important nutritional contributions; help the individual to create meal plans that use these foods.

■ Encourage the elderly person to limit the consumption of foods of low nutrient density (sweets, snack foods) and high-fat items. Fresh or water-pack canned fruits can be used for desserts and snacks. Steaming, microwaving, or baking foods with little or no added fat is preferable to frying.

■ Encourage the elderly person to accumulate at least 30 minutes of moderate-intensity exercise most days of the week. The entire 30 minutes of exercise does not have to be carried out at one time. Instead, physical activity can be performed in three or more sessions of at least 10 minutes in duration. Walking, gardening, and water aerobics are examples of physical activities that can be useful in weight control.

Underweight

Individuals with health or dentition problems or loss of the senses of smell and taste are especially likely to be underweight. If the cause of poor intake can be determined, it is possible to tailor interventions and teaching to the needs of the individual. Try the following suggestions:

■ Try small, frequent feedings rather than three large meals a day if anorexia or severe weakness is present.

■ Be aware of potential side effects of drugs taken regularly (see Appendix H). If medication usage appears to be decreasing the appetite, then the physician may be able to substitute another drug or reduce the dosage. Toxicity often develops in the older adult at lower dosages than in younger adults, and use of multiple drugs increases the risks of adverse effects.

■ Assess the individual for the presence of constipation, which may cause anorexia.

■ Special diets (low-cholesterol, low-sodium, etc.) may seem tasteless to the individual. Consider liberalizing diet restrictions if intake is poor because the therapeutic diet is unappealing.

■ If intake is poor because of declining senses of taste and smell, experiment with low-sodium seasonings such as herbs, spices, salt-free seasoning mixes, and lemon juice to enhance the flavors of foods. Present food in an attractive manner: appealing color combinations, a variety of textures if tolerated by the individual, and not overcooked so that it loses its color or texture.

- If food intake is inadequate because of poverty, refer the person to social services for assistance in obtaining food stamps and other financial assistance. Encourage participation in the National Nutrition Program for the Elderly, which provides meals at group feeding sites.

- Encourage the individual to eat with others whenever possible. Group feeding sites (e.g., daily lunches served at senior citizen centers), church functions, or other social activities offer opportunities for socialization. Eating in a social setting can improve appetite.

- If periodontal disease is responsible for poor intake, arrange for the individual to obtain proper dental care, including well-fitted dentures, if needed.

- Involve elderly individuals in the planning of menus for extended care facilities or group feeding sites. Attempt to accommodate the culture(s) and preferences of the participants as much as possible.

- Light the dining area well so that food can be clearly seen.

- Provide assistance in eating, if necessary. This may range from opening packages of condiments to feeding the person. Plates with high outer rims make it easier for the elderly with physical handicaps to scoop up food. Patience and sensitivity when feeding the individual help preserve dignity and improve intake.

- Instruct the individual in food purchasing and simple food preparation techniques, if appropriate. Elderly men who have never cooked until late in life are especially vulnerable to nutritional deficits. The county extension home economist is a good resource for food purchasing and preparation materials.

- If mobility is a problem, then arrange transportation to the grocery store or to feeding sites for the elderly (contact the local agency on aging) or arrange for home-delivered meals.

Coping with altered gastrointestinal function

To reduce the risk of constipation, hemorrhoids, and diverticulosis:

- Encourage intake of at least 25 to 30 g fiber daily (see Appendix B). Cooked whole grains (oatmeal, brown rice, bulgur, etc.) and cooked, canned, or very ripe raw fruits and vegetables are good choices if there is difficulty chewing.

- Increase physical activity as tolerated because this stimulates gastrointestinal motility.
- Encourage consumption of prunes and prune juice (which contain a natural laxative) regularly if they are acceptable to the individual. Avoid regular use of laxative medications, on which the individual may become dependent.

If achlorhydria is present, then the individual may need supplements of vitamin B_{12} and calcium because absorption of these nutrients is impaired by the lack of gastric acid.

Preventing or delaying the progression of osteoporosis

Encourage a calcium intake of 1,200 mg/day (see Figure 3-4), especially in elderly women. If lactose intolerance is present, substitute cheese, acidophilus milk, yogurt, or buttermilk for milk because these products are lower in lactose than regular milk. Also, lactase enzyme–treated milk is available in some markets, or oral lactase supplements are available to take with milk. Use a calcium supplement (e.g., calcium citrate) if dietary calcium intake cannot be maintained at the recommended level. (Box 5-2 provides guidelines for improving absorption of calcium from the diet or supplements.) Vitamin D is needed for the absorption of calcium. The recommended intake of vitamin D is higher for the elderly than for any other groups of individuals (10 µg/day through 70 years, and 15 µg/day after age 70). If vitamin D–fortified milk or another reliable dietary source (see Appendix A) is not consumed daily, the individual may need a supplement. In addition, regular weight-bearing exercise (at least 20 to 30 min/day, most days of the week) helps to preserve bone.

Medications can reduce the resorption of bone, but the choice of medication is individualized based on the individual's health history. Hormone replacement therapy (estrogen) reduces both bone loss and risk of coronary heart disease (CHD) in postmenopausal women but also appears to increase the risk of endometrial and breast cancer. Thus, for women at high risk for these types of cancer (or those who have already had breast cancer), other therapies may be preferable. Bisphosphonates such as alendronate reduce bone resorption without affecting the rates of CHD or breast or endometrial cancer. Raloxiphene is a nonestrogenic drug that binds to the estrogen receptor. It has some properties similar to

---

Box 5-2   Improving Calcium Absorption

Obtain adequate vitamin D. Vitamin D–fortified milk and breakfast cereals and exposure of skin to sunlight several times a week (using appropriate sunscreen) are good sources.

Consume milk or other lactose-containing dairy products if lactose tolerance is not a problem. Lactose improves calcium absorption.

Avoid excessive intake of phosphorus, which competes with calcium for absorption. Limit meat intake to 5 to 6 oz daily and carbonated drinks to 8 to 12 oz daily.

Limit sodium intake to 2 to 4 g daily because high-sodium diets interfere with calcium absorption.

Avoid excessive protein intake, which increases calcium losses.

Increase calcium intake if diet is high in oxalate (e.g., spinach and other deep green vegetables), phytates (e.g., bran and whole grains), or fiber, all of which inhibit calcium absorption.

Increase calcium intake if achlorhydria is present, and consume calcium with orange juice or other acidic foods. Acid in the upper gastrointestinal tract improves absorption, and an alkaline upper gastrointestinal tract impairs absorption.

Increase calcium intake if using corticosteroid or anticonvulsant medications, which decrease calcium absorption.

Avoid smoking, consumption of more than one to two alcoholic drinks per day (1 drink = 1 oz distilled spirits, 5 oz wine, or 12 oz beer), or excess caffeine intake, which promote bone loss.

---

estrogen (reduction in bone loss and CHD risk) but it also has antiestrogenic effects so that it causes no increase in cancer risk and might even reduce the incidence of breast cancer.

Decreasing the risk of complications during illness

Dehydration is especially likely to occur in the ill elderly person because body water is reduced with aging (from about 55% of body weight in young adults to about 45% in people over 60). Therefore, any given volume of body fluids represents a greater percentage of body water in the elderly person than it does in the younger adult. Diarrhea, vomiting, or a febrile illness often produces dehydration in the older adult. The sensation of thirst may be diminished in old age, and immobility may hinder the elderly in getting fluids to drink, further contributing to the risk of dehydration. Some older adults have a narrow margin of safety in their state of hydration because renal or cardiac impairments make them vulnerable to fluid overload. Caregivers should adhere to the following guidelines to prevent dehydration in the elderly patient:

- Assess state of hydration regularly.
- Evaluate fluid intake of the patient receiving tube feedings or total parenteral nutrition. More fluid may be needed than is included in the nutrient solutions. Extra fluid can be administered orally, as an irrigant for the feeding tube, or intravenously.
- Encourage intake of a minimum of 1500 ml fluid per day, unless a fluid restriction is needed. If the individual has difficulty remembering how much fluid has been consumed, it may help to fill a pitcher with the needed amount at the beginning of the day, place it in an accessible location, and instruct the person to drink it all by the end of the day.

Decreasing the risk of visual loss

All adults should include reliable sources of vitamin C and zinc in their diets daily (see Appendix A) to protect the lens and retina of the eye. Good sources of the carotenoids lutein and zeaxanthin (spinach, kale and other leafy greens, broccoli, brussels sprouts, corn, pumpkin, and celery) are needed on a regular basis. Carrots and most vitamin supplements are not a rich source of these carotenoids.

Selected bibliography

Blumberg J: Nutritional needs of seniors, *J Am Coll Nutr* 16:517, 1997.

Col NF et al.: Individualizing therapy to prevent long-term consequences of estrogen deficiency in postmenopausal women, *Arch Internal Med* 159:1458, 1999.

Duffy VB, Backstrand JR, Ferris AM: Olfactory dysfunction and related nutritional risk in free-living, elderly women, *J Am Dietet Assoc* 95:879, 1995.

Ebeling PR: Osteoporosis in men: new insights into aetiology, pathogenesis, prevention and management, *Drugs & Aging* 13:421, 1998.

Evans WJ, Cyr-Campbell D: Nutrition, exercise, and healthy aging, *J Am Dietet Assoc* 97:632, 1997.

Heaney RP: Age considerations in nutrient needs for bone health: older adults, *J Am Coll Nutr* 15:575, 1996.

Jensen GL, Rogers J: Obesity in older persons, *J Am Dietet Assoc* 98:1308, 1998.

Nutrition interventions manual for professionals caring for older Americans: executive summary, Washington, DC, 1992, Nutrition Screening Initiative.

Roubenoff R, Giacoppe J, Richardson S, Hoffman PJ: Nutrition assessment in long-term care facilities, *Nutr Rev* 54:S40, 1996.

Saltzman JR, Russell RM: The aging gut. Nutritional issues, *Gastroenterol Clin N Am* 27:309, 1998.

Tripp F: The use of dietary supplements in the elderly: current issues and recommendations, *J Am Dietet Assoc* 97(suppl 2):S181, 1997.

Physical Fitness and Athletic Competition

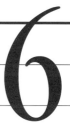

A nutritious diet and exercise are among the major factors contributing to physical fitness and health. Habits that promote physical fitness should be developed during childhood and maintained throughout life.

Physical Activity and the General Population
Physical Fitness

Regular physical activity has many health benefits, including reducing the risk of morbidity and mortality related to heart disease, lowering blood pressure in individuals with hypertension, decreasing the risk of developing non–insulin-dependent diabetes and colon cancer, slowing the rate of bone loss and thus reducing the risk of osteoporosis, and improving psychological well-being. Unfortunately, about 60% of American adults are extremely sedentary, participating in no regular physical activity. Women are less active than men, and Hispanics, Native Americans, and African-Americans are more sedentary than Caucasians. Sedentary habits begin to develop early in life. Activity levels decrease in adolescence, and girls become more inactive than boys.

The American College of Sports Medicine (ACSM, 1998a) has made recommendations for the amount and type of exercise needed to maintain optimal cardiorespiratory fitness, body composition, muscular strength, endurance, and flexibility in healthy adults. Three types of exercise are included: (1) aerobic exercise to enhance cardiorespiratory function, (2) resistance exercise to improve muscular strength and maintain the fat free mass, and (3) flexibility training to maintain full range of motion. Recommendations for aerobic exercise to maintain fitness of the cardiac

---

Box 6-1   Aerobic Exercise for Cardiorespiratory Fitness

Recommendation*

Frequency: at least 3 to 5 days a week

Intensity for a fit adult: 65-90% of maximum heart rate (HR_{max})

HR_{max} = 220 beats/min − age in years

Adults who are very unfit can begin with lower intensity exercise (55-64% of HR_{max}).

Time (duration): at least 20 to 60 min

Exercise can be carried out continually or in bouts no shorter than 10 minutes each.

Example

36-year-old female who exercises 5 days a week

HR_{max} = 220 − 36 = 184 beats/minute

Range of desirable intensity

65% × 184 beats/minute = 120 beats/minute

90% × 184 beats/minute = 166 beats/minute

Her goal should be to maintain her heart rate between 120 and 166 beats/minute.

---

*American College of Sports Medicine position stand. The recommended quantity and quality of exercise for developing and maintaining cardiorespiratory and muscular fitness, and flexibility in healthy adults, *Med Sci Sports Exerc* 30:975, 1998.

and respiratory systems are summarized in Box 6-1. Exercise sessions should total at least 20 to 60 minutes, either in one continuous session or in separate bouts lasting no less than 10 minutes each. Exercise of low intensity needs to be performed for longer time periods (the upper end of the time range) to obtain benefit, whereas hard exercise can be carried out for shorter periods of time (the lower end of the range). The percentage of the maximum heart rate (HR_{max}) achieved during exercise can be used to judge the intensity of the exercise (Table 6-1). Any activity that uses large muscle groups, can be maintained continuously, and uses aerobic capacity can be used to develop and sustain cardiovascular fitness (see Intervention and Teaching). Frail, elderly individuals may not tolerate long or intense aerobic exercise. For these individuals, the goal should be to obtain aerobic exercise at least 3

Table 6-1   Intensity of Exercise Based on the Percentage of HR_{max} Achieved

Intensity	% of HR_{max}
Very light	<35
Light	35-54
Moderate	55-69
Hard	70-89
Very hard	≥90
Maximum	100

From American College of Sports Medicine position stand. The recommended quantity and quality of exercise for developing and maintaining cardiorespiratory muscular fitness and flexibility in healthy adults. *Med Sci Sports Exerc* 30:978, 1998.

days per week for at least 20 minutes per session at low intensity. Walking is an excellent low-intensity exercise for ambulatory elderly individuals; however, arthritis and other diseases causing restriction of mobility, incontinence, weakness, and poor balance may impair exercise ability in the elderly. People who are unable to walk may be able to perform seated exercises in water (with water providing increased resistance) or to use seated stepping machines or devices for arm and leg ergometry.

For a well-rounded exercise program, resistance and flexibility training should be performed at least 2 to 3 days per week. Resistance training consists of at least 8 to 12 repetitions (10 to 15 for elderly or very frail individuals) of 8 to 10 different exercises that condition the major muscle groups (e.g., weight training). Flexibility training stretches the major muscle groups. In the frail elderly, resistance and balance training should precede aerobic training, to ensure that aerobic exercise can be done without increased risk of injury.

The health benefits resulting from physical activity exist on a continuum. An exercise program such as that described previously is optimal for achieving fitness; however, sedentary individuals can obtain benefits with an increase in physical activity, even if no formal exercise program is followed. Both children and adults need to obtain at least 30 minutes of moderate-intensity activity on most, and preferably all, days of the week. The activity can be accumulated in bouts of no less than 10 minutes each or in a single episode lasting 30 or more minutes.

Exercise and Weight Reduction

Exercise facilitates weight reduction in at least two ways. First, it tends to cause fat loss, even with little or no reduction in kcal intake. Second, regular aerobic exercise prevents the decline in resting energy expenditure, which often occurs as weight is lost. This decline in resting energy expenditure can undermine weight loss efforts, even for individuals who follow low-kcal diets closely.

Nutrition for Vigorous Activity and Competition
Nutrient Needs
Protein

It is commonly believed that markedly increased amounts of certain nutrients, particularly protein, are needed to build muscle mass; however, this is not the case. The protein RDA for adults is 0.8 g/kg/day. Adults doing strenuous exercise may need about 1 g/kg/day (a total of about 75 g for the man who weighs 75 kg [165 lb]). This amount is easily obtained in the average North American diet, which provides 80 to 110 g/day.

Kilocalories

Caloric needs vary because of differences in physical activities and the intensity of exercise. Increased caloric needs resulting from exercise can be met through a diet of regular foods. Fat should provide no more than 30% of the kcal, and carbohydrate should provide approximately 55%, with emphasis placed on complex carbohydrates (fibers and starches, found primarily in grains, legumes, vegetables, and fruits).

Vitamins and minerals

A balanced diet almost always provides all necessary vitamins for men and women, and no evidence supports the idea that supplemental vitamins improve athletic performance. B vitamin needs increase during vigorous activity, but they will be met by the increased caloric intake needed during heavy exercise.

Vigorous exercise increases iron needs, and iron deficiency is prevalent among female athletes. Distance runners are especially likely to have iron deficiency. Possible reasons that have been suggested include increased losses of iron in perspiration during prolonged physical activity, damage to red blood cells in the capillaries of the soles of the feet during running, and increased gastrointestinal blood loss, which is known to be more common in runners than in the general population. Iron deficiency impairs physical performance by interfering with energy production and allowing lactate accumulation in muscle, which makes the muscle fatigue more quickly.

Creatine

Creatine phosphate is an important energy source for exercising muscle. Theoretically, increasing the muscle creatine levels should prolong the athlete's ability to perform high-intensity exercise. For this reason, many athletes use creatine supplements. Some laboratory studies suggest that creatine supplements improve performance on short-term, high-intensity tasks, but the benefit of creatine on tasks of longer duration and in real athletic events has not been determined. Carbohydrate increases uptake of creatine by the muscle, so the athlete who chooses to take this supplement needs an adequate carbohydrate intake.

The Female Athlete Triad

Physically active females, especially those in sports or dance activities where low body weight is desirable, are at risk for a syndrome known as the *female athlete triad*. The components of the triad are eating disorders, amenorrhea, and osteoporosis. When individuals lose excessive body weight, they become anovulatory and amenorrheic. As the cyclic hormonal stimulus for bone deposition is disrupted, more mineral is mobilized from the bone than is deposited.

Diet for Athletic Events

Carbohydrate loading

Carbohydrate loading is a technique of manipulating the athlete's diet and exercise regimens to increase muscle glycogen stores and thus to increase endurance during competition. Carbohydrate loading is of benefit primarily to athletes in endurance events lasting at least 1 to 2 hours (e.g., marathon running, long-distance cycling, cross-country skiing). Although strong evidence suggests that carbohydrate loading can improve endurance in men, the data regarding its effects in women are less clear. Carbohydrate loading could be harmful in individuals with diabetes and hypertriglyceridemia, and they should undertake carbohydrate loading only under medical supervision. Whether carbohydrate loading is safe for preadolescent and adolescent athletes is unknown. Water stored with the glycogen can make the muscles feel stiff and swollen. A technique for carbohydrate loading is described in the Intervention and Teaching section later in this chapter.

Preevent meal

The timing and composition of the last meal before athletic competition can influence performance. It is particularly important that the stomach not be extremely full at the time of the event because this diverts blood flow to the mesentery and may impair performance. See Intervention and Teaching later in this chapter for specifics of the preevent meal.

Fluid and electrolyte replacement

Adequate replacement of fluid losses during exercise not only improves physical performance but also helps to maintain the health and safety of the exercising individuals. Losses from perspiration are primarily water; sweat electrolyte levels are lower than those in plasma. There is little need for carbohydrate-electrolyte sport drinks when physical activity lasts less than 1 hour. Water and the normal diet are sufficient to replace perspiration and insensible losses.

Nutritional Care

The objectives of care are for individuals to: (1) establish a lifelong habit of regular aerobic exercise and a nutritionally balanced diet to promote health and physical fitness, (2) avoid nutritional deficiencies, and (3) attain optimal athletic performance in a manner consistent with maintaining good health and nutritional status.

Assessment

Assessment is summarized in Table 6-2.

Intervention and Teaching

Encouraging regular aerobic exercise

Emphasize benefits of exercise, which vary with age and physiologic state. Some of these benefits are:

■ *All age groups:* reduced risk of obesity, increased endurance and muscle tone, feeling of well-being

Table 6-2   Assessment in Physical Fitness and Athletic Competition

Areas of Concern	Significant Findings
Inadequate Energy (kcal) Intake	*History* Energy intake low; frequent dieting to achieve and maintain low "competitive" weight; physiologic state requiring ↑ kcal: childhood, adolescence, pregnancy, lactation; extremely strenuous exercise habits (e.g., distance running); possible eating disorder *Physical Examination* ↓ Body fat, athletic performance; TSF <5th percentile; weight for height <90% of standard or BMI <18.5, (for children or adolescents, weight more than 1 percentile marking < that for height, i.e., if height is at 50th percentile, weight should be at least at the 25th); amenorrhea; delayed growth and development (children and adolescents)
Inadequate Protein Intake	*History* Frequent dieting, kcal intake so low that protein consumed is utilized for energy; physiologic state requiring ↑ protein: childhood, adolescence, pregnancy, lactation *Physical Examination* Edema; delayed growth and development (children and adolescents); thinning of hair, changes in hair texture *Laboratory Analysis* ↓ Serum albumin, transferrin, or prealbumin, lymphocyte count

Continued

Table 6-2   Assessment in Physical Fitness and Athletic Competition—cont'd

Areas of Concern	Significant Findings
Inadequate Mineral Intake	
Fe	*History*
	Intake <RDA by diet history or food record, GI blood loss, especially in distance runners
	Physical Examination
	Pallor; ↓ athletic performance
	Laboratory Analysis
	↓ Hct, Hgb, MCV, MCH, MCHC, serum Fe; ↑ serum transferrin or total iron-binding capacity
Volume Fluid Deficit	*History*
	Failure to replace fluid losses by drinking during and after athletic endeavors; fluid restriction in an attempt to achieve competitive weight; use of diuretics to achieve competitive weight or produce dilute urine in an effort to confound drug testing
	Physical Examination
	Dry, sticky mucous membranes; poor skin turgor; thirst; disorientation; weakness; hypotension
	Laboratory Analysis
	↑ Serum sodium, Hct, BUN, serum osmolality

■ *Childhood and adolescence:* establish habit of regular exercise
■ *Adulthood:* reduced risk of heart disease, hypertension, type 2 diabetes, gout, gallstones, and osteoporosis
■ *Pregnancy:* less constipation
■ *Elderly:* same as adulthood; delay loss of muscle mass and strength; less constipation; can be an opportunity for social contact

Recommend exercises that use large muscle groups rhythmically and that can be maintained continuously. Examples of aerobic activities are running or jogging, walking, hiking, swimming, ice or roller skating, bicycling, cross-country skiing, rope skipping, or rowing. Certain activities, such as those requiring running or jumping and those associated with overuse (e.g., marathon training), have great potential for injury. The beginning exerciser, pregnant women, and the elderly should be especially cautious if they choose these activities. The individual can monitor his or her heart rate during exercise in order to estimate the aerobic benefit. (It is recommended that pregnant women not exceed a heart rate of 140 beats/minute.) If the health care provider helps the individual devise an exercise plan that is tailored to his or her needs and schedule, this increases the likelihood that the exercise program will be sustained (Box 6-2).

Individuals who do not wish to participate in a formal exercise regimen need encouragement to obtain 30 minutes or more of moderate-intensity exercise every day. Examples of moderate-intensity exercises include walking at a rate of 4 mph (6.7 km/hr), pushing a stroller at a rate of 3 mph (5 km/hr), bicycling at a rate of 10 mph (16.7 km/hr), water aerobics, raking leaves, house painting, and playing golf (carrying or pulling clubs). In carrying out these moderate-intensity activities for 30 minutes, an individual weighing 75 kg (165 lb) uses approximately 150 kcal/day or 1000 kcal/week.

Maintaining good health and nutrition in the vigorously exercising individual

Preventing nutritional deficiencies

■ *Kilocalories:* Maintain sufficient kcal intake to prevent underweight. Complex carbohydrates (starches) are especially good kcal sources for the athlete.
■ *Protein:* Maintain intake of at least 1 g/kg (adults) or the RDA (for children and pregnant and lactating women).

Box 6-2   Motivation for Physical Activity

Physical activity is more likely to be initiated and maintained if the individual:

- Perceives a personal benefit.
- Chooses an enjoyable activity.
- Feels competent and safe in doing the activity.
- Can easily access the activity on a regular basis.
- Can fit the activity into the daily schedule.
- Believes the activity does not generate excessive financial or social costs.
- Experiences a minimum of negative consequences (injury, loss of time, negative peer pressure, etc.).
- Recognizes the need to balance the use of labor-saving devices (e.g., power lawn mowers) and sedentary activities (e.g., watching television) with greater physical activity.

Adapted from Physical activity and cardiovascular health, NIH Consensus Statement 13:1, 1995.

- *Iron:* Individuals participating regularly in vigorous physical exercise should be instructed in a diet that includes good sources of iron (legumes, meats, whole and enriched grains; see Appendix A), as well as vitamin C, which promotes iron absorption. Female athletes and distance runners, particularly, may have difficulty maintaining adequate iron nutriture and may need a supplement. Absorption of iron from the supplement will be best if it is taken between meals or at bedtime and with fluids other than coffee, tea, or milk.

Preventing and treating eating disorders

Coaches, trainers, and all other individuals working with female athletes need to be aware of the prevalence and signs of the female athlete triad. The triad can impair athletic performance and increase morbidity and mortality among athletes, and these facts can be used to help motivate the athlete and coaching staff to avoid unhealthy weight control practices. Guidelines for recognizing and treating eating disorders are described in Chapter 8.

Optimizing athletic performance during competitive events
Carbohydrate loading

Carbohydrate loading can be achieved by reducing the amount of exercise performed for approximately 3 days before the athletic competition, while increasing carbohydrate intake to at least 8 to 10 g/kg body weight (65% to 80% of kcal consumed). Most carbohydrates should be complex, to avoid increasing serum triglyceride levels excessively. Table 6-3 gives an example of a diet for carbohydrate loading for an athlete needing approximately 2800 kcal; it can be modified to meet the caloric needs of athletes needing more or fewer kcal.

Preevent meal

On the day of the event, the athlete should: (1) consume the last solids 2 to 4 hours before the event to allow time for gastric emptying, (2) consume a light (150 to 500 kcal) high-carbohydrate meal to improve gastric emptying and avoid high-fat foods because they delay gastric emptying, (3) avoid simple sugars in the 30- to 45-minute period before vigorous exercise (except immediately before exercise, see #4) because sugars stimulate release of insulin and might result in hypoglycemia, and (4) consume sugars or other easily digested carbohydrate 5 to 10 minutes before exercise to provide readily available energy and improve performance. Consumption of simple sugars just before exercise begins will not result in hypoglycemia because glucagon and catecholamines are released as exercise begins, and they will counteract insulin's effect.

Carbohydrate during and after exercise

During intense exercise lasting longer than 1 hour, consumption of carbohydrate at a rate of approximately 30 to 60 g/hr can improve endurance and performance. The carbohydrates can be either sugars or starches. Use of carbohydrate-containing beverages allows carbohydrate intake to be combined with fluid replacement. Drinking 600 to 1200 ml/hr of a solution that provides 4 to 8 g of carbohydrate/100 ml (e.g., a sport drink or fruit juice diluted half strength) will replace fluid losses and provide the needed carbohydrate.

Following intense exercise, muscle glycogen stores need to be replaced. This process is encouraged by consumption of carbohydrate during the post-exercise period at a rate of 1 g/kg body weight

Table 6-3   Sample Food Guide for Carbohydrate Loading

Food Group (No. Servings)	Food	Carbohydrate (g)
Breakfast		
Fruit (2)	Grapefruit, 1 whole	30
Grain (2)	Bran cereal, 1 cup	30
Fruit (1)	Banana, 1 small	15
Milk (1)	Skim milk, 1 cup	12
Grain (2), fat (1)	Bagel, 1, with 2 tbsp low-fat cream cheese	30
—	Sugar, 1 tsp, in decaffeinated tea	4
Lunch		
Meat (2)	Black bean soup, 2 cups	61
Grain (3)	Corn tortillas, 3	45
Vegetable (1), fat (1)	Mixed greens, 1 cup raw, with 2 tbsp reduced fat dressing	5
Fruit (3)	Grapes, 1 cup	45

Grain = bread, cereal, rice, and pasta group.
Milk = milk, cheese, and yogurt group.
Meat = meat, poultry, fish, dry beans, eggs, and nuts group.

(approximately 1 cup cooked pasta and 1 cup fruit juice for an adult) every two hours during the waking hours, or a total of approximately 7 to10 g/kg during the 24-hour period after exercise.

Replacing fluids and electrolytes lost during exercise

Individuals should consume nutritionally balanced diets with adequate fluid intake during the 24-hour period before the athletic event, to ensure that hydration is adequate. About 2 hours before vigorous exercise, they should drink about 500 ml (about 17 fluid oz) of fluid to ensure that they are well hydrated and to allow time for excretion of any excess water before the event. Cool fluids (15° to 22° C, or 59° to 72° F) are recommended because they are more

Table 6-3   Sample Food Guide for Carbohydrate
Loading—cont'd

Food Group (No. Servings)	Food	Carbohydrate (g)
Dinner		
Grain (6)	Spaghetti, 3 cups	90
Vegetable (2), meat (1)	Spaghetti sauce with meat, 1½ cups	10
Vegetable (2)	Broccoli, steamed, 1 cup	10
Vegetable (1)	Beans, Italian, ½ cup	5
Grain (1)	Roll, 1	15
—	Sugar, 1 tsp, in decaffeinated tea	4
Snacks		
Grain (2)	Granola bar, reduced fat, 1	30
Fruit (1)	Apricots, dried, 8 halves	15
Grain (2)	Pretzels, 1½ oz.	30
Milk (1)	Fruit yogurt, 8 oz	46
TOTALS	2855 kcal	532 g carbohydrate (75% of kcal)

rapidly emptied from the stomach than warm beverages. If exercise continues more than 1 hour, use of a beverage with 0.5 to 0.7 g sodium/l (e.g., a sport drink) may be of value in improving palatability, enhancing fluid retention, and preventing the hyponatremia that can occur if excess plain water is consumed. Thirst is not a reliable indicator of fluid needs during or after competition. The athlete should begin drinking early in the event and continue to do so at regular intervals in amounts that will replace fluid losses, or the maximum amount tolerated if the individual cannot ingest enough to replace fluid losses. Weighing before and after exercise is a guide to the amount of fluid replacement needed during and after the event. Voluntary fluid intake after exercise is often inadequate to replace losses in perspiration. The athlete needs a minimum of 480 ml (16 oz) to replace each 0.45 kg (1 lb) lost, but it may be necessary to consume as much as 150% of fluid losses to obtain adequate rehydration. Sugar-containing beverages such as juices and sport drinks help to provide the carbohydrate needed for muscle glycogen synthesis. Alcohol and caffeine-containing drinks, on the other hand, are not desirable as rehydration solutions because they promote fluid loss through diuresis.

SELECTED BIBLIOGRAPHY

American Academy of Pediatrics, Committee on Sports Medicine and Fitness: Promotion of healthy weight-control practices in young athletes, *Pediatrics* 97:752, 1996.

American College of Sports Medicine position stand. The female athlete triad, *Med Sci Sports Exerc* 29:i, 1997.

American College of Sports Medicine position stand. The recommended quantity and quality of exercise for developing and maintaining cardiorespiratory and muscular fitness, and flexibility in healthy adults, *Med Sci Sports Exerc* 30:975, 1998a.

American College of Sports Medicine position stand. Exercise and physical activity for older adults, *Med Sci Sports Exerc* 30:992, 1998b.

Burke LM. Nutrition for post-exercise recovery, *Australian J Sci Med Sport* 29:3, 1997.

Clarkson PM, Haynes EM: Exercise and mineral status of athletes: calcium, magnesium, phosphorus, and iron, *Med Sci Sports Exerc* 27:831, 1995.

Convertino VA, Armstrong LE, Coyle EF, et al: American College of Sports Medicine position stand. Exercise and fluid replacement, *Med Sci Sports Exerc* 28:i, 1996.

Hawley JA, Burke LM: Effect of meal frequency and timing on physical performance, *Br J Nutr* 77 (suppl 1):S91, 1997.

Hawley JA, Schabort EJ, Noakes TD, Dennis SC: Carbohydrate-loading and exercise performance: an update, *Sports Med* 24:73, 1997.

Jones DA, Ainsworth BE, Croft JB, et al: Moderate leisure-time physical activity: who is meeting the public health recommendations? A national cross-sectional study, *Arch Fam Med* 7:285, 1998.

Pate RR, Pratt M, Blair SN, et al: Physical activity and public health: A recommendation from the Centers for Disease Control and Prevention and the American College of Sports Medicine, *JAMA* 273:402, 1995.

Williams MH, Branch JD: Creatine supplementation and exercise performance: an update, *J Am Coll Nutr* 17:216, 1998.

OBESITY AND EATING DISORDERS

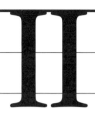

A person who is in **energy balance** matches energy (calorie) intake and energy expenditure so that body weight is maintained at a constant level. Being in positive energy balance, or consuming more calories than needed, results in weight gain and can lead to overweight and obesity. On the other hand, negative energy balance—consuming fewer calories than needed or increasing the amount of physical activity to use more energy—results in weight loss. Negative energy balance is desirable in the obese or over-weight individual, but it becomes a concern when a person who is of normal weight or underweight exhibits excessive preoccupation with body weight and frequently or continually tries to lose weight. In the latter case, an eating disorder may exist. Both the obese individual and the individual with an eating disorder are at risk for significant emotional and physical health problems.

Obesity and Weight Control

7

Obesity is increasing in prevalence in most developed countries. The National Heart, Lung, and Blood Institute (1998) estimates that 55% of all adults are now overweight or obese. In addition, overweight and obesity affects one third of children between 5 and 14 years of age. Because of the prevalence of obesity and the health risks associated with it, it is probably the most serious nutritional problem in the United States.

Pathophysiology
Diagnosis of Obesity and Overweight

In the clinical setting, several practical methods are used to determine whether obesity is present:

1. *Calculation of the body mass index (BMI).* This is one of the simplest methods, and the BMI correlates well with health risks from obesity. A chart for determining BMI can be found inside the back cover of this book, or BMI can be calculated as shown in Box 7-1.
2. *Comparison of weight with tables of ideal body weight (IBW) or desirable weight for height* (see Appendix C).

    % of IBW = (Actual body weight ÷ ideal body weight) × 100

    Overweight is considered to be 110% to 120% of the desirable or ideal body weight (IBW). With this method, obesity can be divided into three degrees: (1) mild, 120% to 140% of IBW, (2) moderate, 141% to 200% of IBW, and (3) severe or morbid, more than 200% of IBW.
3. *Measurement of abdominal girth.* Visceral, or abdominal, fat (the so-called ''apple'' shape, or android fat pattern) is a predictor of cardiovascular disease risk. Fat in the hips and thighs (''pear'' shape, or gynecoid fat pattern), on the other hand,

---

Box 7-1   **Body Mass Index (BMI)**

BMI Calculation

BMI = weight in kg ÷ (height in m)^2

or

BMI = [weight in lb ÷ (height in inches)^2] × 704.5

BMI Classification

Normal	18.5-24.9
Overweight	25-29.9
Obese	30 or more*

Example

Weight 85 kg (187 lb), height 1.68 m (5′6″)

BMI = 85 ÷ 1.68^2 = 30.1 (obese)

Classifications are from the National Heart, Lung, and Blood Institute: *Clinical guidelines on the identification, evaluation, and treatment of overweight and obesity in adults,* National Institutes of Health, Washington, DC, 1998.
*Obesity can be further divided, based on severity: grade I obesity (mild), BMI 30-34.9; grade II obesity (moderate), BMI 35-39.9; and grade III obesity (extreme), BMI 40 or more.

is much less likely to be associated with health risk. The waist/hip ratio can be used as an indicator of visceral fat. It is measured with the individual standing, and the circumference of the body is measured at the narrowest part of the waist and at the widest part of the hips. A ratio greater than 0.8 for women or 0.95 for men indicates excessive abdominal fat. The National Heart, Lung, and Blood Institute (1998) has suggested that the waist circumference alone be used as an indicator of abdominal fat. Men are considered at high risk if the waist circumference is >102 cm (40 in), and women are at high risk if the waist circumference is >99 cm (35 in).

4. *Measurement of subcutaneous fat.* It is estimated that as much as 50% of the fat can be found in the subcutaneous area. Therefore, skinfold (fatfold) measurements can be an indicator of the amount of body fat. Measurement of skinfolds in several parts of the body can give a more accurate indication of the amount of body fat than measurement of a single site. Durnin and Wormsley (1974) have published tables for estimation of

body fat of men and women of various ages, based on the sum of the biceps, triceps, subscapular, and suprailiac skinfolds. Much variability can occur between skinfold measurements performed by two different examiners. To reduce error, only well-trained individuals should measure skinfolds.

Etiology

Most cases of obesity are multifactorial in etiology. Some of the factors are:

Environment

Most cases of obesity in developed countries seem to result from the widespread availability of appealing food and a lifestyle with little physical activity. Familial influences (e.g., using food as a reward, withholding dessert until the plate is clean) help develop eating habits that contribute to obesity.

Energy expenditure

Energy expenditure can be divided into three parts: **resting energy expenditure (REE), thermic effect of food (TEF),** and the energy expended in physical activity (see Chapter 2). REE, the energy required for vital body processes such as operation of the heart and lungs, accounts for 60% or more of energy expenditure for most individuals. REE appears to be normal in the obese. TEF, the energy required for digestion, absorption, and disposition of the nutrients in food, is normally about 10% of the total energy expenditure. The obese have been reported to have low TEF, but this abnormality accounts for very few calories and probably is insufficient to be the cause of most cases of obesity. Physical activity, the most variable component of energy expenditure, accounts for about 20% to 30% of the daily energy expenditure for most individuals. The obese tend to be more sedentary than normal-weight people, but this is balanced by the fact that the obese require more energy to perform the same tasks as normal-weight individuals.

Genetics

Children of obese parents are three to eight times as likely to be obese as children of normal-weight parents, even if they are not reared by their natural parents. Some individuals may have an inherited metabolic makeup that allows them to store fat more efficiently than other individuals do. The discovery of **leptin,** the product of the *ob* gene, has encouraged many researchers to believe that a potentially treatable genetic defect causing obesity will be found in humans. Leptin is released by adipose tissue, and it appears to provide a mechanism for the adipose tissue to communicate with the central nervous system and contribute to the control of food intake and energy metabolism (Figure 7-1). Leptin levels are high in most obese individuals, so obese people apparently have no defect in leptin formation. It may be that the obese are resistant to the effects of leptin. At this point, however, no abnormalities in leptin or its metabolism have been found that could explain most cases of human obesity.

Neuroendocrine

Neuroendocrine disorders are responsible for less than 1% of all cases of obesity. Hypothyroidism, Cushing's syndrome, and polycystic ovary syndrome can lead to obesity, but severe obesity is uncommon in these disorders. Prader-Willi syndrome, associated with excessive appetite, inappropriate food-seeking behaviors, and mental retardation, can lead to massive obesity, but it is quite rare.

Psychology

Overeating may occur as a response to loneliness, grief, or depression. Overeating may also result from a learned response to external cues such as food advertising or the fact that it is mealtime, rather than the internal cue of hunger.

Physiology

Energy expenditure declines with aging, and thus body weight often increases during middle age.

Health Risks Associated with Obesity

Obesity is associated with numerous health risks, which are summarized in Table 7-1. Health risks increase progressively with the severity of obesity. In the past, moderate weight gain with aging was believed to be associated with little health risk, but recent data indicate that the risk of death from heart disease and cancer is increased in women who gain 10 kg (22 lb) or more after the age of 18. The lowest risk was reported in nonsmokers who were at least 15% below average weight (those who had a BMI <19). Weight gain in adult men also increases their health risks.

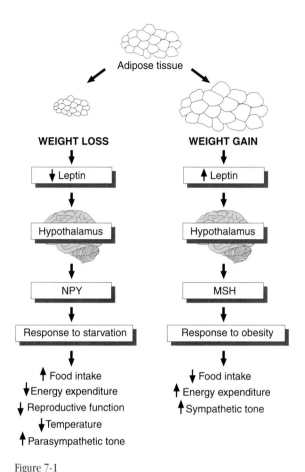

Figure 7-1

Leptin provides a mechanism so that the body can maintain
stable fat stores. The adipose, or fat, tissue releases leptin.
A loss of body fat (weight loss or starvation) reduces leptin
release, and an increase in body fat enhances leptin production. It is believed that the binding of leptin to receptors
in the hypothalamus, a brain region known to be involved
in regulation of body weight, causes the release of neurotransmitters that induce responses aimed at keeping the fat
stores relatively unchanging (e.g., increased or decreased
appetite). Neuropeptide Y (NPY) is released in response
to decreased levels of leptin, and melanocyte-stimulating
hormone (MSH) is released in response to increased leptin.
(Modified from Friedman JM: Leptin, leptin receptors, and the control of body
weight, *Nutrition Reviews* 56(2):S40, 1998. © 1998 International Life Sciences
Institute, Washington, D.C.)

Table 7-1   Health Problems Caused or Worsened by Obesity

Type of Problem	Disease, Symptom, or Difficulty
Cardiovascular or respiratory	Hypertension, coronary heart disease, varicose veins, pickwickian syndrome*
Endocrine or reproductive	Non–insulin-dependent diabetes mellitus, amenorrhea, infertility, preeclampsia
Gastrointestinal	Gallstones, fatty liver
Musculoskeletal and skin	Osteoarthritis, skin irritation and infections, especially in fat folds, striae
Malignancies	Cancer of the colon, rectum, prostate, gallbladder, breast, uterus, and ovaries
Psychosocial	Social discrimination, poor self-image†

*Hypoventilation and lethargy caused by decreased chest movement resulting from excessive weight on the chest.
†Varies by cultural and racial group; blacks are more accepting of obesity and overweight than whites.

Weight cycling, or "yo-yo" dieting, occurs when individuals repeatedly lose and regain weight. There is some concern that this process may accelerate arteriosclerosis or aggravate other health problems, but conclusive data are lacking. The health risks of obesity are so great that the obese should not avoid trying to lose weight because of fears of weight cycling.

Treatment and Nutritional Care

The goals of intervention are to: (1) decrease body fat to achieve a weight within 20% of ideal, (2) develop more healthy eating and physical activity habits, (3) prevent loss of lean body mass (LBM) during weight reduction, and (4) maintain weight loss.

Assessment

Assessment is summarized in Box 7-2.

Box 7-2   Assessment in Obesity and Weight Control

Diet History

Usual Nutrient Intake

Include meal and snack patterns; portion sizes; food preparation methods (frying, sauteing, adding butter or margarine as a flavoring); gravies, sauces, and beverages (including alcohol)

Conditions Under Which Eating Occurs

Keeping a food record helps the individual identify occasions that result in eating; it should include whom the individual eats with (alone versus with family or friends); where and when eating occurs (at the table, while watching television, while preparing meals, while studying); feelings that prompt eating (loneliness, boredom, anxiety or depression versus hunger)

Activity Level

Includes presence or absence of regularly scheduled exercise (type, frequency, duration, and intensity); activity required during work, school, housework, or hobbies

---

Intervention

Weight reduction is achieved by consuming fewer kcal than are required to meet energy needs. Methods for achieving weight reduction include diet, behavior modification, increased physical activity, surgery, and drugs. All of these methods are discussed in this chapter.

Establishing a weight goal

In children, the desirable body weight is between the 5th and 95th percentiles of weight for length or height (see Appendix D). For adults, the IBW can be estimated from the table of desirable weights for height (see Appendix C).

A weight that is no more than 20% greater than ideal, or a BMI between 18.5 and 25, is associated with the least health risks.

Especially in the severely obese individual, however, a goal of less than or equal to 120% of the IBW may seem overwhelming. If the obese individual participates in setting personal weight goals, he or she is more likely to be successful in losing weight. Even a modest weight loss can have health benefits (Box 7-3).

Promoting weight loss while maintaining LBM
Energy needs for safe weight loss

To calculate daily kcal needs:

- First determine IBW in kilograms; if IBW is in pounds, divide by 2.2.
- To estimate daily kcal needs for weight maintenance, multiply IBW in kilograms by 20 to 25 kcal if sedentary, 30 kcal if engaged in moderate activity, or 35 to 50 kcal if engaged in unusually heavy activity.
- To determine kcal needs for weight reduction, subtract 500 to 1000 kcal/day from kcal needed for maintenance. This results in loss of 0.5 to 1 kg (1 to 2 lb) per week because 1 lb of body fat is equivalent to approximately 3500 kcal.

> Example: A woman who is 5'5" has an IBW of 100 lb + (5 × 5 lb) = 125 lb (from rule of thumb, p. 37, or see Appendix C).
>
> IBW in kg = 125 lb ÷ 2.2 = 57 kg
>
> Needs for weight maintenance with sedentary lifestyle = 57 kg × 25 kcal = 1425 kcal/day
>
> Needs for weight loss = 1425 kcal/day − 500 kcal/day = 925 kcal/day

Caution: Intakes of less than 800 kcal/day are considered very low-calorie diets (VLCDs) and should not be used except under a physician's supervision. Short individuals and others with very low kcal needs should be encouraged to increase their activity level to encourage weight loss, rather than decreasing their kcal intake to a VLCD.

Balanced low-calorie diets

Balanced, low-calorie diets (LCDs >800 kcal/day) are the best choice for individuals who are less than 30% overweight. These diets, based on common foods chosen from all food groups, are adequate in all (or almost all) nutrients. The Food Guide Pyramid

---

Box 7-3   Potential Health Benefits of a 10 kg
(22 lb) Weight Loss by an Obese Individual

Mortality

20-25% decrease in total mortality
30-40% decrease in mortality from diabetes
40-50% fall in obesity-related cancer deaths

Blood Pressure

10 mmHg decrease in systolic pressure
20 mmHg decrease in diastolic pressure

Angina

Symptoms reduced by 91%
33% increase in exercise tolerance

Serum Lipids

10% decrease in total cholesterol
15% decrease in low density lipoprotein (LDL) cholesterol
30% decrease in triglyceride levels
8% increase in high density lipoprotein (HDL)* cholesterol

Diabetes

>50% reduction in the risk of developing diabetes
30-50% decrease in fasting blood glucose
15% decrease in hemoglobinA_{1c}**

From Jung RT: Obesity as a disease, *Br Med Bull* 53:307, 1997. Used with permission.
*Increases in HDL are inversely related to risk of heart disease.
**Elevated levels are evidence of elevated blood glucose over an extended period of time.

(see Chapter 1) or the *Exchange Lists for Meal Planning* (see Chapter 18) can be used to plan balanced low-kcal diets.

Diets that are low in fat and high in carbohydrate may be more effective for some dieters. Carbohydrate has less than half the kcal of fat (4 kcal/g vs. 9 kcal/g), and metabolism of carbohydrate causes a greater *thermic effect,* or heat loss (and thus loss of kcal), than fat. Also, complex carbohydrates (starches and fibers) are bulky and may help the individual feel fuller and more satisfied than less bulky meals.

Very low-calorie diets

Very low-calorie diets (VLCDs) are those providing 400 to 800 kcal/day; they should be used only as medically directed. Special diet formulas (usually flavored drinks) are available, with the kcal being mostly in the form of high-quality protein. This diet is sometimes called a protein-sparing modified fast. The usual regimen is to follow the VLCD for 12 to 16 weeks, followed by a gradual reinstitution of regular foods over a period of 3 weeks or longer. Losses of 1.5 to 2.3 kg (3.3 to 5.1 lb)/wk occur during the VLCD, with the higher losses occurring in men.

These diets are usually reserved for individuals who are at least 30% overweight. They are designed to preserve LBM, but some LBM is lost during the dieting period. The severely obese not only contain more body fat but also have a greater LBM and thus tolerate severe kcal restriction better than less overweight individuals. Rates of gallbladder disease are reported to be higher among individuals consuming VLCD.

A VLCD should be begun only after a thorough medical examination, and dieters should have regular measurement of serum electrolytes and examinations by a physician. Intake of noncaloric fluids should be at least 2 L/day to prevent dehydration. Unsupervised dieting can lead to dehydration, electrolyte imbalance, elevation of uric acid, fatigue, dizziness, and headache; over the long term, there is a potential for ventricular dysrhythmias as well as binge eating after the severely restricted diet is ended.

Counseling and behavior modification is essential because one half to two thirds of the weight loss is rapidly regained without it; lifestyle modification can reduce the amount of weight regained to about one third of that lost.

Shortcomings of fad diets

Diets that promise quick weight loss are popular. Unfortunately, these diets tend to be undesirable for one or more of the following reasons: (1) they are nutritionally inadequate; (2) they require expensive foods or time-consuming food preparation; (3) they are medically unsafe; (4) they do not help the individual change poor eating habits, and thus the weight lost is usually regained; (5) much of the weight lost is fluid or LBM, rather than fat. Several fad diets are described in Box 7-4.

Behavior modification

Behavior modification, in conjunction with a balanced reduction diet, helps promote lasting weight loss. It should be a part of all weight loss programs. The following techniques are the primary features of behavior modification programs:

- *Self-monitoring:* recording exercise, food intake, and emotional and environmental circumstances at the time of food consumption to provide a basis for planning changes
- *Stimulus control and environmental management:* acquiring techniques to help break learned associations between environmental cues and food intake
- *Positive reinforcement:* a reward system to encourage changes in behavior
- *Contracts:* signed contracts between the therapist and the individual seeking to modify behavior, outlining the consequences if various changes are made or are not made

Box 7-5 provides suggestions for modifying behavior to lose and maintain weight.

Physical activity

Activities involving gross movements of large muscles promote fat loss while conserving LBM. Aerobic exercise is especially effective in reducing visceral fat. Many individuals on weight reduction diets find that, after an initial period of weight loss, their weight plateaus. The primary reason is that energy expenditure decreases as weight decreases. An increase in physical activity can prevent this plateau from occurring. For best results, the dieter must exercise most days of the week, expending a total of at least 1500 kcal a week (Table 7-2).

Although a regular exercise regimen is invaluable, increasing energy expenditure in the activities of daily living can be even more important in promoting and maintaining weight loss. For example, park farther from the door, use stairs rather than the elevator, and bicycle or walk rather than driving when possible.

Medications

Most medications used for weight loss suppress the appetite through effects on the central nervous system. Serotonin-reuptake

---

Box 7-4   Selected Fad Weight-Reduction Diets

High-Protein "Ketogenic" Diets

Examples: Quick Weight Loss Diet, Scarsdale Diet, Dr. Atkins' Diet Revolution, Stillman Diet

Comments: These diets are very low in carbohydrate to induce ketosis. They often result in rapid weight loss caused by diuresis associated with excretion of ketones; the "water weight" lost is quickly regained.

Nutritional inadequacies: These diets are frequently low in folic acid and fiber, and sometimes in vitamins C and A and riboflavin; they are often high in saturated fat and cholesterol.

Diets Relying on Particular Foods or Hormones Purported to Help "Burn Fat" or Alter the Metabolism

Examples: Beverly Hills Diet, Grapefruit Diet, Simeon Diet

Comments: Neither grapefruit nor any other food or combination of foods helps to burn fat. The Simeon plan includes injections of human chorionic gonadotropin (hCG), which is alleged to accelerate fat loss, but the 500 kcal diet that accompanies the hCG is actually responsible for the weight loss seen with the diet.

Nutritional inadequacies: The Beverly Hills Diet allows only specified fruits for the first 10 days, then a few other foods are gradually added. It is inadequate in protein, Fe, Ca, Zn, and other nutrients. The 500 kcal Simeon diet plan is inadequate in almost all nutrients.

Food Substitutes (Diet Drinks or Foods Substituted for Regular Meals)

Examples: Ultra Slim Fast

Comments: These diets are low in kcal and monotonous. They often result in weight loss, but they do nothing to help the dieter retrain his or her eating habits, and the weight lost is usually rapidly regained.

Nutritional inadequacies: Fiber

Box 7-5 Modifying Behavior To Promote Weight Loss or Maintenance

1. Chew food slowly, and put utensils down between bites.
2. Never shop for food on an empty stomach.
3. Make out a grocery shopping list before starting, and do not add to it as you shop.
4. Leave a small amount of food on your plate after each meal.
5. Fill your plate in the kitchen at the start of the meal; do not put open bowls of food on the table.
6. Eat in only one or two places (e.g., the kitchen and dining room table).
7. Never eat while involved in any other activity, such as watching television.
8. Do not eat while standing.
9. Keep a diary of when and where you eat and under what circumstances (e.g., boredom, frustration, anxiety). Be aware of problem circumstances, and substitute another activity for eating.
10. Keep low-calorie snacks available at all times.
11. Reward yourself for weight loss (e.g., buy new clothes, treat yourself to concert tickets or a trip). Establish a stepwise set of goals with a reward for achieving each goal.
12. If you violate your diet on one occasion, do not use that as an excuse to go off the diet altogether. Acknowledge that setbacks happen, and return to your weight control program.
13. When confronted with an appealing food, remember that this will not be your last chance to have the food. Content yourself with a small portion.

inhibitors such as fluoxetine (Prozac) and sertraline (Zoloft) increase brain levels of the neurotransmitter serotonin by reducing its uptake by nerve terminals. Sibutramine (Meridia) inhibits the reuptake of both serotonin and norepinephrine; it not only suppresses appetite but also increases energy expenditure. Phenylpropanolamine (in over-the-counter products such as Acutrim and Dexatrim) is another product that suppresses appetite and increases

Table 7-2   Energy Expenditure in Selected Activities

| Activity | Kcal/ kg/min | Kcal used during 20 min of exercise | |
		60 kg (132 lb) person	90 kg (198 lb) person
Bicycling, <16 km/h (<10 mph), leisure riding	0.07	80	120
Bicycling, 19 km/h (12 mph), moderate effort	0.13	156	234
Dance, aerobic, low impact	0.08	96	144
Running 8 km/h (5 mph)	0.13	156	234
Swimming, slow freestyle	0.13	156	234
Walking, 4.8 km/h (3 mph)	0.06	72	108
Walking, 6.4 km/h (4 mph)	0.07	80	120

From Ainsworth B, et al: Compendium of physical activities: classification of energy costs of human physical activities, *Med Sci Sports Exer* 25(1):71-80, 1993.

energy expenditure. Orlistat (Xenical) is a new medication that acts in a different way, by inhibiting the release of gastric and pancreatic lipases and thereby blocking the digestion and absorption of approximately one third of the fat consumed.

Weight loss medications are usually used in conjunction with other methods (low-kcal diets, exercise programs, behavior modification) to stimulate weight loss. Medications increase the likelihood that the obese will lose at least 10% of their initial body weight, and therefore they reinforce the effects of lifestyle changes designed to promote weight loss; however, the total amount of weight loss caused by medications by themselves is only moderate—2 to 10 kg (4 to 22 lb) in most reports—and the weight loss plateaus after about 6 months. Weight regain is common after medications are stopped. Because obesity is a long-term problem, there is little benefit from short-term use of medications. Long-term use of medications is currently recommended only for carefully

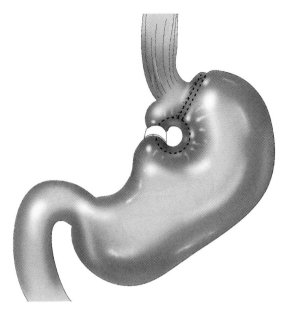

Figure 7-2
Vertical banded gastroplasty.

selected patients, particularly those who have obesity-related health problems, and not in the general obese population.

A Chinese herb regimen has been promoted as a stimulant of weight loss. It has been associated with the development of renal failure (Chinese-herb nephropathy) and renal carcinoma in several individuals (Cosyns, 1999) and consequently is not recommended.

Surgery

An individual with a BMI >40, or a BMI >35 and a serious obesity-related complication, who has failed to lose weight via more conventional methods may be considered for obesity surgery. The most common surgeries are two procedures that limit the capacity of the stomach to store food. In gastroplasty (gastric stapling; Figure 7-2), the stomach is partitioned so that the food enters a small pouch (30 to 60 ml) and the individual quickly feels full. In gastric bypass (Figure 7-3), the reservoir is connected to the

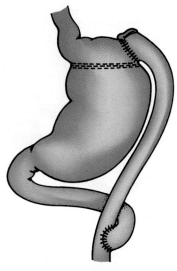

Figure 7-3
Roux-en-Y gastric bypass. The stomach is stapled completely
horizontally; the jejunum is resected from the duodenum
and connected to the upper gastric pouch; the distal duodenal stump is connected to the jejunum to permit drainage
of intestinal secretions.

jejunum, bypassing the distal stomach and the duodenum. Individuals lose weight both because of restricted intake and because
of moderate malabsorption of nutrients following the surgery.

Ninety percent of individuals undergoing gastric bypass lose at
least 50% of their excess weight, but candidates for surgery are very
obese, and therefore only 30% to 50% will achieve a body weight
less than 125% of ideal. Weight loss usually ceases within 12 to 18
months after surgery. Losses of 50% of the excess weight or more
may be maintained for as long as 10 to 15 years, however,
especially by individuals who have had the bypass procedure. The
bypass procedure is reported to be especially effective for
individuals who crave carbohydrates because simple carbohydrates
are likely to aggravate **dumping syndrome,** a common side effect
of gastric bypass or gastrectomy. The symptoms of dumping

syndrome include dizziness, sweating, nausea, weakness, tachycardia, and diarrhea. The syndrome occurs because of the speed with which stomach contents pass into the small bowel. A large load of simple carbohydrates in the diet increases the osmotic concentration of the bowel contents and draws fluid from the tissues into the bowel lumen. This reaction causes rapid reduction in blood volume (thus producing symptoms of weakness, tachycardia, sweating, and faintness) and can result in watery stools.

Specific diet and behavior modifications are required following gastric partitioning. These are discussed under Teaching.

Teaching

Preventing development of overweight and obesity

It is easier to prevent weight gain than to reduce excess weight. The following points are useful in helping adults avoid weight gain:

- Health risks are increased even at moderate degrees of overweight.
- Anticipate the likelihood of weight gain with aging and make lifestyle changes (increase activity level and improve eating habits) to prevent it.
- Be alert to times when weight gain is likely (when quitting smoking, undergoing unusual stress, or in the perimenopausal period, for example), and plan strategies in advance to prevent weight gain.

Achieving fat loss while maintaining LBM and retraining eating habits

Weight control is a lifelong process. After weight loss is accomplished, weight maintenance becomes the goal. Instead of thinking of weight control in terms of dieting, which is a temporary practice, the individual must think of it as a lifestyle change. He or she can never return to old eating habits, or the weight will be regained. This change is achieved through wise eating practices, increases in physical activity, and behavior modification. These measures must be practiced until they become routine for the individual.

Low-calorie diet

There are a variety of ways to plan a low-kcal diet based on common foods. Most adults or adolescents can learn to use the

Exchange Lists for Meal Planning available from the American Diabetes Association and the American Dietetic Association, which allow flexibility and are easier than calorie counting. Some individuals may find that counting fat grams is an easier way to control intake (although simply restricting fat and not total calories has not been found to be effective in promoting weight loss). Individuals may want to use other diet plans that are found in magazines or books or supported by various commercial or community organizations. Box 7-6 provides guidelines for evaluating weight loss programs.

One teaching technique for preschool and young school-age children is the "traffic light" plan. Foods less than 20 kcal/serving are green, or GO, foods and can be used freely. Green foods include seasonings and a few vegetables, such as asparagus. Yellow foods are the primary foods in the diet; they can be eaten with CAUTION. Examples are corn, oranges, baked chicken, skim milk, and English muffins. Red, or STOP, foods are high in kcal. No more than 4 servings of red foods are to be eaten per week. Some examples of red foods are scalloped potatoes, fruit in heavy syrup, fried chicken, whole milk, and doughnuts.

Box 7-6   Characteristics of a Safe and Effective Weight Control Program

1. The diet plan includes more than 800 kcal/day.
2. The diet plan includes foods from all food groups. A plan that relies on regular foods, rather than special proprietary products, is likely to be more effective in retraining eating habits. Very few servings from the fats, oils, and sweets group should be included.
3. No magical "fat-burning" or appetite-reducing products are recommended.
4. Claims for weight loss are no more than an average of 1 kg (~2 lb)/week.
5. Exercise is encouraged.
6. Behavior changes are incorporated.
7. The plan can be adapted to the lifestyle of the individual.
8. The cost of the plan is reasonable.

Some general suggestions for the person who is trying to lose weight are:

- Weighing or measuring foods initially is helpful in learning to recognize portion sizes.
- High-fiber foods take longer to consume than low-fiber ones, and satiety (fullness or satisfaction) may be achieved with fewer kcal when consuming high-fiber foods.
- Decrease use of fats, the most concentrated source of kcal. Use lean meats or skinless poultry, and eat no more than 6 oz (about the size of two decks of cards) daily. Broil, bake, or steam rather than frying foods. Use herbs, spices, lemon juice, or other low-kcal seasonings rather than butter, margarine, olive oil, or salt pork. Choose skim milk and dairy products made with skim milk. Limit foods with "hidden" fat, such as doughnuts, pie crust, croissants, muffins, and other quick breads. Choose fruit ices, fresh fruit, or low-fat cookies (gingersnaps, Newtons) rather than ice cream, cake, pie, or higher fat cookies.
- Do not expect rapid, easy weight loss. Weight gain is usually a gradual process, and so is weight reduction. When lapses occur, do not become depressed; simply resume proper eating habits and physical activity patterns.
- Include occasional high-calorie treats in the eating plan. This approach helps to prevent feelings of deprivation that may lead to binge eating and reduces guilt over indulging in a favorite high-calorie food. It may be necessary to eat high-calorie favorite foods under the supervision of a counselor, health care provider, or trusted family member or friend initially, to avoid losing control.

Physical activity

An aerobic exercise program carried out almost every day (see Interventions) promotes weight loss and maintenance. It can be just as important to increase energy expenditure during daily activities: choose a parking space farther away from the door, walk or bike instead of driving whenever possible, use manual instead of power appliances and tools, and use stairs rather than escalators and elevators.

Behavior modification

Behavior modification helps the individual to learn new behaviors, acquire skills in self-monitoring and cognitive restructuring, and develop strategies for maintaining weight loss, such as keeping records of foods eaten and of physical activity if weight is regained, practicing controlled intake of problem foods, and using available support systems (family, friends, and other weight loss veterans).

The individuals who are most successful in losing weight and maintaining weight loss tend to be those who develop personalized methods of controlling food intake and increasing energy expenditure. As an example, overly rapid food consumption is one cause of overeating. The feeling of satiety takes 20 minutes or more to develop in a hungry person, and the person who eats a meal in less time may overeat simply because he or she does not yet feel full. To slow the eating rate, the individual can eat with friends or family and talk with them during meals, lay utensils down after each bite, chew each bite thoroughly, and eat many leafy salads and other bulky foods. Box 7-5 lists other behavior modification techniques.

Consuming a more healthful diet

Obese individuals are often found to have poor diets, frequently skipping breakfast and consuming many foods low in minerals and vitamins. The eating habits established during weight loss and maintenance efforts should change the quality of the diet in a positive way. The following are specific teaching points for those who are practicing weight control:

- All foods can be eaten in moderation; however, calorie-rich extras with little nutritional value (butter, margarine, salad dressings, sugar, candy, syrups, jams, desserts, pastries, soft drinks, and fruit drinks) should be minimized. Concentrate on foods that provide large amounts of nutrients compared with the energy they contribute.
- Individuals consuming less than 1200 kcal/day usually need a vitamin-mineral supplement because of the difficulty in maintaining adequate nutrient intake within their kcal restriction.
- Omitting meals often makes the individual so hungry that he or she overeats at the next meal.

Seeking support

Support and reinforcement improve the chance of success. Support can come from group or individual counseling through hospital outpatient departments, dietitians or psychologists in private practice, lay-led community groups, family members, and friends.

Maintaining good nutritional habits following obesity surgery

The following measures will help the individual receive optimal benefits from the surgery while avoiding complications:

- Alteration of eating behaviors during the first two postoperative years is essential. During this time, the effects of surgery reinforce dieting endeavors by decreasing the amount the individual can comfortably eat. After this point, the surgery, particularly gastroplasty, has less benefit. The individual should adopt techniques to slow the rate of eating (see Box 7-5), avoid kcal-dense foods (fats, pastries, candy and sweets, and sweetened beverages), and eat regular, small meals.
- Nausea and vomiting are the most common problems, and gastrointestinal obstruction is a possibility postoperatively. Initial feedings are usually liquids or blended, strained foods. Over the first 6 to 8 weeks after surgery, the diet can be progressed to soft and then regular foods. Measures to reduce nausea and vomiting include chewing foods well, eating slowly, and eating small meals.
- Symptoms of dumping syndrome can be alleviated by avoiding concentrated sweets, eating slowly, and avoiding liquids during mealtime (after the initial postoperative period).

Maintenance of weight loss

Unfortunately, regain of lost weight is common among the obese. Maintenance of weight loss is improved if the individual continues in a program providing ongoing dietary counseling to reinforce new food habits and develop strategies for dealing with temptations to overeat, regular physical activity, and behavior therapy. Preferably, this program would continue indefinitely.

SELECTED BIBLIOGRAPHY

Cosyns JP, et al.: Urothelial lesions in Chinese-herb nephropathy, *Am J Kidney Dis* 33:1011, 1999.

Durnin JV, Wormsley J: Body fat assessed from total body density and its estimation from skinfold thickness: measurements on 481 men and women aged from 16 to 72 years, *Br J Nutr* 32:77, 1974.

Franz MJ: Managing obesity in patients with comorbidities, *J Am Dietet Assoc* 98(Suppl 2):S39, 1998.

Hill JO, Peters JC: Environmental contributions to the obesity epidemic, *Science* 280:1371, 1998.

Jensen GL, Rogers J: Obesity in older persons, *J Am Dietet Assoc* 98:1308, 1998.

Kolanowski J: Surgical treatment for morbid obesity, *Br Med Bull* 54:433, 1997.

Manson JE, et al.: Body weight and mortality among women, *N Engl J Med* 333:677, 1995.

National Heart, Lung, and Blood Institute: *Clinical guidelines on the identification, evaluation, and treatment of overweight and obesity in adults,* National Institutes of Health, Washington, DC, 1998.

National Task Force on the Prevention and Treatment of Obesity: Long-term pharmacotherapy in the management of obesity, *JAMA* 276:1907, 1996.

National Task Force on the Prevention and Treatment of Obesity: Weight cycling, *JAMA* 272:1196, 1994.

Riches RM, et al.: Reduction in visceral adipose tissue is associated with improvement in apolipoprotein B-100 metabolism in obese men, *J Clin Endocrinol Metab* 84:2854, 1999.

Rauh-Pfeiffer A, Kelleher D, Duggan C: Obesity and low-fat diets in pediatrics, *Curr Opin Pediatrics* 10:329, 1998.

Rippe JM, Hess S: The role of physical activity in the prevention and management of obesity, *J Am Dietet Assoc* 98(suppl 2):S31, 1998.

Scheen AJ, Lefebvre PJ: Pharmacological treatment of obesity: present status, *Int J Obes Relat Metab Disord* 23 (suppl 1):47, 1999.

Eating Disorders

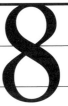

Anorexia nervosa and bulimia nervosa are eating disorders most commonly diagnosed in adolescent and young adult females. The prevalence of these eating disorders among females is about 8 to 10 times higher than among males. Even though the disorders are commonly diagnosed in the young, they may persist throughout life.

Pathophysiology
Characteristics of Eating Disorders

Anorexia nervosa and bulimia nervosa have distinguishing characteristics, as described as follows and in Table 8-1; however, it is relatively common for a combination of these two disorders to exist in the same individual. Moreover, the person who has one of these disorders may later develop the other. A person with anorexia nervosa, for example, may recover sufficiently to maintain a stable body weight but may continue to practice the bingeing and purging behaviors associated with bulimia.

The characteristics of anorexia nervosa include excessive thinness (refusal to maintain weight at or above 85% of the expected weight for height and age); body image disturbances (e.g., misperceptions of body size or shape or denial of the degree of underweight present); serious fear of gaining weight or becoming fat, even though underweight; and amenorrhea for at least three menstrual cycles in a girl or woman who has previously menstruated. Fat accounts for approximately 17% to 27% of the body weight in most healthy women, and amenorrhea is likely when the body fat falls below 17%.

Bulimia is characterized by recurrent (at least twice a week for 3 months) binge eating, defined as eating much more during some period of time than a normal person would and feeling a loss of control over her or his behavior at the same time. In the purging

Table 8-1   Distinguishing Between Anorexia Nervosa
and Bulimia

Characteristic	Anorexia Nervosa	Bulimia
Age of onset (years)	12 to mid-30s; two peaks: 13-14 and 17-18	17-25
Attitude toward therapy	Denial that a problem exists	Often extremely secretive about bulimic behaviors, but willing to accept help once the problem is admitted
Body weight	15% or more below usual or desirable body weight	May be at or only slightly below desirable body weight
Metabolic	Amenorrhea; inability to maintain body temperature in heat or cold stress	Irregular menses, amenorrhea in fewer than 20%
Gastrointestinal	Decreased gastric emptying; constipation; elevated hepatic enzymes	Parotid enlargement; dental enamel erosion; esophagitis; Mallory-Weiss tears
Cardiovascular	Bradycardia; hypotension; dysrhythmias	Ipecac poisoning (tachycardia, cardiac dysrhythmias)
Skeletal	Decreased bone density (correlated with degree of underweight)	

form of this order, bulimic individuals regularly induce vomiting or use laxatives or enemas to prevent weight gain. They may also exercise heavily or fast frequently. In the nonpurging form of bulimia, fasting and heavy exercise are quite common.

The American Psychiatric Association (1995) has established criteria for two other eating disorders related to anorexia nervosa and bulimia nervosa. These are "binge eating disorder" and "eating disorder not otherwise specified." The binge eating disorder (BED) involves binge eating episodes without compensatory behaviors such as purging or exercise. People with BED eat so much within a two-hour period that they are uncomfortable, and they often eat alone when they binge because of their embarrassment over their behavior. Binge eating in BED occurs at least twice a week, and bingeing is followed by feelings of guilt, depression, or disgust. Eating disorders not otherwise specified (EDNOS) are similar to bulimia nervosa except binges occur less often than twice a week. The person vomits after even small amounts of food. EDNOS is similar to anorexia nervosa in the restrained eating pattern, but people with EDNOS manage to maintain a normal body weight and regular menses even though they have lost a large amount of weight. Frequently, people with EDNOS chew and spit out food. Depending on the severity and type of symptoms, these two eating disorders are treated similarly to anorexia nervosa or bulimia nervosa.

Etiology of Eating Disorders

The causes of eating disorders are not fully understood. Cultural factors (e.g., the abundance of food in developed countries coupled with society's emphasis on thinness as desirable and beautiful) probably play a role. A period of restricted eating for the purpose of trying to lose weight often triggers both anorexia nervosa and bulimia. It has been reported that people who diet very stringently may be as much as 18-fold more likely to develop eating disorders as people who have never dieted, and even those who have made only moderate attempts at dieting may be at 5-fold greater risk of eating disorders. Family dysfunction may contribute to development of the disorders (Patton et al., 1999). Families of individuals with eating disorders have been described as overprotective, rigid, lacking in conflict resolution skills, and displaying a lack of confidence in the affected individual. As a result, the children may grow up to be dependent, unassertive, excessively reliant on the approval of others, and low in self-esteem. Abnormal eating behaviors are often initiated as a response to feelings of insecurity and a distorted perception of the importance of body shape and size in determining self-worth. Behavioral theorists also note that anorexia nervosa is reinforced by the attention it receives. The individual becomes the center of attention and manipulates the environment through his or her behavior.

Treatment

Treatment of eating disorders can include individual psychotherapy, group therapy, family psychotherapy, and behavioral therapy. Bulimics, in particular, appear to have a high incidence of depression. Antidepressant medications are sometimes used in therapy. Drugs from the category of selective serotonin reuptake inhibitors, which increase brain serotonin (a neurotransmitter that inhibits eating), have also been used in an effort to prevent binge eating. Substance abuse is common among bulimics, and thus careful screening for alcohol and drug abuse is needed before they begin any pharmacotherapy.

Treatment may occur on an inpatient or outpatient basis. Some indications for hospitalization are: (1) loss of 25% or more of body weight; this state is often life-threatening, and hospitalization for nutritional support and intensive psychiatric therapy is usually necessary; (2) presence or likelihood of serious electrolyte imbalance as a result of an inability to cope with daily living without use of laxatives, diuretics, diet pills, or self-induced vomiting; (3) family tensions necessitating separation of the affected individual and family; (4) severe depression with strong potential for suicide; and (5) inability or unwillingness to cooperate during outpatient therapy.

Nutritional Care

Goals of care are for the individual to change weight gradually, change eating behaviors in an incremental manner until food intake patterns are normal, separate eating behaviors from feelings and psychologic issues, learn to maintain a weight that is healthful without using abnormal food- and weight-related behaviors, and develop more effective coping skills to deal with stress and conflict.

Assessment

Individuals with eating disorders may be deficient in any or all nutrients, depending on the extent of their illness. The nutritional problems addressed in Table 8-2 are the most common ones. With the exception of electrolyte disorders, nutritional deficits are more common in anorexia nervosa than in bulimia.

Intervention

A team approach to intervention is usually the most successful technique. The team usually includes, at a minimum, a physician experienced in treating eating disorders, a therapist if the physician does not serve in this role, a dietitian, and a nurse. The team works together with the patient and family to develop and assess the plan of treatment. Care of the patient includes nutrition assessment and correction of nutritional deficits and electrolyte abnormalities; individual and family counseling; nutrition teaching; modeling of healthful eating and activity patterns, coping strategies, and assertiveness skills; pharmacologic intervention in some cases; and monitoring the patient's status and responses to therapy.

Restoring weight

Restoring body weight should be a major goal in the early treatment of eating disorders. Weight gain, on its own, may improve symptoms of depression, irritability, social withdrawal, and menstrual and other endocrine abnormalities. The long-term goal is for weight to be at least 85% to 90% of that expected for height. Gradual changes in weight and in eating behaviors are usually less stressful to the patient than sudden, sweeping changes. Enteral tube feeding or total parenteral nutrition (TPN; see Chapters 9 and 10) is normally reserved for severe, life-threatening malnutrition and is never used as a punishment for failing to eat. Tube feeding or TPN adds to the feeling of loss of control and can delay recovery.

Establishing a dietary plan

Anorexia nervosa

■ Dietary rehabilitation usually begins with 800 to 1200 kcal/day, and the calorie allowance is increased gradually to promote a weight gain of approximately 0.5 to 1 kg (1 to 2 lb) per week.
■ Patient food preferences should be accommodated as much as possible, especially early in treatment. People with anorexia usually have foods that are considered "bad" or are feared.

Table 8-2   Assessment in Eating Disorders

Areas of Concern	Significant Findings
Fluid and Electrolyte Imbalance	*History* Self-induced vomiting; laxative or diuretic abuse *Physical Examination* Poor skin turgor; weakness; signs of self-induced vomiting: parotid salivary gland enlargement, dental enamel erosion, esophagitis, upper GI bleeding (Mallory-Weiss tears), hoarseness or sore throat; tachycardia, cardiac dysrhythmias (ipecac poisoning, potassium [K$^+$] deficits); anal irritation (laxative abuse) *Laboratory Analysis* Signs of prolonged or frequent vomiting: ↓ serum K$^+$, ↓ serum Cl$^-$; metabolic alkalosis (blood pH >7.45, HCO$_3^-$ >26 mEq/L); stools turn red upon addition of NaOH (caused by presence of phenolphthalein, an ingredient in some laxatives); ↑ BUN (dehydration)
Protein-Calorie Malnutrition (PCM)	*History* Severely restricted food intake (especially over a period of several months or even years); self-induced vomiting; frequent and prolonged periods of physical exercise *Physical Examination* Weight <90% of standard for height; BMI <19 or <5th percentile for age; triceps skinfold <5th percentile; amenorrhea (can also result from psychologic stress); edema; thinning of hair, changes in hair texture

Table 8-2   Assessment in Eating Disorders—cont'd

Areas of Concern	Significant Findings
Protein-Calorie Malnutrition (PCM)—cont'd	*Laboratory analysis* ↓ Serum albumin, transferrin, or prealbumin; ↓ lymphocyte count
Mineral Deficiencies	
Zinc (Zn)	*History* Severely restricted food intake; self-induced vomiting; laxative or diuretic abuse *Physical Examination* Impaired sense of taste; alopecia *Laboratory Analysis* ↓ Serum Zn
Copper (Cu)	*History* Severely restricted food intake; self-induced vomiting; laxative or diuretic abuse *Laboratory Analysis* ↓ Serum Cu; ↓ Hct, Hgb, white blood cell count
Calcium (Ca)	*History* Severely restricted food intake; amenorrhea *Physical Examination* Skinfold measurements <5th percentile *Laboratory Analysis* Radiographic evidence of osteopenia

Including these foods in the diet early in treatment may cause excessive stress. These foods can be introduced later in treatment, when the patient has developed trust that the health care team will not let her lose control of her eating and gain excessive weight.

■ Adequate calcium should be provided in the diet, or a calcium supplement should be used, to allow for bone remineralization.

■ Patients usually deny hunger. They need adequate supervision to prevent the overuse of chewing gum, diet soft drinks, and foods modified to be low in calories, which may help them to avoid feelings of hunger.

■ Patients frequently try to increase energy expenditure with exercise. They need guidelines and supervision to ensure that the amount of exercise is not excessive.

Bulimia nervosa

■ Establishing a pattern of regular eating, with dieting being discouraged, is the first step in therapy. Weight maintenance is the initial goal. Only after bulimic behaviors are under control will it be safe for the individual to undertake a weight reduction diet, if weight needs to be lost.

■ The patient needs to avoid becoming excessively hungry. Bulimic individuals have a great fear of losing control of eating, and excessive hunger can lead to a loss of control. A diet plan with meals or snacks approximately every three hours (i.e., three meals and two to three snacks a day) reduces the risk of hunger. A diet with adequate fiber and fat also helps to promote satiety.

■ The patient needs education and supervision to help her avoid unhealthy weight control strategies and excessive focus on body weight. Weights should be measured only at scheduled intervals, usually no more than once a week. Excessive exercise and strategies such as calorie or fat gram counting need to be identified and corrected.

■ The patient should be helped to include forbidden or "bad" foods in the diet, using behavioral strategies (see Chapter 7). Health care providers can help the individual to plan ways to control stimuli and to plan ahead for situations that have resulted in bingeing in the past.

■ Dietary record-keeping is an essential part of care. The patient and the health care team review the records for evidence of progress and of potential problems.

Monitoring progress and behavior

All weights should be obtained at the same time of day and after the individual has voided. Weighing should be done in the same light clothes (i.e., gown) each time. The return of spontaneous menses is a key milestone in the nutritional rehabilitation of the anorectic individual.

During intensive inpatient therapy, the individual should be observed closely to protect her and maximize therapy. Examples of behaviors that undermine treatment include absenting herself from group activities after meals to vomit, diluting tube feeding formulas to reduce caloric intake, surreptitiously wearing weights during weight measurement, failing to void before daily weight measurement, or hiding uneaten food.

Outpatients have increased responsibility for self-monitoring. Individuals should weigh themselves only at scheduled intervals, usually once weekly, to interrupt unhealthy weighing behaviors accompanying their intense fear of weight gain. Individuals record their dietary intakes, as well as any episodes of vomiting and diuretic or laxative use. Health professionals and the affected individual evaluate these records for signs of progress and to plan strategies for dealing with problems.

A system of contingencies for failing to follow the treatment plan and rewards for successfully adhering to the plan are established. Usually the patient is involved in establishing the contingencies and rewards. Contingencies are often the withholding of desired privileges, and rewards may be the receipt of the same privileges.

Teaching

Controlling eating behaviors and avoiding binge eating

The patient can be taught to maintain control of eating behaviors by practicing the following habits:

- Identify activities that can serve as distractions when temptations or negative emotions prompt a desire to binge, such as engaging in hobbies, taking a walk, telephoning friends, doing yardwork or housework, shopping (not at a grocery store), or exercising.
- Identify cues or stimuli that lead to overeating and alter these stimuli. For instance, if overeating is most likely to occur in the kitchen, avoid eating in the kitchen and instead eat only in the dining room.

- Learn what an appropriate serving size is (using scales, measuring cups, or food models), and eat that amount. Many individuals with eating disorders have spent most of their lives either eating almost nothing or gorging. They may have little knowledge of normal serving sizes.
- Eat slowly; bingeing is associated with rapid food intake.
- Eat at regular meal times. Skipping meals and becoming excessively hungry may trigger bingeing.
- Avoid repeated helpings of food. At meals, serve the food and then put leftovers away before beginning to eat. At parties, sit as far from the food as possible.
- Plan ahead for events when excessive kcal intake can be expected. For instance, if the individual plans to go out for pizza with friends, she or he can reduce food intake throughout the day to compensate.
- Limit alcohol intake because it adds kcal and may reduce control over behavior.

Increasing self-esteem and coping skills

The individual can be helped to develop a better self-image, greater assertiveness, and better problem-solving techniques through group or individual therapy. Professionals provide positive reinforcement for progress made toward weight goals and improving self-esteem and interactive skills. The patient and the health care team should recognize that setbacks are normal and should be accepted calmly. Social situations are often very stressful to people with an eating disorder. They need to learn healthy ways to cope with interpersonal interaction, rather than focusing on food.

Principles of a nutritious diet

Most individuals with anorexia nervosa and bulimia have misconceptions about food and nutrition. It may have been several years since they consumed a balanced diet. They need help in recognizing and selecting a nutritious diet. The goal is to establish the habit of eating a nutritious diet while maintaining a balance with energy expenditure so that it will not be necessary to resort to unhealthy practices such as self-induced vomiting to control weight. The Food Guide Pyramid (see Chapter 1) can be used in teaching. The diet should be moderate in protein (12% to 20%) and fat (less than 30%), with the balance of kcal coming from carbohydrate. Changes should be made gradually to avoid increasing stress. Foods that are most feared (usually those likely to be associated with bingeing) should be introduced only after recovery is well under way. The person with an eating disorder needs to learn a new approach to food intake, focusing on the nutritional contributions and other desirable characteristics of foods, rather than on the energy content.

SELECTED BIBLIOGRAPHY

Diagnostic and statistical manual of mental disorders, ed 4, Washington, DC, 1995, American Psychiatric Association.

Greeno CG, Wing RR, Marcus MD: How many donuts is a "binge"? Women with BED eat more but do not have more restrictive standards than weight-matched non-BED women, *Addict Behav* 24:299, 1999.

Kleifield EI, Wagner S, Halmi KA: Cognitive-behavioral treatment of anorexia nervosa, *Psychiatr Clin N Am* 19:715, 1996.

Neumark-Sztainer D, Story M: Dieting and binge eating among adolescents: what do they really mean? *J Am Dietet Assoc* 98:446, 1998.

Patton GC, et al.: Onset of adolescent eating disorders: population based cohort study over 3 years, *BMJ* 318:765, 1999.

Powers PS: Initial assessment and early treatment options for anorexia nervosa and bulimia nervosa, *Psychiatr Clin N Am* 19:639, 1996.

Rock CL, Curran-Celentano J: Nutritional management of eating disorders, *Psychiatr Clin N Am* 19:701, 1996.

NUTRITION SUPPORT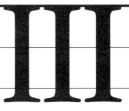

Nutrition support refers to the "provision of specially formulated and/or delivered parenteral or enteral nutrients to maintain or restore optimal nutritional status."[1] **Enteral feedings** are those given into the gastrointestinal tract, either by mouth or by tube. **Parenteral,** or intravenous, **feedings** may be given via a central venous catheter or peripheral vein. Enteral feedings are preferred over parenteral feedings if they are at all feasible. It is commonly said, "If the gut works, use it." Enteral feedings are generally less expensive and, in selected groups of patients, may pose less risk for development of sepsis than parenteral feedings. Enteral feedings may help to prevent atrophy of the intestinal mucosa and "translocation" of microorganisms from the intestinal lumen across the intestinal wall. Studies in humans have not yet clearly demonstrated that enteral feedings maintain intestinal structure or prevent bacterial translocation better than parenteral feeding. Nevertheless enteral feedings have some theoretical physiologic advantages. Enteral feeding stimulates the release of gastrointestinal hormones involved in nutrient metabolism and allows the liver "first-pass" extraction of nutrients, before they are presented to other tissues. The liver plays an important role in metabolism of many nutrients, control of blood glucose, storage of carbohydrates as glycogen, and protein synthesis. Patients who require parenteral feedings also are often given enteral feedings, even if only small amounts of enteral feedings are tolerated, in order to receive the benefits of both types of feedings.

The choice of route and type of nutrition support are based on the individual patient's needs. Figure III-1 shows an example of a decision tree that might be used for determining the appropriate form of nutrition support.

Nutrition support is a specialized treatment modality, and multidisciplinary groups of health care professionals have been

---

[1]A.S.P.E.N. Board of Directors: Definition of terms used in A.S.P.E.N. guidelines and standards, *J Parenter Enter Nutr* 19:1, 1995.

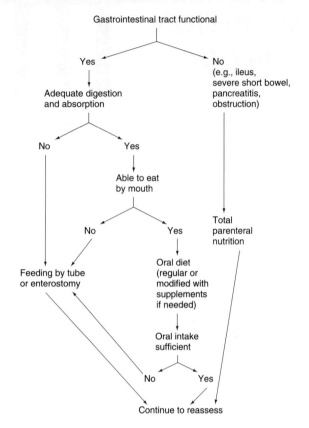

Figure III-1
Determining the optimal form of nutrition support. Caregivers continually reassess the individual and change the type of nutrition support as needed.

developed to deliver this treatment in the safest, most efficacious, and most cost-effective manner possible. These groups are called nutrition support services or teams. They often include one or more physicians, nurses, dietitians, and pharmacists (and sometimes other professionals such as physical therapists and social workers) with advanced skills in nutrition assessment and delivery of nutrition support.

Enteral Nutrition

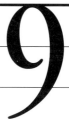

Enteral feedings can be delivered in three ways: (1) oral diets of regular or modified foods, (2) nutritional supplements given by mouth, and (3) tube feedings.

Modified Diets

Modified diets are used by individuals with specific difficulties in consuming, digesting, absorbing, or metabolizing foods usually included in regular, unmodified diets. Some typical modified diets are summarized in Appendix J. Additional information is given in the chapters in Section IV.

Oral Supplements

Oral supplements are useful for individuals who can digest and absorb nutrients. They are most effective for people who are consuming some foods but cannot take in enough because of anorexia or increased metabolic demands resulting from trauma, burns, infection, or other causes.

Types of Supplements

Some individuals prefer home-prepared foods such as shakes and eggnogs. Commercial formulas, or medical nutrition products, that contain protein, carbohydrates, fat, vitamins, and minerals may also be used (Table 9-1). Generally, products for oral consumption should provide at least 1.5 kcal/ml, because it is difficult to take in adequate amounts of more dilute products. Some medical nutrition products are in the form of fortified bars, soups, or puddings.

Modular products (Table 9-2) providing kcal (carbohydrates, lipids, or protein) can be added to such foods as cooked or dry cereals, mashed potatoes, applesauce, juices, tea, coffee, shakes,

Text continued on p. 200

Table 9-1   Enteral Feeding Formulas

Product* and Manufacturer	Kcal/ml	Osmolality (mOsm/kg H$_2$O)	Pro/CHO/Fat (g/L)	Approximate ml Needed to Meet Vitamin DV**
Polymeric Formulas				
Oral Supplements, Lactose-Free Unless Stated that They Contain Milk				
Boost High	0.75	640	47/135/3	1066
Protein Powder (in water)[1]				
Boost High	1.09	950	79/180/6	1064
Protein Powder (in skim milk)[1]				
Carnation Instant Breakfast (in milk)[2]	0.92	661-747	48/147/18	1065
Forta Shake (in milk)[3]	1.2	808	72/147/36	1000
NuBasics Drink[2]	1.0	500-520	35/132/37	1000
NuBasics 2.0	2.0	750	80/196/106	750
NuBasics Plus[2]	1.5	710	52/176/65	650
NuBasics VHP[2]	1.0	490	62/113/33	1050
Resource[4]	1.06	430	37/143/38	1890
Resource Plus[4]	1.5	600	56/202/53	1400

Tube or Oral, Standard Protein, Lactose-Free, Low-Residue

Boost[1]	1.01		43/17/18	960
Deliver 2.0[1]	2.0	640	75/200/102†	1000
Ensure[3]	1.06	555	37/167/25	948
Ensure Plus[3]	1.5	690	55/200/53	1420
IsoSource[4]	1.2	360	36/142/34†	1500
IsoSource HN[4]	1.2	330	44/133/34†	1500
Osmolite[3]	1.06	300	37/151/35†	1887
Osmolite HN[3]	1.06	300	44/144/35†	1321
Pediasure[3] (children)	1.0	335	30/110/50†	1000-1300
TwoCal HN[3]	2.0	690	84/216/89†	947

Tube or Oral, High-Protein, Lactose-Free, Low-Residue

Boost High Protein (liquid)[1]	1.01	650	61/139/23	1000
Boost Plus[1]	1.52	670	61/190/57	800
Promote[3]	1.0	340	62/130/26†	1000

Pro, protein; *CHO*, carbohydrate; *DV*, daily value.

*This is only a representative sample of the available products and is not meant to imply endorsement of these products.

**DV are for adults, unless product is designed for children. Children's formulas are for ages 1 to 10 years.

†Contains MCT (medium-chain triglyceride).

Manufacturers: [1]Mead Johnson & Co, Evansville, IN; [2]Nestlé Clinical Nutrition, Deerfield, IL; [3]Ross Products, Columbus, OH; [4]Novartis, Minneapolis, MN; [5]Nutrition Medical, Minneapolis, MN; [6]B Braun+McGaw, Irvine, CA.

Continued

Table 9-1 Enteral Feeding Formulas—cont'd

Product and Manufacturer	Kcal/ml	Osmolality (mOsm/kg H$_2$O)	Pro/CHO/Fat (g/L)	Approximate ml Needed to Meet Vitamin DV
Tube or Oral, Lactose-Free, Fiber-Containing				
Ensure with Fiber[3]	1.06	500	37/169/26	948
Kindercal[1] (children)	1.06	310	34/135/44†	<950
Nutren Junior with Fiber[2] (children)	1.0	350	30/128/42†	<1000
Pediasure with Fiber[3] (children)	1.0	335	30/114/50†	1000-1300
Promote with Fiber[3]	1.0	380	62/138/14†	1000
Tube Only, Standard Protein, Lactose-Free, Low-Residue				
Comply[1]	1.5	460	60/180/61†	830
Isocal[1]	1.06	270	34/135/44†	1890
Isocal HN[1]	1.06	270	44/124/45†	1180
Nutren 1.0[2]	1.0	300	40/127/38†	1500
Nutren 2.0[2]	2.0	720	80/196/106†	750
Tube Only, Lactose-Free, Fiber-Containing				
FiberSource[4]	1.2	390	42/168/40†	1500
Jevity[3]	1.06	300	44/155/35†	1321
Nutren 1.0 with Fiber[2]	1.0	310	40/127/38†	1500
Ultracal[1]	1.06	310	44/123/45†	1250

Elemental Formulas, Lactose-Free, Low-Residue

At Least 50% of Nitrogen from Peptides and Hydrolyzed Proteins

Criticare HN[1]	1.06	650	38/220/5	1890
Peptamen[1]	1.0	270	40/127/39†	1500
PRO-Peptide[5]	1.0	270	40/127/39†	1500
PRO-Peptide for Kids[5]	1.0	360	30/138/38†	1000
Reabilan[2]	1.0	350	32/132/41†	2000
Reabilan HN[2]	1.3	490	58/158/54†	1500
Subdue[1]	1.01	330	50/127/34†	1185
Vital High Nitrogen[3]	1.0	500	42/185/11	1500

Nitrogen Primarily from Free Amino Acids

L-Emental[5]	1.0	630	38/210/3	2000
L-Emental Pediatric[5]	0.8	360	24/130/24†	1000–1170
Vivonex Pediatric[4]	0.8	360	24/130/24†	1000–1170
Vivonex TEN[4]	1.0	630	38/210/3	2000

Condition-Specific Formulas

AIDS/HIV/Malabsorption

Advera[3]	1.28	700	60/216/23†	1184
Lipisorb liquid[1]	1.35	630	57/161/57†	1180

AIDS/HIV, acquired immunodeficiency syndrome/human immunodeficiency virus infection.

Manufacturers: [1]Mead Johnson & Co, Evansville, IN; [2]Nestlé Clinical Nutrition, Deerfield, IL; [3]Ross Products, Columbus, OH; [4]Novartis, Minneapolis, MN; [5]Nutrition Medical, Minneapolis, MN; [6]B Braun+McGaw, Irvine, CA.

Continued

Table 9-1   Enteral Feeding Formulas—cont'd

Product and Manufacturer	Kcal/ml	Osmolality (mOsm/kg H$_2$O)	Pro/CHO/Fat (g/L)	Approximate ml Needed to Meet Vitamin DV
Condition-Specific Formulas—cont'd				
Glucose Intolerance				
Choice dm[1]	1.06	440	45/106/51†	1000
DiabetiSource[4]	1.0	360	50/90/49	1060
Glucerna[3]	1.0	355	42/96/54	1422
Glytrol[2]	1.0	380	45/100/48†	1400
Hepatic Encephalopathy				
Hepatic-Aid II[6]	1.2	560	45/172/37	NA
NutriHep[2]	1.5	690 (unflavored)	40/290/21†	1500
Pulmonary Disease or Ventilator Dependence				
NutriVent[2]	1.5	330 (unflavored)	68/100/94†	1000
Oxepa[3] (ARDS)	1.5	493	62/106/94†	947
Pulmocare[3]	1.5	475	63/106/93†	947
Respalor[1]	1.52	580	76/148/71†	1420

Renal Failure

Magnacal Renal[1] (dialysis)	2.0	570	75/200/101†	<1000
Nepro[3] (dialysis)	2.0	665	70/222/96	947
Renalcal[2] (pre-dialysis)	2.0	600	34/290/82†	1000
		(unflavored)		
Suplena[3] (pre-dialysis)	2.0	600	30/255/96	947

Stress/Critical Illness/Trauma

Alitraq[3]	1.0	575	52/165/16†	1500
Crucial[2]	1.5	490	94/135/68†	1000
Impact[4]	1.0	375	56/130/28†	1500
Impact with Fiber[4]	1.0	375	56/140/28†	1500
Immun-Aid[6]	1.0	460	80/120/22†	2000
IsoSource VHN[4]	1.0	300	62/130/29	1250
Optimental[3]	1.0	540-580	51/138/28	1422
Perative[3]	1.3	385	67/177/37†	1155

Wound Healing—Surgery, Pressure Ulcers, Burns

Promote[3]	1.0	340	62/130/26†	1000
Promote with Fiber[3]	1.0	380	62/138/28†	1000
Protain XL[1]	1.0	340	57/129/30†	1250
Replete[2]	1.0	300	62/113/34†	1000
Replete with Fiber[2]	1.0	310	62/113/34†	1000

NA, not applicable; *ARDS*, adult respiratory distress syndrome.
Manufacturers: [1]Mead Johnson & Co, Evansville, IN; [2]Nestlé Clinical Nutrition, Deerfield, IL; [3]Ross Products, Columbus, OH; [4]Novartis, Minneapolis, MN; [5]Nutrition Medical, Minneapolis, MN; [6]B Braun+McGaw, Irvine, CA.

Table 9-2   Modular Components for Enteral Feeding

Product and Manufacturer	Nutrient Content
Protein Modules	
Casec[1]	0.9 g protein/g powder
Elementra[2]	0.75 g protein/g powder
ProMod[3]	0.75 g protein/g powder
Carbohydrate Modules	
Moducal[1]	3.75 kcal/g powder
Polycose liquid[3]	2.0 kcal/ml
Polycose powder[3]	3.8 kcal/g powder
Fat Modules	
MCT Oil[1]	8.3 kcal/g or 7.7 kcal/ml
Microlipid[1]	4.5 kcal/ml

MCT, Medium-chain triglycerides.
Manufacturers: [1]Mead Johnson & Co, Evansville, IN; [2]Nestlé Clinical Nutrition, Deerfield, IL; [3]Ross Products, Columbus, OH.

soups, salad dressings, and sandwich fillings. Modular carbohydrates are especially versatile because they can be added to most soft foods or liquids without altering their flavor or texture.

Delivery of Oral Supplements

Individuals should sip liquid supplements slowly, taking 180 to 360 ml over 15 to 45 minutes. Liquid supplements contain readily digested carbohydrate. As a result, they can cause dumping syndrome, with abdominal cramping, weakness, tachycardia, and diarrhea, if they are consumed rapidly. Liquid supplements taste best if they are chilled or served over ice. Modular products may be added to any meal or snack.

Enteral Tube Feedings

The following are some reasons for enteral tube feedings:

■ Inability to consume adequate food because of mechanical problems with eating, psychologic disorders, or unconsciousness; tube feedings may be used to supplement or replace oral feedings; examples: head and neck tumors, esophageal stricture or obstruction, coma, anorexia of chronic illness, anorexia nervosa, hyperemesis gravidarum, and neurologic disorders interfering with swallowing

■ Increased nutritional requirements that may not be met by oral feedings alone; examples: severe trauma, burns, congenital heart disease

■ Maldigestion or malabsorption requiring unpalatable modified formulas or making continuous feedings necessary to maintain adequate nutritional status; examples: pancreatic or biliary insufficiency, short-bowel syndrome, inflammatory bowel disease, and protracted diarrhea with malnutrition

Types of Tube Feeding Formulas

Polymeric or intact protein formulas

When the gastrointestinal (GI) tract is functional, **polymeric** nutritionally complete **formulas** can be used. These contain proteins such as casein or lactalbumin; carbohydrates in the form of sugars, hydrolyzed starches, or dextrins; and varying amounts of fat. Most commercially prepared formulas are lactose-free because lactose intolerance is common among older adults and individuals with malabsorption. Fiber is included in some polymeric formulas, as an aid to the control of bowel function. Dietary fiber passes into the colon, where it can be partially or fully fermented by gut bacteria. Insoluble forms of fiber such as wheat bran and psyllium increase the fecal mass and thus reduce the likelihood of constipation. Soluble forms of fiber such as modified guar gum may decrease serum cholesterol and postprandial blood glucose concentrations. They are fermented to short-chain fatty acids (SCFAs) by colonic bacteria. The SCFAs are absorbed along with sodium and water in the colon, and evidence suggests that this action reduces the likelihood of diarrhea.

The fat in polymeric formulas is usually in the form of vegetable oils or a combination of vegetable oils and **medium-chain triglycerides (MCTs).** MCTs contain fatty acids 8 to 12 carbons in length. They are used as a calorie source because they are easily digested and absorbed, compared with the long-chain triglycerides (LCTs) found in vegetable oils.

Fat digestion and absorption

Fat is a key nutrient to consider when planning enteral feedings for the patient with impaired digestion or absorption. LCTs in particular require adequate lipase (an enzyme that removes fatty acids from the glycerol backbone of the triglyceride), bile salts, and absorptive area in the small intestine (see Figure 1-4). The following ingredients are necessary for absorption of fat:

- *Lipase:* LCTs are too large to be absorbed intact. Usually the two outer fatty acids are removed, leaving the inner fatty acid attached to glycerol and creating a monoglyceride (one fatty acid attached to glycerol). Lipase is released in the mouth and the stomach, and these lipases may be important in infancy. Most fat digestion in adults and older children is performed by lipase released by the pancreas, however. Release of pancreatic lipase is likely to be low in individuals with diseases of the pancreas such as cystic fibrosis and pancreatitis. Because MCTs are smaller and more water-soluble than LCTs, lipase activity is less important with MCTs.

- *Bile salts:* Bile salts (produced in the liver and stored in the gallbladder) combine with fatty acids and monoglycerides to form **micelles.** Bile salts can cause micelle formation because they have both water-soluble and fat-soluble components. The fatty acids and the fat-soluble part of the bile salt are in the center of the micelle, and the water-soluble portion of the bile salt and the glycerol portion of the monoglycerides are on the outer part of the micelle. Micelles are soluble enough in water to carry the long-chain fatty acids through the unstirred water layer that lies just over the intestinal mucosal cells. Medium-chain fatty acids are smaller and more soluble in water than long-chain fats, and they do not require thorough micelle formation to pass through the unstirred water layer.

- *Bowel surface area for absorption:* The jejunum is responsible for much of the fat absorption, and the ileum is needed for bile salt reabsorption. Reabsorbed bile salts are returned to the liver for reuse. Conditions such as surgical removal of the jejunum, inflammatory bowel disease, or radiation damage to the bowel can interfere with fat absorption. Ileal resection or damage impairs bile salt reabsorption and can deplete the body's pool of bile salts. Because absorption of MCTs is less dependent on bile salts than absorption of LCTs, MCTs can be useful in treating fat malabsorption that occurs when bowel surface area is diminished.

The absorption of MCTs is more similar to the absorption of protein and carbohydrate than that of LCTs (see Figure 1-4). Not only is micelle formation less important for MCTs than for LCTs, but also MCTs do not have to be packaged as chylomicrons in order to be soluble enough to enter the circulation. Fatty acids from MCTs are released directly from the intestinal cells into the blood, just as the amino acids and monosaccharides are.

Elemental formulas

Many individuals with maldigestion and malabsorption tolerate polymeric formulas, particularly those containing MCTs; however, **elemental** or oligomeric ("pre-digested") **formulas** are also available. These formulas contain protein hydrolysates, peptides, and/or free (crystalline) amino acids (see Table 9-1). Free amino acids were originally believed to be more easily absorbed than peptides, but it is now known that free amino acids have no advantage over peptides. Peptide-containing formulas may be appropriate for selected patients with short bowel syndrome or other malabsorptive disorders. These formulas are more expensive than the polymeric ones.

Disease- or condition-specific formulas

Specialized formulas have been developed for many different disease or metabolic conditions, including acquired immune deficiency syndrome (AIDS), glucose intolerance or diabetes, hepatic encephalopathy, pulmonary disease, renal failure, trauma and critical illness, and wound healing (see Table 9-1). Although these formulas are usually based on sound theoretical principles, many of them have not yet been tested in such a way that their effects on therapeutic outcomes can be determined. They are almost always more expensive than formulas for general use. Therefore, it is important to evaluate patients carefully to determine whether there is a real need for a specialized product. These condition-specific products can be characterized in the following manner:

- *AIDS and severe malabsorption:* concentrated in kcal, low in fat or very high in MCT to reduce fat malabsorption
- *Glucose intolerance:* moderate to low carbohydrate content, fiber-containing to reduce blood glucose response to feeding, high in monounsaturated fatty acids to reduce the risk of heart disease
- *Hepatic encephalopathy:* concentrated in kcal to allow fluid restriction, low protein, high in branched-chain amino acids and low in aromatic and ammonia-forming amino acids, low in sodium

- *Pulmonary disease:* concentrated in kcal to allow fluid restriction; moderate to low in carbohydrate to reduce carbon dioxide production, contain MCT to enhance fat absorption; some are fortified with antioxidants to reduce oxidative damage during oxygen therapy; Oxepa contains fish oils to reduce the inflammatory response
- *Renal disease:* concentrated in kcal to allow fluid restriction, predialysis products are low in protein with emphasis on essential amino acids, dialysis products are moderate to high in protein to replace losses, moderate to low in vitamins A and D and high in folic acid and vitamin B_6, restricted in sodium and potassium
- *Stress and critical illness:* high protein; some are enriched in glutamine to maintain skeletal muscle and the normal gut barrier and arginine to improve immune function and wound healing; most are rich in vitamins C and E, B vitamins, zinc, and copper—needed in healing, some contain fish oils to reduce the inflammatory response
- *Wound healing:* high protein, rich in zinc and vitamins needed for healing

Other formula characteristics

Caloric density

Many formulas provide 1 kcal/ml because adults need approximately 1 ml water per kilocalorie consumed; however, calorie-dense formulas containing 1.5 to 2 kcal/ml are available for individuals needing fluid restrictions. The hydration status of patients receiving these concentrated formulas must be closely monitored, with more free water given as required.

Osmolality

Osmolality refers to the number of osmotically active particles per kilogram of water in a solution. A formula is considered to be isotonic or isosmolar if its osmolality is similar to that of plasma (300 mOsm/kg). It is hypertonic or hyperosmolar if its osmolality is greater than that of plasma. It was once thought that hyperosmolar solutions were a common cause of diarrhea. For this reason, formulas were diluted to quarter- or half-strength when tube feedings were initiated, and the strength was gradually increased. It is now recognized that hyperosmolality by itself is unlikely to cause diarrhea and that use of diluted formula only delays the delivery of adequate nutrients to the patient. In some patients with other causes for diarrhea, use of a hyperosmolar formula might worsen diarrhea, however.

Tube Feeding Sites, Selection of Tubes, and Tube Placement

Routes for tube feedings

Tube feedings may be given into the esophagus, stomach, or small intestine. Figure 9-1 illustrates the gastric and intestinal locations. Nasogastric (NG) and nasoduodenal (ND)/nasojejunal (NJ) tubes are often used for short-term feedings, and esophagostomy, gastrostomy, and jejunostomy are frequently chosen for long-term feedings. Percutaneous endoscopic gastrostomies (PEGs) are especially popular because they can be performed without general anesthesia. Jejunostomy tubes can also be inserted via PEG tubes.

Esophagostomy (inserted via an esophageal stoma)

- *Advantages:* Allows use of virtually all of the GI tract for digestion; bypasses oral surgery or obstruction
- *Disadvantages:* May be difficult to hide stoma in some clothing; usually cannot bypass esophageal obstruction

Nasogastric (NG) tubes (or orogastric in infants)

- *Advantages:* Tube easily inserted; allows use of almost all of the GI tract
- *Disadvantages:* Tube easily dislodged, especially with altered sensorium; potential for pulmonary aspiration and for development of sinusitis and otitis media

Nasoduodenal (ND) or nasojejunal (NJ) tubes

- *Advantages:* Theoretically decreases the likelihood of pulmonary aspiration, although clinical investigations to date have not found a significant difference in rates of aspiration between gastric and small bowel feedings; useful in individuals with delayed gastric emptying
- *Disadvantages:* More difficult to insert tube than NG; bypasses the stomach, a barrier to infection; usually necessitates continuous feedings given with a pump; can cause dumping syndrome; tube easily dislodged; potential for development of sinusitis and otitis media

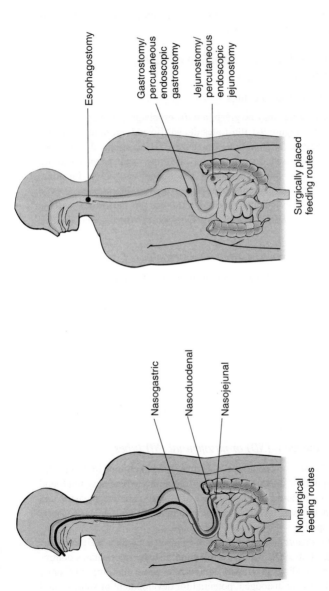

Figure 9-1
Types of enteral feeding routes.
(From Rolin Graphics, in Grodner M, Long Anderson S, DeYoung S: *Foundations and clinical applications of nutrition: a nursing approach*, ed 2,

Esophagostomy

Gastrostomy/percutaneous endoscopic gastrostomy

Jejunostomy/percutaneous endoscopic jejunostomy

Surgically placed feeding routes

Nasogastric

Nasoduodenal

Nasojejunal

Nonsurgical feeding routes

Gastrostomy

- *Advantages:* More difficult to dislodge tube than NG; usually has a larger diameter than NG, allowing use of more viscous formulas (e.g., home blended); easily hidden by clothing; conventional surgical gastrostomies can bypass esophageal obstruction, but placement of PEG tubes requires a patent esophagus
- *Disadvantages:* Potential for irritation of skin around insertion site caused by leakage of gastric secretions

Jejunostomy

- *Advantages:* Same as for ND/NJ; can bypass upper GI obstruction; more difficult to dislodge tube than ND/NJ
- *Disadvantages:* Requires surgical insertion; potential for erosion of skin around insertion site from leakage of intestinal contents (containing digestive enzymes); bypasses the stomach, a barrier to infection; usually requires continuous feedings given via pump; feedings can cause dumping syndrome

Types of feeding tubes

Nonreactive tubes are soft, nonirritating tubes made of polyurethane, silicone rubber, or similar materials. Tubes for NG and ND/NJ feedings range in size from 5 to 12 French (F) (1 F ≈ 0.34 mm). Insertion of these pliable tubes is sometimes difficult, but stylets are available to facilitate insertion. Nonreactive tubes can be left in place for several weeks. Some tubes have weighted tips designed to facilitate ND/NJ intubation and to help to maintain the tube's position in the intestine; however, studies suggest that unweighted tubes actually pass through the pyloric sphincter more readily than weighted ones and that tube position is better maintained with unweighted tubes.

Polyethylene (PE) and polyvinylchloride (PVC) tubes range from 5 to 18 F in size. They are stiffer than nonreactive tubes and require no stylets for insertion. These tubes harden during use. To avoid GI perforation, they should be replaced every 3 to 4 days. They tend to irritate the nose and throat more than nonreactive tubes. PE and PVC tubes are initially cheaper than nonreactive ones, but the need for frequent replacement may make them more expensive in the long run.

Insertion of NG and ND/NJ tubes (Figure 9-2)

1. Select an appropriately sized tube. Generally, 8 F tubes, often called "small-bore" or "fine-bore," are suitable for adults and

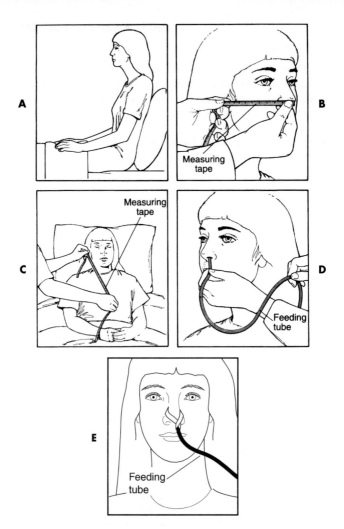

Figure 9-2

Insertion of a feeding tube. **A,** Place the patient in the Fowler's position before tube insertion, if possible, so that gravity can facilitate passage of the tube. **B** and **C,** Measure the distance nose to ear and then to xiphoid process and calculate length of tube needed. **D,** Encourage patient to sip fluids or chew ice chips while the tube is gently advanced. **E,** Tape tube securely in place.

(A-D, From Beare PG, Myers JL, eds: *Principles and practice of adult health nursing,* St Louis, 1990, Mosby. E, Redrawn from Beare PG, Myers JL, eds: *Principles and practice of adult health nursing,* St Louis, 1990, Mosby.)

children. If blended-tube feedings or other thick fluids are to be used, then a 10 to 12 F tube may be needed. Most infants can use 6 or 8 F tubes, but premature infants may need 5 F tubes.

2. Explain the procedure to the individual. Patients may be reassured by the information that tube insertion is not painful, although it may cause gagging. Have the person sit up, if possible, and lean the head forward.

3. Determine the length of tube to be inserted. For adults:

> Length for NG insertion = {[nose to ear to xiphoid process measurement (cm) − 50 cm] ÷ 2} + 50 cm

For children, one suggested method is:

> Length for NG insertion = 6.7 + 0.226 (height in cm) + 3 cm
> + distance from distal tip to feeding pores on tube (cm)

4. Lubricate the tip of the tube with water-soluble lubricant. Gently advance the tube through the nostril parallel to the roof of the mouth and then down the esophagus. Inhalable nasal decongestants used before tube insertion can make the process more comfortable. The patient can help by sipping fluids, unless they are contraindicated, or swallowing while the tube is being advanced.

5. If the individual begins to cough or choke during the insertion, the tube may be in the trachea. Remove it and try again.

6. When the proper length of tube has been inserted, secure the tube to the nose with tape.

7. If ND/NJ placement is desired, insert a sufficient length of tubing (85 cm appears adequate for most adults). Prokinetic agents such as metoclopramide or erythromycin administered before insertion of the tube increase the likelihood that the tube will pass spontaneously through the pylorus. A variety of techniques has also been recommended by experienced practitioners, including rotating the tube while advancing it through the stomach, placing the individual in the right lateral decubitus position, and insufflation of air into the stomach while advancing the tube. Fluoroscopic or endoscopic techniques may be used to place the tube if the aforementioned techniques are unsuccessful, but they increase the cost of the procedure.

8. Confirm tube placement before administering feedings.

Methods of confirming tube placement

■ *Abdominal radiograph:* This method is accurate but adds to the cost of care and exposes the patient to radiation.

■ *pH of fluid obtained from the tube:* If it is ≤4 in patients not receiving gastric acid inhibitors or <5.5 in patients who are receiving acid inhibitors, then the tube tip is likely to be in the stomach. (Intestinal secretions usually have a pH >6, and respiratory tract fluids usually have a pH >5.5 [Metheny et al., 1994]). Some tubes are equipped with pH monitoring systems. The esophagus can have an acid pH, which may cause confusion between esophageal and gastric placement; however, other clues can help in identifying esophageal placements: it may be especially difficult to aspirate fluid out of a tube with its tip in the esophagus, a large portion of the tube may be outside the body (but a tube inserted to the proper length may be coiled in the esophagus), and belching may occur immediately after air is injected into the tube.

Delivery of tube feedings

Continuous feedings

Continuous feedings, feedings delivered over the entire day or some portion of the day (usually 10 to 12 hours), are used in certain circumstances:

■ Duodenal or jejunal feedings because continuous feedings reduce the risk of dumping syndrome.
■ Decreased absorptive area (chronic diarrhea, short-bowel syndrome, acute radiation enteritis, and severe malnutrition with atrophy of the villi) because continuous feedings may increase the total amount tolerated.
■ Some cases of severe stress with normal GI function (Burn patients, for instance, have been found to have less diarrhea and more adequate intake if given continuous, rather than intermittent, feedings.)

Although continuous NG or gastrostomy feedings may be beneficial in certain situations, they keep the gastric pH continuously high and have been associated with increased risk of pneumonia in very ill patients. It is suggested that the less acid gastric pH allows increased growth of bacteria and yeast in the stomach and that these organisms can colonize the trachea and cause pneumonia. Transpyloric feedings (delivered into the small bowel) may be preferable to intragastric feedings in extremely ill patients. To reduce the risk of pneumonia during tube feedings, use aseptic or scrupulously clean technique in administering tube feedings and administer feedings in closed feeding sets. It has long been taught that gastric residuals should be aspirated from the feeding tube and measured on a regular schedule; however, the nonreactive tubes tend to collapse when suction is applied to them and often do not yield accurate residuals. Moreover, regular aspiration of residuals increases the likelihood of clogging the tube. Therefore, aspiration of residuals is not always practiced at the present time. Instead, the patient is monitored frequently for gastric distension, bloating, and increase in abdominal girth.

Intermittent feedings

Feedings given every 2 to 4 hours are preferred for certain patients:

- Confused individuals who, if left unattended, are in danger of dislodging the tube.
- Stable long-term patients, especially outpatients, in whom continuous feedings interfere with normalization of lifestyle.

Intermittent feedings are usually better tolerated if given by slow drip rather than by rapid bolus infusion. Usually 300 to 400 ml can be tolerated several times daily if each feeding is infused over at least 30 minutes. Abdominal discomfort, diarrhea, tachycardia, and nausea during or shortly after feedings signal that the flow is too rapid or the volume too large.

Promoting comfort

The most common complaints of tube-fed individuals are thirst, being deprived of tasting food, sore nose or throat, and dry mouth. Comfort can be increased by the following methods:

- Encourage intake of food and fluids if not contraindicated. (Many people are initially afraid that they cannot eat while the tube is in place.)
- Provide adequate fluid. Most formulas for adults provide 1 kcal/ml. This ratio may not provide adequate fluid for some patients. If the individual cannot drink fluid and is not fluid restricted, then provide extra water by tube. For example, irrigate the tube after each feeding or every 4 to 6 hours with 30 to 60 ml or more of water.
- Provide regular mouth care and stimulation of saliva flow. Important comfort measures include rinsing the mouth with water or mouthwash; brushing the teeth; sucking hard candy or

chewing gum in moderation, if not contraindicated; and gargling with warm salt water to relieve sore throat.
- Use nonreactive tubes, and use the tube with the smallest possible diameter.
- Tape the tube in place securely so that it does not move back and forth.

Assessing Response to Nutrition Support

Anthropometric measurements, physical assessment, and hematologic and biochemical measurements are used in assessing response to nutrition support (Table 9-3).

Preventing and Correcting Complications of Enteral Nutrition

Enteral nutrition support is sometimes perceived as less risky than total parenteral nutrition, but tube feedings are associated with several serious and challenging complications. Measures for the prevention or correction of tube feeding complications are described in Table 9-4.

Malnourished individuals receiving either enteral or parenteral feedings are at risk of developing the **refeeding syndrome.** One major contributor to the refeeding syndrome is hypophosphatemia. As muscle and fat are lost in starvation, fluid and minerals, including phosphorus, are also lost. During refeeding, especially with high-carbohydrate feedings, insulin levels rise and cellular uptake of glucose, water, phosphorus, potassium, and other nutrients is stimulated. Serum levels of phosphorus subsequently fall, which can lead to cardiac dysrhythmias, congestive heart failure, hemolysis, muscular weakness, seizures, acute respiratory failure, and a variety of other complications, including sudden death. Hypokalemia, hypomagnesemia, and vitamin (thiamin) deficiency may occur for similar reasons. Glucose intolerance and fluid overload often accompany the refeeding syndrome. Caregivers should be aware of patients who are at risk for refeeding syndrome, especially those with kwashiorkor or marasmus (see Chapter 2), anorexia nervosa, morbid obesity with recent massive weight loss, and prolonged fasting. In these individuals, it is especially important to monitor blood levels of electrolytes, phosphorus, glucose, and magnesium carefully, particularly during

Text continued on p. 219

Table 9-3   Assessing Response to Nutrition Support

Parameter	Frequency of Measurement*	Purpose/Comments
Anthropometric Measurements		
Weight	Daily	Indicator of efficacy, patient should have steady gain; use usual or IBW for guide to desirable weight; a gain of >0.1-0.2 kg (0.25-0.5 lb) a day usually indicates fluid retention
Skinfolds, AMC	Weekly	Indicator of efficacy
Length or height (pediatrics only)	Monthly	Indicator of efficacy; see growth charts (Appendix D) for expected growth pattern
Physical Assessment		
State of hydration	Daily	Overhydration: check for edema of dependent body parts, shortness of breath, rales in lungs, fluid intake consistently >output; dehydration: look for poor skin turgor, dry mucous membranes, complaints of thirst, output >intake (measure stool volumes if liquid), >10% difference between blood pressure when lying and standing

Continued

IBW, Ideal body weight.
*These are suggested frequencies only. Individual patients may need more or less frequent assessment.

Table 9-3 Assessing Response to Nutrition Support—cont'd

Parameter	Frequency of Measurement*	Purpose/Comments
Physical Assessment—cont'd		
Gastrointestinal motility (tube-fed individuals)—i.e., presence of bowel sounds, signs of abdominal distension, passage of flatus or stool, nausea or vomiting	Every 2-4 hr during initiation of feedings; every 8 hr when stable	Indicators of GI motility and feeding tolerance
Hematologic and Biochemical Measurements		
Serum glucose and electrolytes	Daily until stable, then 2-3/wk	Indicates whether intake is adequate or excessive
BUN	1-2/wk	Increased: inadequate fluid intake, renal impairment, or excessive protein intake; decreased: inadequate protein intake is possible

Serum Ca, P, Mg	1-2/wk	Ensure stability, avoid refeeding syndrome
Complete blood count	1/wk	Indicator of adequacy of Fe, protein, folic acid, and vitamin B_{12}; see Chapter 2 for more information
Serum triglycerides (during TPN)	After each ↑ in lipid dosage; 2-3/wk when stable	Elevated levels indicate inadequate lipid clearance and possibly a need for reduction in lipid dosage
Serum albumin, transferrin, or prealbumin	1/wk	Indicator of efficacy in maintaining or improving protein nutriture

BUN, Blood urea nitrogen; *Ca*, calcium; *P*, phosphorus; *Mg*, magnesium; *Fe*, iron.

Table 9-4   Management of Tube Feeding Complications

Complication	Possible Cause	Suggested Intervention
Pulmonary aspiration*	Feeding tube in esophagus or respiratory tract	Confirm proper placement of tube before administering any feeding; check placement at least every 4-8 hr during continuous feedings
	Regurgitation of formula	Consider giving feedings into small bowel rather than stomach; keep head elevated 30 degrees during feedings; stop feedings temporarily during treatments such as chest physiotherapy; tint formula with food coloring to make it easier to detect formula in the respiratory tract
Diarrhea	Antibiotic therapy	Antidiarrheal medications may be ordered if the possibility of infection with *Clostridium difficile* has been ruled out; *Lactobacillus* or *Saccharomyces boulardii* are sometimes given enterally in an effort to establish benign gut flora
	Hypertonic medications (e.g., KCl or medications containing sorbitol)	Dilute enteral medications well; evaluate sorbitol content of medications
	Malnutrition/hypoalbuminemia	Use continuous rather than bolus feedings; consider a formula with MCT and/or soluble fiber

	Bacterial contamination	Use scrupulously clean formula preparation and administration techniques; refrigerate home-prepared, reconstituted, or opened cans of formula until ready to use, and use all such products within 24 hr
	Predisposing illness (e.g., short-bowel syndrome, inflammatory bowel disease, AIDS)	Use continuous feedings; consider a formula with MCT and/or soluble fiber
	Lactose intolerance	Use a lactose-free formula
	Fecal impaction	Perform digital examination to rule out fecal impaction with seepage of liquid stool around the obstruction
	Intestinal mucosal atrophy	Consider use of formula containing soluble fiber and MCT
Constipation	Lack of fiber	Fiber-containing formula may be helpful, unless contraindicated; stool softeners may be ordered
Tube occlusion	Administration of medications via tube	Avoid crushing tablets and administer medications in elixir or suspension form whenever possible; irrigate feeding tube with water before and after giving medications; never mix medications with enteral formulas because this may cause clumping of formula

Continued

MCT, Medium-chain triglycerides.

*Signs and symptoms of pulmonary aspiration include tachypnea, shortness of breath, hypoxia, and infiltrate on chest radiographs.

Table 9-4   Management of Tube Feeding Complications—cont'd

Complication	Possible Cause	Suggested Intervention
Tube occlusion —cont'd	Sedimentation of formula	Irrigate tube with water† every 4-8 hr during continuous feedings and after every intermittent feeding; one study found less clogging of polyurethane than silicone rubber tubes; irrigate tubes well if gastric residuals are measured, since gastric juices left in the tube may cause precipitation of formula in the tube; instilling pancreatic enzyme into the tube may clear some occlusions
Delayed gastric emptying	Serious illness, diabetic gastroparesis, prematurity, surgery, high-fat content of formula	Consult with physician regarding whether feedings can be administered into the small bowel, a lower-fat formula can be used, or metoclopramide can be administered to stimulate gastric emptying

†Fluids such as cranberry juice or Coca-Cola are sometimes used as irrigants, in the mistaken belief that they are better than water at preventing tube occlusion. Research has shown cranberry juice to be inferior to and Coca-Cola no better than water.

the first week of refeeding, keep careful records of fluid intake and output, record weight daily, and monitor heart rate frequently. Severely malnourished patients are often bradycardic. With overfeeding and an increase in the intravascular volume, heart rate increases; a rate of 80 to 100 beats/minute in a previously bradycardic patient may be a sign of significant cardiac stress.

Home Care

Teaching of the individual and family who are going to deliver tube feedings at home includes:

- Clean technique
- Caring for the access device (feeding tube and, if applicable, feeding stoma site)
- Checking for residual volumes, if applicable
- Preparation of the enteral formula, if necessary
- Safe administration of the formula, including operation of the enteral feeding pump if one is used
- Signs and symptoms of complications; measures to take if these occur
- Self-monitoring; for example, weighing regularly and evaluating state of hydration

SELECTED BIBLIOGRAPHY

Ahmed W, et al: The rates of spontaneous transpyloric passage of three enteral feeding tubes, *Nutr Clin Pract* 14:107, 1999.

Beckstrand J, et al.: The distance to the stomach for feeding tube placement in children predicted from regression on height, *Res Nurs Health* 13:411, 1990.

Bleicher G, et al.: Saccharomyces boulardii prevents diarrhea in critically ill tube-fed patients. A multicenter, randomized, double-blind placebo-controlled trial, *Intensive Care Med* 23:517, 1997.

Chen MYM, Ott DJ, Gelfand DW: Nonfluoroscopic, postpyloric feeding tube placement: number and cost of plain films for determining position, *Nutr Clin Pract* 15:40, 2000.

Faries MB, Rombeau JL: Use of gastrostomy and combined gastrojejunostomy tubes for enteral feeding, *World J Surg* 23:603, 1999.

Frankel EH, et al: Methods of restoring patency to occluded feeding tubes, *Nutr Clin Pract* 13:129, 1998.

Guenter P, Jones S, Ericson M: Enteral nutrition therapy, *Nurs Clin N Am* 32:651, 1997.

Hanson R: Predictive criteria for length of nasogastric tube insertion for tube feeding, *J Parenter Enter Nutr* 3:160, 1979.

Klein S, et al.: Nutrition support in clinical practice: review of published data and recommendations for future research directions. Summary of a conference sponsored by the National Institutes of Health, American Society for Parenteral and Enteral Nutrition, and American Society for Clinical Nutrition, *Am J Clin Nutr* 66:683, 1997.

Lipman TO: Grains or veins: Is enteral nutrition really better than parenteral nutrition? A look at the evidence, *J Parent Enter Nutr* 22:167, 1998.

Lord LM: Enteral access devices, *Nurs Clin N Am* 32:685, 1997.

Metheny N, et al.: pH testing of feeding-tube aspirates to determine placement, *Nutr Clin Pract* 9:185, 1994.

Patchell CJ, et al.: Reducing bacterial contamination of enteral feeds, *Arch Dis Child* 78:166, 1998.

Salasidis R, Fleiszer T, Johnston R: Air insufflation technique of enteral tube insertion: a randomized, controlled trial, *Crit Care Med* 26:1036, 1998.

Stechmiller JK, Treloar D, Allen N: Gut dysfunction in critically ill patients: a review of the literature, *Am J Crit Care* 6:204, 1997.

Parenteral Nutrition

10

Total parenteral nutrition (TPN), or delivery of all nutrients by intravenous infusion, is usually recommended when oral or tube feedings are expected to be contraindicated or inadequate for more than 5 to 7 days. TPN is most commonly used for one of two reasons:

1. The gastrointestinal (GI) tract is unable to digest or absorb adequate nutrients. Examples include intractable vomiting, severe diarrhea, prematurity, some cases of abdominal trauma, prolonged ileus, and massive small bowel resection.
2. There is a need for bowel rest. Examples include enteral fistulae and acute inflammatory bowel disease that does not respond to other therapies.

In most instances, TPN is contraindicated when the gastrointestinal tract is functional, enteral feedings are expected to be adequate within 5 days, or death from the underlying disease is imminent.

Feeding with TPN alone is associated with atrophy of the intestinal villi and impaired absorption when feedings are resumed. The intestinal mucosa's ability to act as a barrier to microorganisms is impaired, and in animal studies there is increased risk of translocation, or movement of bacteria through the intestinal wall into the bloodstream and to other organs. When the patient can tolerate them, small amounts of food help to prevent villous atrophy. Soluble fiber, short-chain fatty acids, and the amino acid glutamine are factors that are being explored in relation to maintaining mucosal integrity in patients receiving nutrition support.

Routes for Parenteral Nutrition

There are several possible routes for TPN delivery.

Peripheral Venous Catheters

These catheters are usually inserted in the upper extremities.

■ *Advantages:* Few mechanical complications, other than the risk of superficial phlebitis
■ *Disadvantages:* Requires good peripheral venous access, which limits its long-term use; not usually useful for home TPN; may be difficult to deliver adequate kcal to stressed individuals or those with high kcal needs because peripheral veins do not tolerate solution concentrations >900 mOsm/kg, which limits dextrose concentrations to about 10%

Central Venous Catheters

Central venous catheters (CVCs) are usually inserted into the superior or inferior vena cava via the subclavian, internal or external jugular, or femoral veins.

■ *Advantages:* Allow use of extremely hypertonic solutions (≥1800 mOsm/kg); appropriate for long-term and home use; long-term catheters are not easily dislodged because their proximal ends are tunneled under the skin and have cuffs that adhere to the subcutaneous tissues (Figure 10-1); multilumen CVC catheters reduce the risk of drug incompatibilities when more than one medication is given at once and allow for blood sampling via the CVC; the Groshong catheter has a one-way valve that prevents blood reflux into the catheter, eliminating the need for frequent flushing of the catheter with a heparinized solution
■ *Disadvantages:* Complications include pneumothorax, air embolism, central vein thrombosis, superior vena cava syndrome, catheter-related sepsis, and catheter embolization (rare)

Subcutaneous Infusion Ports

The subcutaneous infusion port is an implanted reservoir with a catheter attached. Before each infusion, a noncoring needle is inserted through the skin and into the septum on the port.

■ *Advantages:* Useful for intermittent therapy (e.g., chemotherapy, selected patients needing intermittent TPN); require no flushing or site care when not in use; lower infection rates than standard catheters in several studies

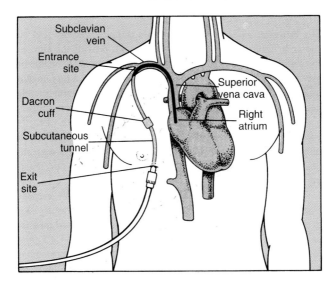

Figure 10-1
Hickman central venous catheter. The proximal end is tun-
neled under the subcutaneous tissue to increase stability.
A Dacron cuff on the catheter provides a roughened surface,
which encourages subcutaneous tissue to adhere to the
catheter and further secure it.
(From Beare PG, Myers JL, eds: *Principles and practice of adult health nursing,*
St Louis, 1990, Mosby.)

- *Disadvantages:* Requires a needle to access the port; risk of
  extravasation of infusate if the needle slips out of the port

Peripherally Inserted Central Catheters

Peripherally inserted central catheters (PICCs) are long Silastic or
polyurethane catheters threaded through peripheral veins into large
central veins.

- *Advantages:* Allow delivery of very hypertonic solutions without
  the risk of pneumothorax; less costly than central venous catheter
  placement; can be used for long-term patients and at home
- *Disadvantages:* Complications include phlebitis (and potential
  central vein thrombosis), catheter-related sepsis, and catheter
  fracture (with potential for embolization)

Composition of TPN Solutions

The estimated nutrient needs of stable patients needing TPN are shown in Table 10-1. Crystalline amino acids provide the nitrogen (protein) needed. Specialized amino acid solutions are available for use in renal and hepatic failure, severe injury, and premature infants. Glucose is usually a major kcal source, but neither adults nor children can oxidize glucose more rapidly than approximately 5 mg/kg/minute. If glucose is infused at a faster rate, then the excess is used to form lipids. Thus, a 70 kg adult should receive no more than about 500 g glucose daily. If caloric needs are greater than this, then lipid emulsions can be used to meet 30% to 50% of the energy needs.

Lipid emulsions are available as 10%, 20%, and 30% preparations, containing 10, 20, or 30 g fat/100 ml and providing 1.1, 2.0, or 3.0 kcal/ml, respectively. It is recommended that lipid infusion be limited to 2.5 g/kg/day for adults and no more than 4 g/kg/day for children. Lipid emulsions may be administered separate from or mixed with the glucose-amino acid solutions. When lipids are mixed with glucose and amino acids, the solution is known as a total nutrient admixture or *3-in-1* solution. If lipids are not needed to supply energy (and if the patient receives little or no lipid via the enteral route), then IV lipid emulsions are given in small amounts to prevent essential fatty acid deficiency (EFAD). When used to prevent EFAD, lipids may be given only 3 to 4 days a week. Lipid emulsions support the growth of *Candida* and many bacteria better than glucose-amino acid solutions do and thus should be administered with scrupulous aseptic technique.

Carnitine, a derivative of the amino acid lysine, stimulates passage of long-chain fatty acids into the mitochondria so that they can be oxidized as an energy source. Carnitine is found in foods of animal origin and is synthesized by healthy adults and children, but TPN solutions do not normally contain carnitine. Infants and long-term TPN patients may not synthesize adequate amounts of carnitine. Signs of deficiency include cardiomyopathy, muscle weakness, lethargy, hypoglycemia, encephalopathy, delayed growth, and seizures. Carnitine supplements are available to be given orally or added to TPN solutions when deficiency is suspected or anticipated.

Administration of TPN

TPN may be infused continuously or cyclically. Cyclic TPN is usually infused for several hours, then discontinued until the

Table 10-1 Estimated Daily Nutrient Needs of TPN Patients[a]

Component	Adults	Term Infants	Children over 1 yr
	(per kg per day)	(per kg per day)	(per kg per day)
Amino acids (g)	0.8-1 (maintenance) 1.2-2 (catabolic)	2-2.5	1.5-2 (children) 0.8-2 (adolescents)
Energy (kcal)[b]	25-30	90-120 (<6 mo) 80-100 (6-12 mo)	75-90 (1-7 yr) 60-75 (7-12 yr) 30-60 (>12-18 yr)
	(total)	(per kg per day)	(per kg per day)
Electrolytes and Minerals			
Na (mEq)	≥60	2-3	3-4
K (mEq)	≥60	1-2	2-4
Mg (mEq)	8-20	0.3-0.7	0.2-0.3
Ca (mg)	200-300	60-70[c]	20-60
Phosphate (mg)	600-1200	50-55[c]	40-45

From American Medical Association Department of Foods and Nutrition: *J Parenter Enteral Nutr* 3:258, 1979; Greene HL, et al: *Am J Clin Nutr* 48:1324, 1988; National Advisory Group on Standards and Practice Guidelines for Parenteral Nutrition: Safe practices for parenteral nutrition formulations, *J Parent Ent Nutr* 22:49, 1998.

[a]Amounts of constituents must be individualized; the levels listed are "usual" ranges.

[b]It is common to count only nonprotein kcal (glucose and lipids) in calculating the energy delivered, especially in children and catabolic adults. The goal is for the amino acids to be used for tissue synthesis rather than energy. Glucose monohydrate, used in IV solutions, contains 3.4 kcal/g.

[c]Calcium and phosphate not to exceed 500-600 mg/L and 400-450 mg/L, respectively, to prevent precipitation.   *Continued*

Table 10-1   Estimated Daily Nutrient Needs of TPN Patients—cont'd

Component	Adults (total)	Term Infants (per kg per day)	Children over 1 yr (per kg per day)
Electrolytes and Minerals—cont'd			
Zinc (mg)	4	0.25 <3 mo 0.10 >3 mo	0.05 (max. 5/day)
Copper (mg)	0.8-1	0.02	0.02 (max. 0.3/day)
Chromium (µg)[d]	10-12.5	0.20	0.20 (max. 5/day)
Manganese (µg)[e]	60-100	1.0	1.0 (max. 50/day)
Selenium (µg)	20-60[f]	2-3	2-3 (max. 40/day)
Vitamins (Per Day)			
A (IU)	3300	2300	2300
D (IU)	200	400	400
E (IU)	10	7	7
K (µg)	200	200	200
C (mg)	100	80	80
Thiamin (mg)	3	1.2	1.2

Vitamins (Per Day)—cont'd		
Riboflavin (mg)	3.6	1.4
Niacin (mg)	40	17
Pyridoxine (B$_6$) (mg)	4	1
Pantothenic acid (mg)	15	5
Folate (μg)	400	140
Vitamin B$_{12}$ (μg)	5	1
Biotin (μg)	60	20

From American Medical Association Department of Foods and Nutrition: *J Parenter Enteral Nutr* 3:258, 1979; Greene HL, et al: *Am J Clin Nutr* 48:1324, 1988; National Advisory Group on Standards and Practice Guidelines for Parenteral Nutrition: Safe practices for parenteral nutrition formulations, *J Parent Ent Nutr* 22:49, 1998.

[d]Omit in patients with renal dysfunction.
[e]Excreted in bile; omit in patients with obstructive jaundice.
[f]Recommended for long-term adult TPN patients.

next day (e.g., 12 hours on TPN, then 12 hours off). Cyclic TPN allows the long-term patient more flexibility and freedom and may improve liver function. In administering either continuous or cyclic TPN:

- Examine TPN solutions and lipid emulsions for precipitation, separation, or signs of contamination (e.g., fungal growth) before hanging them.
- Handle TPN solutions, administration sets, and the peripheral or central catheter with aseptic technique.
- Use a filter on TPN infusion lines to reduce the risk of lipid embolism, infusion of particulate matter, and infection. A filter with 0.22 μm pores can be used for amino acid-glucose mixtures, and a filter with 1.2 to 5 μm pores can be used for lipid-containing solutions. Administer TPN within 10% of the ordered rate. A constant infusion rate minimizes rapid changes in blood glucose and insulin levels. A flow rate too low can result in hypoglycemia and inadequate nutrient delivery. A flow rate too high can cause hyperglycemia and excessive delivery of kcal, protein, fluid, and other nutrients.
- Some clinicians recommend that the rate be tapered before TPN is discontinued. For instance, the rate may be reduced 50% for 1 to 2 hours before stopping the infusion. The patient receiving large doses of glucose usually secretes large amounts of insulin, and tapering the TPN infusion rate helps to prevent hypoglycemia from occurring by allowing insulin levels to begin to decline.

Assessing Response to TPN

Anthropometric measurements, physical assessment, and hematologic and biochemical measurements are used in assessing response to nutrition support (see Table 9-3).

Preventing and Correcting Complications of Parenteral Nutrition

Table 10-2 summarizes complications of parenteral nutrition and lists measures for their prevention or correction. The refeeding syndrome, which can occur in malnourished patients given either enteral or parenteral nutrition, is described in Chapter 9.

Table 10-2 TPN Complications

Complication	Signs/Symptoms	Prevention/Intervention
Catheter-related sepsis	Fever, chills, glucose intolerance, positive blood culture; bacterial colony counts in blood aspirated from the catheter 5-10 times higher than in blood obtained from a peripheral site	Maintain an intact dressing, change if contaminated by vomitus, sputum, etc.; use aseptic technique whenever handling catheter, IV tubing, and TPN solutions; hang a single bottle of TPN no longer than 24 hr, lipid emulsion no longer than 12 hr; a 0.22 μm filter can be used with TPN not containing lipids or a 1.2 μm filter with solutions that contain lipids; salvage of infected catheters has been attempted with an "antibiotic lock" by placing a concentrated antibiotic solution in the catheter for 12 hr
Air embolism	Dyspnea, cyanosis, tachycardia, hypotension, possibly death	Use Luer-lok system or secure all connections well; Groshong catheter, which has valve at tip, may reduce risk of air embolism; use an inline 0.22 μm air-eliminating filter if solutions do not contain lipids or 1.2 μm or larger if solutions contain lipids; have patient perform Valsalva's maneuver during tubing changes; if air embolism is suggested, place patient in left lateral decubitus position and administer oxygen; immediately notify physician, who will attempt to aspirate air from the heart

Continued

Table 10-2 TPN Complications—cont'd

Complication	Signs/Symptoms	Prevention/Intervention
Central venous thrombosis	Unilateral edema of neck, shoulder, and arm; development of collateral circulation on chest; pain in insertion site	Follow measures to prevent sepsis; repeated or traumatic catheterizations are most likely to result in thrombosis; treatment usually includes anticoagulation; if symptoms are not too severe, the catheter might be left in place; if symptoms are severe, thrombolytic therapy and/or catheter removal may be necessary
Catheter occlusion or semiocclusion	No flow or sluggish flow through the catheter; or infusion through the catheter possible, but blood cannot be aspirated from the catheter	Flush catheter with heparinized saline if infusion is stopped temporarily; if catheter appears to be occluded, attempt to aspirate the clot; thrombolytic agent may restore patency if clotted or occluded by fibrin sheath; hydrochloric acid, 0.1 N, has been used to clear drug precipitates and 70% ethanol to clear lipid precipitates

Hypoglycemia	Diaphoresis, shakiness, confusion, loss of consciousness	Do not discontinue TPN abruptly, taper rate over several hours; use pump to regulate infusion so that it remains ±10% of ordered rate; if hypoglycemia is suggested, then administer oral carbohydrate; if oral intake is contraindicated or patient is unconscious, a bolus of IV dextrose may be used
Hyperglycemia	Thirst, headache, lethargy, increased urination	Monitor blood glucose frequently until stable; TPN is usually initiated at a slow rate or with a low dextrose concentration and increased over 2-3 days to avoid hyperglycemia; the patient may require insulin added to the TPN if the problem is severe

Preparing the Patient and Family for Home Parenteral Nutrition

Preparation for home TPN is a multidisciplinary process, usually involving the physician, nurse, and dietitian. In many instances, the pharmacist and social worker are also involved. Topics that must be covered in patient teaching include the following:

- Sterile technique
- Caring for the access device, including irrigation and heparinization of the catheter and dressing changes
- Making additions to the TPN solution (if necessary)
- Initiating, administering, and discontinuing the TPN infusion, including operation of the infusion pump
- Signs and symptoms of complications and management of those complications; self-monitoring (e.g., monitoring of blood glucose, regular weighing, checking body temperature as needed, evaluating state of hydration, etc.)

SELECTED BIBLIOGRAPHY

Andris DA, Krzywda EA: Central venous access: clinical practice issues, *Nurs Clin N Am* 32:719, 1997.

Didier ME, Fischer S, Maki DG: Total nutrient admixtures appear safer than lipid emulsion alone as regards microbial contamination: growth properties of microbial pathogens at room temperature, *J Parenter Enter Nutr* 22:291, 1998.

Klein S, et al.: Nutrition support in clinical practice: review of published data and recommendations for future research directions, *J Parenter Enter Nutr* 21:133, 1997.

Krzywda EA, Andris DA, Edmiston CE: Catheter infections: diagnosis, etiology, treatment, and prevention, *Nutr Clin Pract* 14:178, 1999.

Ma TY, et al.: Total parenteral nutrition via multilumen catheters does not increase the risk of catheter-related sepsis: a randomized prospective study, *Clin Infec Dis* 27:500, 1998.

National Advisory Group on Standards and Practice Guidelines for Parenteral Nutrition: Safe practices for parenteral nutrition formulations, *J Parenter Enter Nutr* 22:49, 1998.

Orr ME: Vascular access device selection for parenteral nutrition, *Nutr Clin Pract* 14:172, 1999.

Schloerb PR, Henning JF: Patterns and problems of adult total parenteral nutrition use in US academic medical centers, *Arch Surg* 133:7, 1998.

Sheridan RL, et al.: Maximal parenteral glucose oxidation in hypermetabolic young children: a stable isotope study, *J Parenter Enter Nutr* 22:212, 1998.

NUTRITION AND SPECIFIC CLINICAL CONDITIONS

IV

Acute and chronic illnesses are treated in a variety of settings, including acute care hospitals, rehabilitation centers, extended care facilities, clinics, offices of private practitioners, and patients' homes. Whatever the setting, however, nutritional care is an essential part of treatment. In recognition of its importance, nutritional care of medical, surgical, and emotional conditions is often referred to as *medical nutrition therapy*.

Surgery, Trauma, and Burns

Surgery, trauma, and burns are stressors that result in **hypermetabolism,** or increased energy expenditure. Nutritional care is a priority to minimize nutritional deficits during the period of hypermetabolism and to promote repair during convalescence.

Pathophysiology

Major surgery, trauma, and burns are accompanied by a stress response. The stress response is designed to perform two important tasks:

1. Produce adequate energy to meet increased metabolic needs from surgery and injury. Increased secretion of glucagon, epinephrine, norepinephrine, and corticosteroids results in breakdown of glycogen, fat stores, and body proteins, especially skeletal muscles. The net effect in severe injury is increased urinary nitrogen loss, muscle wasting, weight loss, and decreased levels of albumin and other serum proteins.
2. Maintain the blood volume. Antidiuretic hormone (ADH) secretion increases during the stress response, with decreased urine output and retention of fluid. In hypovolemia, increased aldosterone secretion occurs, and sodium and fluid are retained.

The primary period of wound healing lasts from 5 to 15 days in minor surgery to more than one month in major trauma or burns. During this time, the wound has priority needs for kcal, amino acids, and other nutrients needed in healing. Nutritional deficits may impair wound healing.

Treatment

Wound treatment depends on the type, site, and extent of injury. For example, skin grafting is often a part of burn care. Corticosteroids and phenobarbital are commonly used in treatment of head injury, to reduce the inflammatory response and the metabolic rate.

An increasing number of individuals are undergoing organ transplantation (kidney, liver, heart, lung, small bowel, or pancreas). These individuals require long-term immunosuppressive therapy with corticosteroids, cyclosporine, FK506, azathioprine, or antilymphocyte antibody preparations such as OKT_3. Immunosuppressive agents can have major impacts on nutritional status. Both cyclosporine and corticosteroids affect serum lipids; hypertriglyceridemia, hypercholesterolemia, increases in low-density lipoproteins, and decreases in high-density lipoproteins are common (see Chapter 15). Hyperglycemia is another side effect of cyclosporine and corticosteroids. Azathioprine and OKT_3 can cause anorexia and gastrointestinal symptoms such as nausea, vomiting, and diarrhea.

Nutritional Care

The goal of nutritional care is to prevent or correct nutritional deficits that could impair healing. There is much ongoing research related to optimal nutritional support in trauma, sepsis, and burns. Investigators are exploring alternative energy sources (intravenous lipid emulsions with "structured" triglycerides that contain both medium- and long-chain fatty acids, branched-chain amino acids [leucine, isoleucine, and valine], glutamine, or short-chain fatty acids) and nutrients that could potentially promote healing or enhance immune function (arginine, nucleotides, and omega-3 fatty acids).

Assessment

Assessment is summarized in Table 11-1.

Intervention

Providing adequate nutrients to meet the individual's needs for maintenance and anabolism

Fluid and electrolyte needs

Daily maintenance requirements for fluid and electrolytes during stress response are presented in Table 11-2. Needs for fluids and
Text continued on p. 243

Table 11-1 Assessment in Surgery, Trauma, and Burns

Area of Concern	Significant Findings
Protein-Calorie Malnutrition (PCM)	*History*
	Increased needs caused by hypermetabolism from trauma, burns, surgery, fever, sepsis, pneumonia, or other infection; catabolic effects of corticosteroid therapy (used in head injury); weight loss before surgery, especially if >2% in 1 wk, >5% in 1 mo, >7.5% in 3 mo, or >10% in 6 mo; poor intake caused by anorexia (can be caused by pain, malignancy, psychologic factors), intestinal obstruction or ileus, nausea or vomiting, and alcoholism; increased losses caused by resection of small intestine, especially ileum, gastrectomy, fistula, burns (loss of serum proteins through damaged capillaries)
	Physical Examination
	Muscle wasting; triceps skinfold or arm muscle circumference <5th percentile; edema; weight <90th percentile or BMI <18.5
	Laboratory Analysis
	↓ Serum albumin, transferrin, or prealbumin (serum albumin levels may be ≥0.5 g/dl lower than usual because of the hemodilution that occurs during bedrest, the effects of fluid resuscitation, blood loss, etc.); ↓ lymphocyte count; negative nitrogen balance; ↓ creatinine height index

Continued

Table 11-1   Assessment in Surgery, Trauma, and Burns—cont'd

Area of Concern	Significant Findings
Altered Carbohydrate Metabolism	*History* Catabolism caused by trauma; corticosteroid or cyclosporine therapy *Physical Examination* Muscle wasting *Laboratory Analysis* ↑ Serum glucose; glucosuria
Altered Lipid Metabolism (Hypercholesterolemia, Hypertriglyceridemia)	*History* Cyclosporine or corticosteroid use *Laboratory Analysis* ↑ Serum cholesterol, ↑ low-density lipoprotein (LDL) cholesterol, ↓ high-density lipoprotein (HDL) cholesterol, ↑ serum triglycerides
Vitamin Deficiencies C	*History* Increased needs caused by trauma, burns, or major surgery; poor intake caused by anorexia *Physical Examination* Gingivitis; petechiae, ecchymoses; delayed wound healing *Laboratory Analysis* ↓ Serum or leukocyte vitamin C

Table 11-1   Assessment in Surgery, Trauma, and Burns—cont'd

Area of Concern	Significant Findings
Vitamin Deficiencies—cont'd	
B complex	*History*
	Increased needs caused by fever or hypermetabolism; poor intake (same reasons as for PCM)
	Physical Examination
	Glossitis; cheilosis; peripheral neuropathy; dermatitis
K	*History*
	Antibiotic usage
	Physical Examination
	Petechiae, ecchymoses
	Laboratory Analysis
	↑ Prothrombin time
Mineral Deficiencies	
Iron (Fe)	*History*
	Blood loss, acute or chronic, as in stress ulcer, trauma, long-bone fracture; poor intake (same causes as PCM); impaired absorption, especially after gastrectomy
	Physical Examination
	Pallor; koilonychia; tachycardia
	Laboratory Analysis
	↓ Hct, Hgb, MCV, MCH, MCHC; ↓ serum Fe and ferritin; ↑ serum transferrin or total iron-binding capacity

Continued

Table 11-1   Assessment in Surgery, Trauma, and Burns—cont'd

Area of Concern	Significant Findings
Mineral Deficiencies—cont'd	
Zinc (Zn)	*History* Increased losses from burns (loss of albumin to which Zn is bound), fistula drainage, diarrhea or steatorrhea; increased needs for healing of surgical wounds, burns, trauma; poor intake (same reasons as for PCM) *Physical Examination* Hypogeusia, dysgeusia; ↓ tensile strength of wounds; dermatitis *Laboratory Analysis* ↓ Serum Zn
Phosphorus (P)	*History* Aggressive refeeding (especially high-carbohydrate feedings, as in TPN) in malnourished individuals; alcoholism; increased losses or impaired absorption caused by use of antacids (phosphate-binders) as prophylaxis/treatment for stress ulcer, severe diarrhea, or vomiting *Physical Examination* Tremor, ataxia; irritability progressing to stupor, coma, and death *Laboratory Analysis* ↓ Serum P; respiratory alkalosis (↑ blood pH, ↓ blood P_{CO_2})

Table 11-1   Assessment in Surgery, Trauma, and Burns—cont'd

Area of Concern	Significant Findings
Mineral Deficiencies—cont'd	
Magnesium (Mg)	*History*
	Increased losses caused by prolonged vomiting, diarrhea, steatorrhea, fistula drainage; poor intake caused by alcoholism
	Physical Examination
	Tremor; disorientation; hyperactive deep reflexes
	Laboratory Analysis
	↓ Serum Mg
Fluid and Electrolyte Imbalances	
Potassium (K^+) excess	*History*
	Loss of K^+ from damaged cells into extracellular fluid caused by burns (early, usually within first 3 days) or crushing injuries
	Physical Examination
	Irritability; nausea, diarrhea; weakness
	Laboratory Analysis
	↑ Serum K^+
K^+ deficit	*History*
	Increased losses caused by burns (after the fifth day), diarrhea or vomiting
	Physical Examination
	Weakness, ↓ reflexes, intestinal ileus
	Laboratory Analysis
	↓ Serum K^+

Continued

Table 11-1   Assessment in Surgery, Trauma, and Burns—cont'd

Area of Concern	Significant Findings
Fluid and Electrolyte Imbalances—cont'd	
Fluid deficit	*History* Increased losses from burns, persistent vomiting or diarrhea, gastric suction without adequate replacement, fever, tachypnea, fistula drainage, transient diabetes insipidus following head injury, use of radiant warmers or phototherapy (infants); poor intake caused by intestinal obstruction, coma, or confusion, causing failure to recognize or communicate thirst, use of tube feedings (especially in obtunded individual) without adequate fluid (formulas providing 1 kcal/ml may not provide enough fluid for patients with increased losses; more concentrated formulas require especially close monitoring of hydration)
	Physical Examination Poor skin turgor; acute weight loss (can be 5%-10% of usual weight within 3-7 days); oliguria (adult: <20 ml/hr; infant or child; <2-4 ml/kg/hr; infant <6 days: <1-3 ml/kg/hr); hypotension; dry skin and mucous membranes; sunken fontanel (infants)
	Laboratory Analysis Serum Na >150 mEq/L; ↑ serum osmolality, urine specific gravity, Hct, BUN

Table 11-1   Assessment in Surgery, Trauma, and Burns—cont'd

Area of Concern	Significant Findings
Fluid and Electrolyte Imbalances—cont'd	
Fluid volume excess	*History* Head injury *Physical Examination* Decreased urine output because of temporary syndrome of inappropriate antidiuretic hormone secretion (SIADHS) *Laboratory Analysis* Serum Na <126 mEq/L

Table 11-2   Fluid and Electrolyte Requirements

Infants, Children, and Adults	Water (ml)	Na$^+$ (mEq/kg)*	K$^+$ (mEq/kg)*
Infants/Children		2-4	1-3
≤10 kg	100/kg		
11-20 kg	1000 + 50/kg over 10 kg		
>20 kg	1500 + 20/kg over 20 kg		
Adults	35-55/kg	2-3	2-3

*1 mEq Na$^+$ (sodium) = 23 mg; 1 mEq K$^+$ (potassium) = 39 mg.

electrolytes may be higher in times of severe stress. Formulas used in estimating fluid needs in burn patients include:

■ *First 24 hours:* 2 to 4 ml lactated Ringer's solution × wt (kg) × %body surface area (BSA) burned. Give half in first 8 hours and half in remaining 16 hours (Parkland-Baxter formula)

■ *Second 24 hours:* 0.5 ml colloids (plasma, plasma protein fraction [Plasmanate], or dextran) × wt (kg) × %BSA burned plus maintenance fluids (approximately 2000 ml dextrose in water for adults) (Brooke Army formula)

Energy (kilocalorie) needs

Indirect calorimetry is the most accurate method for measuring energy needs. Where it is not available, estimates of energy expenditure are made using the calculations in Chapter 2 (pp. 57-59). If the Harris-Benedict equations are used, the results are often multiplied by "injury factors" (Table 11-3) to estimate total daily energy expenditure.

For newly paraplegic and quadriplegic individuals, the figures for fractures, head injury, or soft tissue trauma (whichever is most appropriate) can be used in the first few weeks after injury. Once

Table 11-3   Estimating kcal Needs in Sick or Injured Patients*

Clinical Condition	Injury Factor†
Fever	$1 + 0.13/°$ C above normal (or $0.07/°$ F)
Elective surgery	1-1.2
Peritonitis	1.2-1.5
Soft tissue trauma	1.14-1.37
Multiple fractures	1.2-1.35
Major sepsis	1.4-1.8
Major head injury	
With steroids	1.4-2.0
Without steroids	1.4
Burns (%BSA‡)	
0%-20%	1.0-1.5
20%-40%	1.5-1.85
40%-100%	1.85-2.05

Modified from Silberman H: *Parenteral and enteral nutrition,* ed 2, New York, 1989, McGraw-Hill. Used with permission of The McGraw-Hill Companies.
*Total energy expenditure = (basal energy expenditure, or BEE) × (injury factor). If W = actual weight in kg, H = ht in cm, and A = age in yr, then
BEE (males) = $66 + (13.7 \times W) + (5 \times H) - (6.8 \times A)$, and
BEE (females) = $655 + (9.6 \times W) + (1.7 \times H) - (4.7 \times A)$
†These are maximum increases; they must be tapered as recovery progresses.
‡Percent of body surface area burned.

they are stable and rehabilitating, adult paraplegics need approximately 27.9 kcal/kg, and quadriplegics need approximately 22.7 kcal/kg. Ideal body weight (IBW) of paraplegics and quadriplegics is 4.5 kg and 9 kg, respectively, less than that of healthy adults of the same height because their muscle mass is less.

Protein needs

Needs for patients in the posttrauma and postoperative periods are approximately 1.2 to 2 g/kg/day for adults and 2 to 3 g/kg/day for children. One method for calculating protein needs in burns is:

Adults: 1 g/kg + (3 g × %body surface area burned)

Children: 3 g/kg + (1 g × %body surface area burned)

Total parenteral nutrition (TPN) or enteral feedings for trauma or surgery patients are sometimes supplemented with the amino acids glutamine and arginine. Evidence suggests that glutamine helps to promote positive **nitrogen balance,** maintain skeletal muscle mass, and maintain the integrity of the gastrointestinal tract in stressed patients. Arginine levels fall in injured patients, and experimental data indicate that arginine stimulates immune function and wound healing.

Vitamin and mineral needs

Needs for most vitamins and minerals increase following trauma; however, caloric needs are also high, and if caloric needs are met, adequate amounts of most vitamins and minerals are usually provided. Vitamin C, vitamin A or β-carotene, and zinc intakes may need special attention, however.

Vitamin C is needed for collagen formation for optimal wound healing. Supplements of 500 to 1000 mg/day should provide adequate vitamin C.

Vitamin A and its precursor, β-carotene, also appear to be important in healing. Furthermore, it is believed that the stressed individual may have an excess of oxidant production. Production of oxidants can be helpful; white blood cells use this method for killing bacteria. However, overproduction of oxidants can damage body cells. An adequate intake of antioxidants (including vitamins A, E, and C and β-carotene) gives some protection.

Zinc increases the tensile strength (the force required to separate the edges) of the healing wound; commonly used supplementation dosages are 6 mg/day IV during acute stress and 4 mg/day IV or

50 to 75 mg/day orally when stable. Additional zinc is needed when there are unusually large intestinal losses; estimated zinc needs are 12.2 mg/L of small bowel fistula drainage and 17.1 mg/kg of stool or ileostomy drainage.

Delivering nutrition support in a safe and effective manner

Intravenous (IV) fluids, glucose, and electrolytes

■ *Indications:* Maintenance of fluid and electrolyte balance in the initial postinjury or postsurgical period; IV glucose-electrolyte solutions are inadequate in kcal and all nutrients except electrolytes and fluid; it is not recommended that they be the sole source of nutrition for more than 5 to 7 days
■ *Example of use:* Immediately after a burn or gastrointestinal (GI) surgery

Oral diet

■ *Indications:* Preferred method of feeding for all individuals; requires GI motility (presence of bowel sounds), fecal output <10 ml/kg/day, unobstructed GI tract
■ *Example of use:* Burns; gastric, gallbladder, or colon surgery
■ *Comments:* Feedings often start with clear liquids (tea, broth, gelatin, Citrotein [Novartis]), advance to full liquids (cream soups, shakes, puddings, custards, commercial liquid supplements [see Chapter 9]), and then progress according to patient tolerance

Enteral tube feedings

■ *Indications:* Same as for oral feedings, except that oral intake is contraindicated or inadequate as a result of upper GI injury or surgery, anorexia, or unconsciousness
■ *Example of use:* Burn patients who cannot consume enough orally; esophageal, mouth, or jaw surgery; coma
■ *Comments:* Ileus and gastric atony are common after head or abdominal injury; if bowel sounds return but gastric emptying is poor, then nasoduodenal feedings may be possible; cardiopulmonary stability is essential before the administration of enteral feedings; intestinal ischemia from low cardiac output or poor oxygen saturation results in loss of epithelial cells of the villi with impaired absorption of all nutrients and secretion of fluid and electrolytes into the intestine; feeding as soon after the injury as possible may reduce the risk of stress ulcer formation

TPN

- *Indications:* Enteral intake unlikely for approximately 7 days as a result of ileus, bowel obstruction, diarrhea, or vomiting; may be indicated even if enteral intake is not expected to be delayed for 7 days if there is severe injury (e.g., major burns) or preexisting malnutrition; may be used as an adjunct to enteral feedings when vomiting or diarrhea limits enteral intake
- *Example of use:* Extensive small intestinal resection, high-output intestinal fistula, multiple organ system failure
- *Comments:* Special care should be taken to prevent catheter infection in burned individuals, whose wounds are likely to be colonized with microorganisms

The techniques for delivering specialized nutrition support are described in Chapters 9 and 10.

Care of patients receiving any of these therapies includes monitoring intake and output; state of hydration; serum levels of electrolytes, albumin, and other nutrition-related parameters; and response to therapy. Caregivers maintain daily food records for patients with oral intake or tube feedings.

Preventing renal lithiasis

Immobile patients are highly susceptible to kidney and bladder stones (lithiasis) because of the release of calcium from the bones. For this reason, a calcium-restricted diet, with one serving or less of dairy products daily, is sometimes prescribed for the person on bedrest. Acid-ash diets (see Chapter 17) are sometimes used to prevent precipitation of calcium stones in the urinary tract. A fluid intake of at least 50 ml/kg will produce dilute urine in which stones are less likely to precipitate.

Alleviating constipation

Immobility following injury or surgery contributes to constipation. The individual who has no dietary restrictions can be encouraged to choose foods rich in fiber (whole grains, legumes, fresh fruits and vegetables). Formulas containing fiber may be of benefit for patients receiving tube feedings (see Chapter 9). A fluid intake of 35 ml/kg or more, as long as it is not contraindicated, will also help produce softer stools.

Teaching

Principles of a nutritious diet

Encourage a diet high in protein (1.2 to 1.5 g/kg, or about 100 g for a person whose ideal body weight is 70 kg [154 lb]) and adequate in kcal, to be maintained throughout the period of convalescence (usually 6 to 12 weeks for major surgeries). Individuals with severe impairment of nutrition as a result of surgery (e.g., massive small bowel resection) or preexisting malnutrition will need to continue a high-protein diet until their weight is at the desirable level and serum proteins are within the reference range. Table 11-4 lists good protein sources; these foods or others high in protein should be consumed daily in sufficient amounts to meet protein requirements.

Supplements rich in protein and kcal (see Tables 9-1 and 9-2) can be used if the person has difficulty consuming enough regular foods. Specialized products are sometimes needed by individuals with pancreatic or intestinal resection. Medium-chain triglycerides (MCTs) are often better absorbed than long-chain triglycerides (LCTs) (see Chapter 9). Complete liquid supplements high in MCTs are available, such as Portagen (Mead Johnson), Crucial (Clintec), or AlitraQ (Ross), or MCT oil can be substituted for the standard LCT oils in food preparation. Supplements of calcium, zinc, and magnesium might also be needed.

Table 11-4   Protein Sources

Food	Serving Size	Protein (g)
Beef, cooked	1 oz (~3″ × 3″ × ¼″)	7
Poultry, cooked	1 oz (1 small chicken drumstick)	7
Canned fish	¼ cup	7
Milk	1 cup	8
Powdered milk, instant	⅓ cup	8
Cheese	1 oz	7
Cottage cheese	¼ cup	7
Egg	1 large	7
Dried beans or peas (kidney, garbanzo, lentils)	½ cup	7
Peanut butter	2 tbsp	8

Monitoring the patient's nutritional status

The patient's nutritional status should be monitored regularly, and he or she should be weighed at least weekly after hospital discharge until weight is stable. Daily weights are needed if the patient's fluid and electrolyte status is precarious (e.g., short-bowel syndrome). The patient and family are instructed to report weight loss or declining nutritional intake to the health care team so that appropriate interventions can be planned.

Diet modifications to promote healing and reduce complications in posttransplant patients

■ Protein intake of 1.2 to 2 g/kg per day for the first few weeks after surgery and 1 to 1.5 g/kg per day after the initial postoperative period is usually sufficient to allow for healing. This diet must be tailored to the patient's needs (e.g., reduced if renal failure develops).

■ Patients who have transplants are often severely malnourished as a consequence of their primary disease (renal or liver failure, short-bowel syndrome, cardiac cachexia, etc.) and have lost weight. Gradual weight gain helps to restore strength and stamina. Ideally, malnutrition is corrected in the pretransplant period, to improve the potential for healing.

■ Hyperphagia stimulated by immunosuppressant drugs and by improved well-being, inactivity, improved absorption, and unhealthy eating behaviors contribute to weight gain posttransplant. Gradual weight loss helps to control both hyperlipidemia and hyperglycemia. An increase in activity, behavioral measures to control eating behaviors, and instruction in healthy food choices are approaches to preventing or correcting unwanted weight gain. A modest reduction in kcal is accomplished by limiting fried foods and high-fat foods such as pastries, whole milk and products made with whole milk, butter, margarine, oils, nuts, chips, and other snack foods. Limiting intake of meats to no more than 5 or 6 ounces daily also reduces fat and energy intake. For additional information, see Chapter 7.

■ Restrict intake of simple sugars (sugar, candies, desserts) to control hypertriglyceridemia and hyperglycemia.

■ Implement a diabetic meal plan if diabetes results from immunosuppressive therapy. It may be possible to correct the problem with a change in immunosuppressive medications or use of oral hypoglycemic agents.

- Limit alcohol intake to 1 or 2 drinks per day or less if hypertriglyceridemia is present.
- Limit cholesterol intake to 300 mg/day, total fat intake to less than 30% of total kcal, and limit saturated fat to no more than 10% of kcal. (Follow the Step-One diet in Chapter 15.)
- Supplements of vitamin D, calcium, and fluoride may help to prevent osteoporosis related to the disease state or corticosteroid therapy. Other measures to reduce osteoporosis include limiting alcohol intake, avoiding smoking, and increasing weight-bearing exercise.

Home tube feeding or TPN

Individuals with short-bowel syndrome as a consequence of bowel resection are likely to experience malabsorption, which may persist for many months, years, or permanently. Some of these individuals can maintain adequate nutritional status with the use of a low-fat, high-protein diet, and some can maintain adequate nutrition with tube feedings of a defined formula diet. Formulas with substantial amounts of MCTs are often better absorbed than those containing large amounts of LCTs. Some individuals have too little absorptive surface to sustain their nutrition and hydration with enteral feedings and require TPN or IV hydration fluids to meet at least part of their needs. Instruction in home tube feeding and TPN is described in Chapters 9 and 10.

SELECTED BIBLIOGRAPHY

Alexander JW, Ogle CK, Nelson JL: Diets and infection: composition and consequences, *World J Surg* 22:209, 1998.

Braga M, et al.: Artificial nutrition after major abdominal surgery: impact of route of administration and composition of the diet, *Crit Care Med* 26:4, 1998.

Cox SAR, et al.: Energy expenditure after spinal cord injury: an evaluation of stable rehabilitating patients, *J Trauma* 25:419, 1985.

Demling RH, DeSanti L: Increased protein intake during the recovery phase after severe burns increases body weight gain and muscle function, *J Burn Care Rehab* 19:161, 1998.

Hunt TK, Hopf HW: Wound healing and wound infection. What surgeons and anesthesiologists can do, *Surg Clin N Am* 77:587, 1997.

King BK, Kudsk KA: Can an enteral diet decrease sepsis after trauma? *Adv Surg* 31:53, 1997.

Mayes T: Enteral nutrition for the burn patient, *Nutr Clin Pract* 12 (1 suppl):S43, 1997.

Raff T, Germann G, Hartmann B: The value of early enteral nutrition in the prophylaxis of stress ulceration in the severely burned patient, *Burns* 23:313, 1997.

Yu YM, et al.: The metabolic basis of the increase in energy expenditure in severely burned patients, *J Parent Ent Nutr* 23:160, 1999.

Gastrointestinal Disorders 12

A variety of disorders that affect the gastrointestinal (GI) tract and its accessory organs, the liver, gallbladder, and pancreas, can impair nutritional status. Effects of these disorders include malabsorption, discomfort associated with eating, anorexia, impaired intake, and food intolerances. Disorders that often have an unfavorable impact on nutritional status are discussed in this chapter.

Esophageal Disorders
Reflux, Obstruction, and Dysfunction
Pathophysiology

Among the problems that can interfere with normal esophageal function are gastroesophageal reflux, esophageal obstruction, and motor dysfunction. In **gastroesophageal reflux disease (GERD)**, reflux of stomach contents into the esophagus occurs, causing esophagitis and heartburn. Ulcer and stricture formation are two possible complications, and long-term GERD can predispose the individual to adenocarcinoma of the esophagus. Reduced lower esophageal sphincter (LES) pressure contributes to GERD. Other contributing factors include impairments of gastric emptying or esophageal peristalsis.

Mechanical obstructions of the esophagus can result from strictures (e.g., from caustic injury caused by ingestion of lye or from GERD) or tumors. **Dysphagia** is a common symptom. Two motor disorders affecting the esophagus are **achalasia,** or incomplete relaxation of the LES after swallowing, and *scleroderma,* a collagen-vascular disease causing proliferation of connective tissue and fibrosis in many organs. Achalasia obstructs the passage of food into the stomach, and dysphagia and regurgitation of food are common symptoms. Carcinoma of the esophagus is a potential long-term sequela. Scleroderma impairs peristalsis and LES closure; symptoms are the same as those of GERD.

Esophageal dysfunction places the patient at risk for pulmonary aspiration, dyspnea, and pneumonia.

Treatment

Antireflux measures include the following: elevation of the head of the bed; cessation of smoking, which reduces LES pressure; avoidance of medications that reduce LES pressure (e.g., anticholinergics, α-adrenergic antagonists, β-adrenergic agonists, calcium channel blockers, opiates, progesterone, and theophylline) if possible; use of antacids; and dietary modification (see the following discussion on nutritional care). Medications to reduce gastric acidity include histamine H_2-receptor antagonists (e.g., cimetidine and ranitidine) and proton pump inhibitors (e.g., omeprazole). Prokinetic medications such as metoclopramide increase LES pressure and promote gastric emptying. Antireflux surgery is a consideration for the patient who does not benefit from medical therapy.

Mechanical dilation may be used in treatment of strictures and achalasia, and surgery, or a combination of surgery and radiation therapy, is usually used in the treatment of esophageal tumors.

Nutritional care

Assessment

Assessment is summarized in Table 12-1.

Intervention and teaching

Preventing or reducing reflux. To reduce the possibility of reflux:

- Consume small, frequent meals.
- Avoid alcohol, fatty foods, peppermint, chocolate, and smoking, which reduce LES pressure.
- Eat the last meal of the day several hours before bedtime, and avoid late-night snacking.
- Keep the head of the bed elevated at least 15 cm (6 in).
- Reduce weight if overweight or obesity is present.

Text continued on p. 259

Table 12-1   Assessment in Gastrointestinal Disorders

Areas of Concern	Significant Findings
Protein-Calorie Malnutrition (PCM)	*History* Decreased food intake caused by a desire to prevent pain associated with eating (e.g., gastroesophageal reflux [GER], gastric ulcer, cholecystitis, pancreatitis), alcohol abuse, nausea and vomiting, anorexia, dysphagia, anticipation of dumping syndrome; increased losses (malabsorption) related to severe diarrhea or steatorrhea (stools greasy or difficult to flush away), pancreatic insufficiency (pancreatitis, cystic fibrosis), short-bowel syndrome, dumping syndrome; increased kcal/protein needs in healing, infection, fever; increased work of breathing (cystic fibrosis); catabolism resulting from corticosteroids *Physical Examination* Muscle wasting; edema; alopecia; triceps skinfold <5th percentile; weight <90% of that expected for height or BMI <18.5; failure to follow individual established pattern on growth charts (children) *Laboratory Analysis* ↓ Serum albumin, transferrin, or prealbumin; ↓ lymphocyte count, ↓ creatinine-height index

Table 12-1   Assessment in Gastrointestinal Disorders—cont'd

Areas of Concern	Significant Findings
Inadequate Fluid Balance	*History* Excessive losses caused by severe vomiting or diarrhea (especially short-bowel syndrome and dumping syndrome); when diarrhea is severe, stools should be weighed or measured to determine output accurately *Physical Examination* Poor skin turgor; dry, sticky mucous membranes; feeling of thirst; acute loss of >3%-5% of body weight; hypotension *Laboratory Analysis* ↑ BUN; ↑ Hct; ↑ serum Na
Vitamin Deficiencies	
A	*History* Decreased absorption as a result of steatorrhea, pancreatic insufficiency, or cholestyramine use *Physical Examination* Drying of skin and cornea; papular eruption around hair follicles (follicular hyperkeratosis) *Laboratory Analysis* ↓ Serum retinol; ↓ retinol-binding protein (indicating PCM, with inadequate protein to manufacture carrier for vitamin A)
E	*History* Decreased absorption as a result of steatorrhea, pancreatic insufficiency, or cholestyramine use

Continued

Table 12-1   Assessment in Gastrointestinal Disorders—cont'd

Areas of Concern	Significant Findings
Vitamin Deficiencies—cont'd	
E—cont'd	*Physical Examination*
	Neuromuscular dysfunction (causing extreme weakness)
	Laboratory Analysis
	↓ Serum tocopherol; hemolysis
K	*History*
	Decreased absorption as a result of steatorrhea or pancreatic insufficiency; decreased production caused by destruction of intestinal bacteria by antibiotic usage (e.g., in hepatic encephalopathy or cystic fibrosis)
	Physical Examination
	Petechiae, ecchymoses
	Laboratory Analysis
	Prolonged prothrombin time (PT)
B_{12}	*History*
	Decreased absorption as a result of gastrectomy (loss of intrinsic factor necessary for absorption), distal ileal disease (e.g., Crohn's disease), or resection (loss of absorptive sites); bacterial overgrowth in the bowel competing for vitamin B_{12} (seen in short-bowel syndrome or gastric resection)
	Physical Examination
	Pallor; sore, inflamed tongue; neuropathy
	Laboratory Analysis
	↓ Serum vitamin B_{12}; ↓ Hct, ↑ MCV

Table 12-1   Assessment in Gastrointestinal Disorders—cont'd

Areas of Concern	Significant Findings
Mineral/Electrolyte Deficiencies	
Calcium (Ca)	*History*
	Decreased intake of milk products caused by lactose intolerance; increased losses as a result of steatorrhea or corticosteroid use
	Physical Examination
	Tingling of fingers; muscular tetany and cramps, carpopedal spasm; convulsions
	Laboratory Analysis
	↓ Serum Ca (severe deficits only); ↓ bone density on radiograph (chronic Ca deficit)
Magnesium (Mg)	*History*
	Inadequate intake as a result of alcoholism; increased losses as a result of steatorrhea or diarrhea, vomiting (e.g., pancreatitis, hepatitis), loss of small bowel fluid (e.g., short-bowel syndrome, fistula formation in inflammatory bowel disease)
	Physical Examination
	Tremor, hyperactive deep reflexes; convulsions
	Laboratory Analysis
	↓ Serum Mg

Continued

Table 12-1   Assessment in Gastrointestinal Disorders—cont'd

Areas of Concern	Significant Findings
Mineral/Electrolyte Deficiencies—cont'd	
Iron (Fe)	*History*
	Blood loss (e.g., inflammatory bowel disease, ulcer); impaired absorption caused by decreased acid within upper GI tract, resulting from gastrectomy or chronic antacid or cimetidine use (as in peptic ulcer); decreased intake (e.g., restriction of protein foods in liver disease)
	Physical Examination
	Koilonychia; pallor, blue sclerae; fatigue
	Laboratory Analysis
	↓ Hct, Hgb, MCV, MCH, MCHC; ↓ serum Fe and ferritin; ↑ serum transferrin
Zinc (Zn)	*History*
	Increased losses as a result of diarrhea/steatorrhea, loss of intestinal fluid (e.g., short-bowel syndrome, high output ileostomy, fistula drainage); decreased intake caused by protein restriction
	Physical Examination
	Anorexia; hypogeusia, dysgeusia; diarrhea; dermatitis
	Laboratory Analysis
	↓ Serum Zn

Table 12-1   Assessment in Gastrointestinal Disorders—cont'd

Areas of Concern	Significant Findings
Mineral/Electrolyte Deficiencies—cont'd	
Potassium (K+)	*History*
	Increased losses caused by diarrhea
	Physical Examination
	Muscle weakness, ileus; diminished reflexes
	Laboratory Analysis
	↓ Serum K+; inverted T wave on ECG
Nutrient Excess	
Iron (Fe)	*History*
	Family history of hemochromatosis
	Physical Examination
	No abnormalities if diagnosed early; later: bronze skin (in areas not exposed to sun)
	Laboratory Analysis
	↑ serum Fe, ↑ ferritin

Coping with dysphagia. Solid foods and thin liquids usually cause the most difficulty. Foods that create a semisolid bolus when chewed are generally best tolerated.

■ Liquids can be thickened with dry infant cereals, mashed potatoes or potato flakes, cornstarch, or yogurt.
■ Try fluids in frozen form (e.g., sherbet or fruit ices).
■ Consult with a speech therapist, who may be able to assist dysphagic individuals in improving their swallowing techniques.
■ Wait until dilation or surgical therapy has been performed before trying to increase oral intake in the person with achalasia; the risk of pulmonary aspiration is high before treatment.

Providing nutrition support as needed. Where esophageal obstruction exists or reflux or dysphagia is severe, impairing intake so much that weight loss occurs or placing the individual at high risk of pulmonary aspiration, tube feedings (via gastrostomy or jejunostomy if esophageal obstruction is present) may be needed. Special care must be taken to reduce the risk of pulmonary aspiration, e.g., frequent monitoring of gastric residual volumes and elevation of the head of the bed. Nasoenteric feedings are generally not used before definitive therapy for achalasia has been provided.

Gastric Disorders
Peptic Ulcer (Gastric and Duodenal Ulcer)
Pathophysiology

Excess acid secretion or disruption of the GI mucosal barrier predisposes the individual to ulcer formation. *Helicobacter pylori,* a bacillus found only on gastric epithelium, is currently believed to be a major factor in the pathogenesis of peptic ulcers, although cigarette smoking, regular use of nonsteroidal antiinflammatory drugs (NSAIDs) such as aspirin, corticosteroid medications, genetic predisposition, and emotional stress may be contributory factors. Gastric ulcers are often associated with pain exacerbated by eating, and duodenal ulcers are associated with pain relieved by eating.

Treatment

Medications that reduce gastric acidity, such as antacids, the histamine H_2-receptor antagonists cimetidine and ranitidine, and proton pump inhibitors (e.g., omeprazole), are often prescribed. Sucralfate and bismuth are specific antiulcer agents. Bismuth and antibiotics are sometimes used in attempts to eradicate *H. pylori,* but recurrence is common. In addition, the person is usually advised to avoid smoking, alcohol, and NSAIDs, which increase gastric acid production or impair the mucosal barrier that protects the GI tract from damage. Stress-reduction techniques may also be of benefit. Endoscopic thermal therapy or injection of a sclerosing agent is used in treatment of some bleeding ulcers, and partial gastrectomy and vagotomy are usually performed only when perforation or uncontrollable bleeding occurs.

Nutritional care
Assessment
Assessment is summarized in Table 12-1.

Intervention and teaching
Dietary practices and other techniques to promote comfort.
Current practice is to restrict only those foods that cause the
individual patient discomfort. For some patients these include
caffeine-containing foods (see Appendix G), decaffeinated coffee,
alcohol, and red or black pepper or other spicy foods. In addition,
small, frequent meals and snacks may help alleviate pain.

Use relaxation and stress-reduction techniques to avoid excessive gastric acid secretion. It is especially important to keep
mealtimes calm. Smoking cessation may also reduce discomfort.

Gastrectomy
Pathophysiology
Partial or total resection of the stomach is sometimes required for
treatment of peptic ulcer or gastric cancer. Two problems are likely
after gastrectomy: fat malabsorption and dumping syndrome. Fat malabsorption results from the bypass of the duodenum by the Roux-en-Y
esophagojejunostomy and other common gastrectomy procedures.
Bacteria multiply within the bypassed duodenum, and the bacteria
deconjugate bile salts, making micelle formation and fat absorption
inadequate (see pp. 201-203 for a discussion of fat absorption).
Dumping syndrome results from the rapid passage of foods into the
small bowel, caused by the loss or bypass of the pyloric sphincter.
Rapid hydrolysis (digestion) of nutrients increases the osmolality
(concentrations of solutes) within the upper small bowel. Fluid from
the plasma and extracellular space is drawn into the bowel to dilute
the hypertonic intestinal contents. Symptoms include nausea, abdominal pain, weakness, diaphoresis (sweating), diarrhea, and weight loss.

Nutritional care
Assessment
Assessment is summarized in Table 12-1.

Intervention
Preventing protein-calorie malnutrition
■ Maintain weight by consuming a high-protein (1.5 to 2 g/kg/day)
and high-kcal diet with moderate fat.

■ Slow gastric emptying and decrease the likelihood of dumping syndrome by reducing gastric distension and osmolality of foods consumed: eat small, frequent meals; limit intake of simple carbohydrates; and never drink beverages with meals.

Supplementation. Calcium and iron may be poorly absorbed postoperatively because these minerals are absorbed best in an acidic environment. Normally, much of their absorption takes place in the duodenum, because that segment of the small intestine is acidified by the entry of the stomach contents. (The pancreas releases bicarbonate and alkaline secretions, creating a basic environment in the jejunum and ileum.) Secretion of gastric acid is greatly reduced postoperatively, which makes the duodenum less acidic. Supplements of calcium and iron help to reduce the risk of osteoporosis and iron-deficiency anemia.

Intrinsic factor and hydrochloric acid, both produced in the stomach, are required for absorption of vitamin B_{12}. Therefore, supplemental vitamin B_{12} (regular injections, high-dose oral supplements, or nasal gel) is usually required for the remainder of the person's life.

Teaching

Dietary modifications and their rationale. To maintain a stable body weight and reduce fat malabsorption, select a high-protein, high-energy diet that is moderate in fat (no more than 30% of total energy intake). To achieve these goals:

■ Use skinned poultry, lean meats, skim or low-fat milk, and dairy products made from skim or low-fat milk.
■ Use plant proteins such as dried beans and peas regularly.
■ Limit fried or fatty foods.

Reduce the likelihood of dumping syndrome with the following measures:

■ Eat small meals and snacks often; six meals a day may be needed.
■ Avoid beverages at mealtime. Drink fluids at least 1 hour before or after meals.
■ Avoid concentrated sweets (e.g., candy, cookies, pies, cakes, jam, jelly, soft drinks, sugared beverages or foods). Although they are high in simple carbohydrates, fresh fruits are often well-tolerated

because of their soluble fiber (pectin) content. They can be used as desserts and snacks.

■ Maintain nonstressful eating practices. Eat slowly in a relaxed setting. Lying down for about 1 hour after meals can also help prevent dumping syndrome.

■ Pectin or guar gum taken with meals and snacks may delay gastric emptying and carbohydrate absorption, reducing the risk of dumping syndrome.

Intestinal Disorders

Nutrients are absorbed at specific sites in the small intestine (see Figure 1-5); therefore, the location and the extent of small intestinal disease or resection determine which nutrients will be affected. Generally, damage to or loss of the duodenum or jejunum is tolerated better than impairment of the ileum. The ileum can absorb most nutrients normally absorbed in the duodenum and jejunum, but these portions of the bowel cannot assume all of the roles of the ileum, such as absorption of vitamin B_{12} (see Chapter 1).

Short-Bowel Syndrome
Pathophysiology

Massive resection of the small bowel, creating **short-bowel syndrome,** severely reduces the area available for the absorption of nutrients. This procedure is sometimes required in Crohn's disease, necrotizing enterocolitis (see Chapter 20), congenital atresias, acute volvulus, strangulated hernias, mesenteric artery occlusion, and similar disorders. Malabsorption and diarrhea are greater if: (1) more than 80% of the small bowel is resected, (2) the ileum is resected, (3) the ileocecal valve is removed, or (4) the unresected bowel is damaged. For at least the first 2 years after massive bowel resection, adaptation occurs via bowel hyperplasia and hypertrophy. This response takes place in phases:

Phase 1: In the immediate postoperative period there are enormous losses of fluids, electrolytes, magnesium, calcium, zinc, and amino acids. In addition to the loss of absorptive area, temporary gastric hypersecretion contributes to fluid and electrolyte losses.

Phase 2: Diarrhea diminishes, along with fluid and electrolyte problems.

Phase 3: The individual achieves a stable weight determined by the amount of bowel remaining.

Treatment

Antidiarrheal and anticholinergic drugs, such as codeine, lopera-mide (Imodium), diphenoxylate with atropine (Lomotil), or glycopyrrolate (Robinul), may be helpful in controlling diarrhea during Phases 1 and 2. If the ileum is removed, large amounts of bile salts may enter the colon and cause diarrhea by stimulating colonic water secretion. At least 100 cm of ileum is required for complete absorption of bile salts. Cholestyramine is sometimes used to bind the bile salts and reduce diarrhea. Some patients with short-bowel syndrome have undergone small bowel transplanta-tion, which procedure may become much more common in the future. Treatment with trophic factors (growth hormone and glutamine) and a low-fat, high-carbohydrate diet has been success-ful in allowing some patients to discontinue or markedly decrease their use of total parenteral nutrition (TPN).

Nutritional care

Assessment

Assessment is summarized in Table 12-1. Massive small bowel resection can be expected to affect absorption of almost every nutrient and to have great potential for causing malnutrition.

Intervention

Replacing losses and preventing malnutrition

Phase 1: Intravenous (IV) support is essential to replace fluids, electrolytes, and other nutrient losses. Most individuals require TPN for at least a few weeks after surgery. It is especially important to replace zinc losses (12 to 17 mg of zinc is lost per kilogram of feces or ileostomy drainage) because wound healing is impaired without zinc, and standard TPN solutions do not contain enough zinc to replace diarrheal losses.

Phase 2: The presence of nutrients within the GI tract is necessary for bowel adaptation to occur. Enteral feedings are often started as soon as the volume of fecal losses decreases to less than 1 L/day. Typically, TPN continues as continuous tube feedings are begun. Small oral feedings may also be started. They are generally low in fat (less than 10 g/day) and fiber and high in starch. White rice, enriched white bread and toast, noodles, macaroni, and peeled boiled or baked potato (all without added milk, cheese, margarine, butter, or other fat) are examples of possible foods.

Phase 3: Oral feedings can be advanced. They should be small and frequent. Fat intake can be increased unless **steatorrhea** worsens. Concentrated sugars, excessive fat, or alcohol consumption may worsen malabsorption. Medium-chain triglycerides (MCTs) may be used for caloric supplementation, but excessive amounts often worsen diarrhea. MCTs can be used in cooking or added to juice or applesauce to increase caloric intake. Lactose, or milk sugar, often causes diarrhea and cramping and should be limited if these problems occur with milk intake. TPN will continue to be required if the individual is unable to maintain adequate nutriture with oral or oral plus enteral tube feedings.

Supplementation

- *Individuals not receiving TPN:* Daily supplements are often necessary, particularly vitamins A and E and iron, calcium, magnesium, and zinc.
- *Severe steatorrhea:* Water-miscible forms of vitamins A and E may be better absorbed than standard fat-soluble forms. Hypomagnesemia and hypocalcemia are common; a low-fat diet combined with supplements of these minerals helps to correct deficiencies. Zinc supplements may also be needed.
- *Absence of the terminal ileum:* Vitamin B_{12} supplements are needed, usually in regularly scheduled injections. Some patients may absorb enough B_{12} if they take large oral doses (1000 μg) daily, and the vitamin is available as a nasal gel.

Emotional support. The effects of massive bowel resection are catastrophic and are likely to be permanent. The individual and family need encouragement and reinforcement, particularly if home TPN or tube feedings are required.

Teaching

Dietary modifications and their rationale. The individual will need instruction in a high-kcal diet with small, frequent feedings. The need for a low-fat diet (Table 12-2) is controversial; some clinicians recommend it in short-bowel syndrome. It appears to be most effective in individuals who still have the colon. Individuals with

Table 12-2   Fat-Restricted Diet

Type of Food	Foods to Include	Foods to Avoid
Milk products	Milk products made with skim milk	Milk products made with 2% or whole milk
Meat and meat substitutes	Lean meat, fish (water packed, if canned), poultry without skin, egg whites	Fried meats, sausage, frankfurters, poultry skins, duck, goose, salt pork, luncheon meats, peanut butter, egg yolk except as allowed*
Breads and cereals	Plain pasta, cereals, whole-grain or enriched bread or rolls	Biscuits, doughnuts, pancakes, sweet rolls, waffles, muffins, high-fat rolls such as croissants
Fruits	All except avocado	Avocado except as allowed*
Vegetables	All if plainly prepared	Fried, au gratin, creamed, or buttered
Desserts	Sherbet made with skim milk, angel food cake, gelatin, pudding made with skim milk, fruit ice	Cake, pie, pastry, ice cream (except for fat free), or any dessert containing fat or chocolate
Sweets	Jelly, jam, syrup, sugar, hard sugar candies, jelly beans, gum drops	Any candy made with chocolate, nuts, butter, or cream

*The following contain 5 g of fat per serving and must be used only in limited amounts. Usually no more than 5 to 6 of these fat servings per day are included in a low-fat diet: 1 tsp butter, margarine, oil, shortening, or mayonnaise; 1 tbsp salad dressing or heavy cream; 1 strip crisp bacon; ⅛ avocado; 6 small nuts; 10 peanuts; 5 small olives; ½ cup "light" ice cream; 1 egg yolk or whole egg.

severe steatorrhea are often more comfortable when they restrict fat intake. MCTs may be added to the diet if increased calories are needed. Lactose intolerance is common, but yogurt, hard cheeses, and milk treated with lactase enzyme are good sources of calcium for lactose-intolerant individuals. Alcohol and caffeine stimulate GI activity and should be avoided for at least 1 year after surgery.

Hyperoxaluria (excessive urinary excretion of oxalates), which may result in formation of urinary stones, occurs in some individuals with steatorrhea because they fail to absorb adequate calcium as a result of formation of calcium soaps with fat in the stool. Normally, calcium binds oxalate in the gut to inhibit oxalate absorption, but excessive fecal calcium losses allow increased amounts of oxalate to be absorbed. A calcium supplement can reduce oxalate absorption. A low-oxalate diet can be used if the calcium supplement does not correct the hyperoxaluria. Foods high in oxalate are nuts; coffee; chocolate; green beans; green, leafy vegetables; beets; rhubarb; eggplant; celery; carrots; artichokes; plums; blackberries; and whole wheat.

Administration of home nutritional support. Some individuals will need instruction in home TPN or tube feedings because these may need to continue at least until maximal adaptation occurs (see Chapters 9 and 10).

Celiac Disease (Nontropical Sprue or Gluten-Sensitive Enteropathy)
Pathophysiology

The exact mechanism of **celiac disease** is unknown, but intestinal villi atrophy because of intolerance of the **gliadin** portion of **gluten** (a protein found in wheat and several other grains). The surface area of the bowel is markedly decreased, and disaccharidase and peptidase activity is lost because these enzymes, which digest carbohydrates and proteins, are found in the intestinal mucosal cells. Diarrhea, steatorrhea, impaired absorption of all macronutrients (carbohydrate, protein, and fat), muscle wasting, weight loss or failure to gain weight (in children), and anemia often occur.

Diagnosis of celiac disease is made through small-bowel biopsy, with microscopic evidence of blunting of the villi; the presence of serum antibodies to gliadin; and response to a trial of a gluten-restricted diet.

Nutritional care

Assessment

Assessment is summarized in Table 12-1.

Intervention and teaching

Gluten-free diet. Permanent removal of gluten from the diet is the only treatment for celiac disease. Following the diet is especially important because GI lymphoma appears to be more common in individuals who fail to do so. This diet is difficult to follow because grain products are so widely used in processed foods. The individual and family need extensive encouragement and reinforcement.

Recommendations for restricting gluten include the following:

■ Avoid wheat, barley, rye, and all products made with these grains. Table 12-3 lists foods to include and to avoid in gluten sensitivity. The use of oats in the diet is controversial. Evidence suggests that oats are tolerated by most adults with celiac disease, but there is insufficient evidence to determine whether oats can safely be included in the diet. Even if oats are well-tolerated, they are often contaminated with wheat during harvest, and thus they are best avoided at the present time.
■ Read labels carefully because gluten-containing grains are added to many products. When it is unclear whether a product contains gluten, use the address on the food label to obtain further information.
■ In restaurants, ask whether unfamiliar foods contain restricted grains.
■ Celiac disease support groups can provide recipes, practical information, and support for the affected individual and the family. Local groups can be located via the national Celiac Sprue Association (see Appendix I).

Inflammatory Bowel Disease (Crohn's Disease and Ulcerative Colitis)

Pathophysiology

Inflammatory bowel disease (IBD) can affect individuals of all ages. In **Crohn's disease** (regional ileitis), inflammation extends through all layers of the bowel wall. It can affect any part of the GI tract but most often affects the terminal ileum. In acute exacerba-

Table 12-3 Diet for Gluten Intolerance

Type of Food	Foods to Include	Foods to Avoid
Milk products	Fresh, dry, evaporated, or condensed milk; whipping cream; sour cream (check vegetable gum used)	Malted milk, some commercial chocolate milk, some nondairy creamers
Meat products	All fresh meats, poultry, and fish	Breaded products; some sausages, frankfurters, luncheon meats, and sandwich spreads
Cheeses	All natural cheeses	Any cheese containing oat gum,* some pasteurized processed cheese
Breads and starches	Potatoes, potato flour, rice, rice flour, wild rice, corn, cornstarch, tapioca, arrowroot starch, soy flour, millet, special gluten-free pasta	Regular pasta products, all products containing wheat, rye, oats,* barley, buckwheat, or triticale (wheat-rye hybrid)
Vegetables	All plain or buttered	Creamed, au gratin, breaded (unless made with gluten-free starch)
Fruits	All fresh, canned, or frozen	Canned fruit pie fillings
Beverages	Wine, instant and ground coffee, tea, distilled spirits	Beer and ale, roasted grain beverages such as Postum
Miscellaneous	Most spices, cider and wine vinegar, all nuts and seeds	Some dry seasoning mixes, curry powder, catsup and mustard, soy sauce; distilled white vinegar

*Evidence suggests that oats may be acceptable for a gluten-free diet, but the safest practice is to exclude them until further data are available.

tions, abdominal pain, fever, nausea, and diarrhea occur. In chronic disease, weight loss, anorexia, anemia, and steatorrhea are common.

In **ulcerative colitis,** congestion, edema, and ulcerations affect the mucosal and submucosal layers of the bowel. It usually involves the rectum and colon and sometimes extends to the ileum. Bloody diarrhea, abdominal and rectal pain, weight loss, and anorexia are common.

Diagnosis is made by barium enema, endoscopy (sigmoidoscopy, colonoscopy, or esophagoscopy), and intestinal biopsy.

Treatment

Drugs that are often used include corticosteroids to decrease inflammation; antidiarrheals, such as diphenoxylate (Lomotil); and antispasmodics, such as tincture of belladonna, to decrease discomfort. Sulfasalazine is used in ulcerative colitis for its antiinflammatory and antimicrobial effects. (See Appendix H for drug-nutrient interactions.) Surgery may be necessary if fistulas, hemorrhage, perforation, or intestinal obstruction occurs. Resection of the colon is often performed after several acute exacerbations of ulcerative colitis because of the risk of development of colon cancer.

Nutritional care

Assessment

Assessment is summarized in Table 12-1.

Intervention and teaching

Diet and other lifestyle modifications

- *Acute disease:* Supportive therapy with intravenous (IV) fluids and a clear liquid diet is often provided. In severe disease, or when a fistula is present, TPN without any oral intake may be used for several weeks in an effort to rest the bowel and promote healing. Enteral tube feedings may also be effective.
- *Chronic disease:* A low-fat diet (see Table 12-2) may be prescribed to decrease steatorrhea, which is common with ileal involvement. A high-protein diet (1.5 to 2 g/kg/day) helps promote bowel regeneration and replace losses.

If areas of intestinal stenosis are present, then a restricted-fiber diet that eliminates berries, raw fruits except banana or avocado, raw vegetables, whole grains, and dried beans or peas is often recommended to reduce the potential for bowel obstruction.

Lactose intolerance is common in Crohn's disease. Some lactose-intolerant individuals can tolerate yogurt, buttermilk, and hard cheeses. Lactase enzyme can be added to milk to hydrolyze the lactose.

Stress can exacerbate inflammatory bowel disease (IBD). Furthermore, chronic disease imposes its own stresses. Development of coping and stress-reduction skills improves quality of life.

Supplementation. The following supplements may be needed:

- Iron if blood loss is sufficient to cause anemia.
- Vitamins A and E, calcium, magnesium, and zinc if steatorrhea is present.
- Vitamin B_{12} if the terminal ileum is involved.

Pancreatic Dysfunction
Pancreatitis (Acute or Chronic)
Pathophysiology

Pancreatitis refers to inflammation, edema, and necrosis of the pancreas as a result of digestion of the pancreas by enzymes normally secreted by the pancreas. Alcoholism, biliary tract disease, trauma, peptic ulcer disease, hyperlipidemia, and the use of certain drugs (glucocorticoids, sulfonamides, chlorothiazides, and azathioprine) may cause pancreatitis. Symptoms include pain in the epigastric region, persistent vomiting, abdominal rigidity, and elevated serum amylase. Malabsorption and decreased glucose tolerance are common in chronic pancreatitis.

Treatment

Anticholinergic agents, such as atropine, may be used to decrease pancreatic secretion. Meperidine is used for pain relief.

Nutritional care
Assessment

Assessment is summarized in Table 12-1.

Intervention and teaching

Acute pancreatitis. The goal of treatment is to avoid pain and reduce inflammation caused by pancreatic stimulation.

- All oral feedings may be withheld during severe attacks. IV fluids and electrolytes are given to replace the massive losses that occur during inflammation. In the past, TPN has often been recommended for individuals with pancreatitis, because it causes little or no stimulation of pancreatic secretion, thus promoting healing. Evidence suggests, however, that jejunal feedings of a low-fat defined formula diet stimulate pancreatic secretion very little and are well-tolerated by most patients with acute pancreatitis.

■ Once pain has subsided, clear liquids by mouth are usually introduced, and the diet is progressed as tolerated. A low-fat (<20% of total calories), high-carbohydrate diet usually causes less pain than an unrestricted diet. MCTs can be added if needed for adequate energy intake. The diet is gradually liberalized as the patient tolerates it.

■ Alcohol is contraindicated because it increases pancreatic damage and pain.

Chronic pancreatitis. The goal of treatment is to promote healing and compensate for the decrease in pancreatic secretion.

■ A high-protein, high-carbohydrate diet with as much fat as can be tolerated promotes healing. Skinned, baked or broiled poultry, lean meats, low-fat cheeses, and vegetable proteins, such as dried beans and peas, provide protein with a low to moderate fat intake.

■ The individual may need to limit fat in the diet if it causes steatorrhea or pain (see Table 12-2). If additional food energy is needed, MCT oil can be used to replace the usual dietary fats in cooking, combined into a shake with milk and ice milk, or served in juice.

■ Pancreatic enzyme replacement may be administered with each meal to improve digestion.

■ Insulin secretion is likely to be impaired. If glucose intolerance is present, then the patient is treated as a diabetic (see Chapter 18).

Supplementation. If fat malabsorption is severe, water-miscible forms of vitamins A and E, as well as supplements of zinc and calcium, may be needed.

Cystic Fibrosis

Pathophysiology

Cystic fibrosis (CF) results from a genetic defect in a cell membrane protein, the cystic fibrosis transmembrane conductance regulator (CFTR), that regulates the passage of chloride out of cells.

Indirectly, this defect disrupts the sodium and water balance across cell membranes. The respiratory system is especially vulnerable to the effects of this disruption because there is not enough water on the airway surface to maintain normal, well-hydrated mucus secretions. Instead, viscous mucus collects in the respiratory tract, which can obstruct the airways and provide a favorable environment for growth of microorganisms. Other areas that are likely to be obstructed by thickened secretions include the pancreatic duct, through which the pancreatic digestive enzymes enter the duodenum, the common bile duct, and the vas deferens of the male reproductive tract. Involvement of the pancreas (and, to a lesser extent, the common bile duct) results in malabsorption, with fat being the nutrient most affected. Consequently, stools tend to be large and bulky and growth failure is common unless aggressive nutritional intervention is initiated. In contrast to most of the body cells, which normally secrete chloride, the sweat glands reabsorb it. The defect in the CFTR results in increased losses of chloride in sweat and provides a key tool for diagnosis of CF. Sweat chloride concentrations greater than 60 mmol/L are indicative of CF.

Treatment

Prevention of atelectasis and respiratory infections is a primary goal of treatment. Daily chest physiotherapy, including percussion and postural drainage, is especially effective. Antibiotics are given as necessary to treat or prevent pneumonia. Inhalation of human recombinant DNase has been effective in improving pulmonary function in clinical trials. Lung transplantation has been performed in some patients with end-stage pulmonary disease. A variety of experimental treatments are under study, including new mucolytics and hydrating agents to liquify secretions and gene therapy to insert normal CFTR in the respiratory tract.

As many as 85% of individuals with CF have pancreatic insufficiency and require pancreatic enzyme replacement with all meals and snacks to correct malabsorption.

Nutritional care

Assessment

Assessment is summarized in Table 12-1.

Intervention and teaching

Promoting optimum growth and preventing malnutrition. Adequate energy intake is needed to compensate for malabsorption, increased work of breathing, and increased needs imposed by infection. Each day, healthy children need about 1000 kcal + 100 kcal per year of life. Depending on the extent of their disease, children with CF may grow well on this number of kcal or may need 120% to 150% of this amount and 2 to 2.5 g protein per day.

A high-protein, moderate to high-fat diet (30%-40% of total kcal) should be encouraged. Some individuals experience abdominal pain and severe steatorrhea with unrestricted fat intake. Adjustment of their pancreatic enzyme dosages usually improves their fat tolerance. MCT oil may be used to increase caloric intake when steatorrhea is severe. If oral intake is inadequate to prevent or correct malnutrition, then enteral tube feedings to supplement oral intake have been found to be beneficial in improving nutritional status. Nasal polyps are common in CF, and therefore nasogastric and nasointestinal tubes may be poorly tolerated. Gastrostomy feedings are an alternative.

Supplementation. Zinc, magnesium, and calcium supplements and water-miscible forms of vitamins A and E may be necessary in individuals with steatorrhea. Food should be generously salted, especially in hot weather, to replace abnormal electrolyte losses in sweat.

Emotional support. Cystic fibrosis is a chronic, incurable disease. The affected person and family need much support to cope with the illness. The disease can be mild to severe, making it difficult to foresee exactly what the individual's functional level and length of survival will be. The median age of survival, currently more than 30 years, is continually increasing with improved treatment. Individuals should be encouraged to participate in all activities compatible with their functional abilities. Support groups may be of great help to the individuals and their families.

Hepatic Diseases
Hepatitis
Pathophysiology

Hepatitis is an inflammation of the liver caused by a virus, toxin, obstruction, parasite, or drug (alcohol, chloroform, or carbon tetrachloride). Symptoms include jaundice, abdominal pain, hepatomegaly, nausea, vomiting, and anorexia. Elevated serum levels of bilirubin, aspartate aminotransferase (AST, or SGOT), alanine aminotransferase (ALT, or SGPT), and lactic dehydrogenase (LDH) are commonly present.

Treatment

If the cause of hepatitis is known, then it should be removed. Rest and nutritional therapy are the primary treatments.

Nutritional care

Assessment

Assessment is summarized in Table 12-1.

Intervention and teaching

Promotion of liver regeneration. A high-kcal, high-protein (70 to 100 g), moderate-fat diet promotes healing. Lean meats, poultry, legumes, and cheese or cottage cheese made with skim or low-fat milk are good protein sources that are low to moderate in fat. Starches, such as pasta, rice, potatoes, cereals, and breads, are good calorie sources. Frequent, small feedings are better tolerated than large feedings. Alcohol is toxic to the liver and should be avoided for at least 1 year.

Supplementation. If steatorrhea is present, then supplemental water-miscible vitamins A and E, calcium, and zinc may be needed.

Cirrhosis and Hepatic Encephalopathy or Coma
Pathophysiology

Cirrhosis occurs following hepatic damage. Causes of damage include alcoholism, biliary tract obstruction, and viral infection. Although the liver is able to regenerate much of the damaged tissue, some fibrous tissue develops, impairing the normal flow of blood, bile, and hepatic metabolites. Portal vein hypertension occurs, with esophageal and gastric varices, GI bleeding, hypoalbuminemia, ascites, and jaundice. Severe liver dysfunction results in intolerance to protein and **hepatic encephalopathy.** Signs of encephalopathy include confusion, increased serum ammonia levels (worsened by high-protein intake), and a flapping hand tremor, with progression to somnolence and coma. Aromatic amino acids (phenylalanine and tyrosine) and methionine appear to contribute to the problem, perhaps by formation of false neurotransmitters in the central nervous system. Intestinal bacteria digest blood in the GI tract, and ammonia released by this process is absorbed into the body, worsening hepatic encephalopathy.

Treatment

Drug therapy includes use of lactulose, which reduces absorption of ammonia from the GI tract, and poorly absorbed antibiotics such as neomycin, which are given orally to destroy intestinal bacteria that produce ammonia.

Nutritional care

Assessment

Assessment is summarized in Table 12-1.

Intervention

Dietary modifications. The goal is to avoid inducing encephalopathy or worsening symptoms, while providing as nutritious a diet as possible.

Alcohol intake must be eliminated. A high-kcal diet (45 to 50 kcal/kg) prevents breakdown of body tissues to meet energy needs (which releases ammonia and other wastes that worsen encephalopathy). Carbohydrates provide most of the kcal. Moderate fat (30% of total energy intake) can be provided unless steatorrhea is present. If steatorrhea occurs, then fat can be reduced. MCTs can be used to increase energy intake where steatorrhea is present.

Protein intake is usually limited to 1 to 1.5 g/kg desirable weight per day unless hepatic encephalopathy is impending. In encephalopathy, protein is often limited to 0.5 g/kg or less. With improvement, intake can be gradually liberalized, with the eventual goal being 1 g/kg/day. Vegetable protein appears to be better tolerated than meat protein by some patients with chronic hepatic encephalopathy. There is some evidence that increased intakes of branched-chain amino acids (BCAAs) are beneficial for selected patients with encephalopathy. Enteral formulas high in BCAAs (Hepatic-Aid II [B Braun-McGaw] and NutriHep [Nestle]) can be taken orally or delivered by tube. BCAA-enriched amino acid solutions are available for use in TPN.

Restriction of sodium intake to 500 to 1500 mg (20 to 65 mEq)/day of sodium helps to control fluid retention and ascites. (See Box 15-1 for sodium-restricted diets.)

Small, frequent feedings are better tolerated than larger, less frequent ones. Soft foods that are low in fiber help prevent bleeding from esophageal varices, which may result in elevated ammonia levels as the blood proteins are absorbed or in shock if severe acute bleeding occurs.

Supplementation. Supplements providing at least two to three times the RDA of B complex vitamins, especially folic acid, are often used. Many individuals with cirrhosis are alcoholics and have followed poor diets; they have poor tissue stores of vitamins.

Teaching

Dietary restrictions and rationale. Alcohol intake must be eliminated because it can increase the liver damage.

If there is no history of encephalopathy and no evidence of encephalopathy developing, then a normal protein diet can be maintained. If the person has had encephalopathy or protein intolerance, then limit protein intake to about 0.5 to 0.7 g/kg dry weight daily. This amount can be gradually increased as tolerated by the patient. Starchy foods such as pasta, rice, potatoes, and breads provide needed calories. Fat can be used to increase palatability and caloric intake unless steatorrhea occurs.

Sodium is moderately limited to 1000 to 2000 mg/day if ascites or edema are present. To achieve this limit, no salt should be added in cooking, and obviously salty foods should be avoided (see Box 15-1).

Multivitamin and mineral supplements are usually given because stores are often inadequate.

Hemochromatosis

Pathophysiology

Hemochromatosis is a genetic disorder in which excessive iron is stored in various organs, especially the liver, pancreas, heart, gonads, skin, and joints, disrupting organ function. Cirrhosis of the liver, bronzing of the skin, and diabetes are likely to occur if the disorder is left untreated. The laboratory evidence of hemochromatosis includes elevated serum iron and ferritin concentrations, saturated iron-binding capacity, and excessive parenchymal iron in liver biopsy tissue.

Treatment

Regular phlebotomy is used to remove excessive iron stores, with the goal being to maintain serum ferritin at 50 $\mu g/L$ or less.

Nutritional care

Assessment

Assessment is summarized in Table 12-1.

Intervention and teaching

Limit dietary iron and its absorption. To limit dietary iron:

- Avoid medicinal iron and iron-containing mineral supplements, breakfast cereals and other foods highly fortified with iron, and use of iron cookware.
- Avoid consuming vitamin C supplements or food sources rich in vitamin C with meals, and avoid supplements with excessive amounts of vitamin C, which can increase iron absorption.
- Choose foods rich in fiber and drink tea, coffee, or milk with meals, to reduce the absorption of iron from the meal.
- Avoid alcohol intake or consume alcohol in very limited amounts. Alcohol potentiates liver damage from hemachromatosis and increases the likelihood of cirrhosis and death.

SELECTED BIBLIOGRAPHY

Barton JC, et al.: Management of hemochromatosis. Hemochromatosis Management Working Group, *Ann Intern Med* 129:932, 1998.

Bernstein CN, Shanahan F: Critical appraisal of enteral nutrition as primary therapy in adults with Crohn's disease, *Am J Gastroenterol* 91:2075, 1996.

Corish C: Nutrition and liver disease, *Nutr Rev* 55:17, 1997.

Dieteman LA, Heizer WD: Nutritional issues in inflammatory bowel disease, *Gastroenterol Clin N Am* 27:435, 1998.

Erdman SH: Nutritional imperatives in cystic fibrosis therapy, *Pediatr Ann* 28:129, 1999.

Han PD, et al.: Nutrition and inflammatory bowel disease, *Gastroenterol Clin N Am* 28:423, 1999.

Huff C: Celiac disease: helping families adapt, *Gastroenterol Nurs* 20:79, 1997.

Jelalian E, et al.: Nutrition intervention for weight gain in cystic fibrosis: a meta analysis, *J Pediatr* 132:486, 1998.

LeLeiko NS, Walsh MJ: The role of glutamine, short-chain fatty acids, and nucleotides in intestinal adaptation in gastrointestinal disease, *Ped Clin N Am* 43:451, 1996.

Lykins TC, Stockwell J: Comprehensive modified diet simplifies nutrition management of adults with short-bowel syndrome, *J Am Dietet Assoc* 98:309, 1998.

McClave SA, Spain DA, Snider HL: Nutritional management in acute and chronic pancreatitis, *Gastroenterol Clin N Am* 27:421, 1998.

Nehra V: New clinical issues in celiac disease, *Gastroenterol Clin N Am* 27:453, 1998.

Scolapio JS, Fleming CR: Short bowel syndrome, *Gastroenterol Clin N Am* 27:467, 1998.

Thompson T: Do oats belong in a gluten-free diet? *J Am Dietet Assoc* 97:1413, 1997.

Cancer 13

It is estimated that at least one third of all cancers in western countries are related to nutrition and diet, and thus dietary changes are an important area for primary prevention. Chapter 1 describes in more detail the recommendations for a diet likely to be low in cancer risk, which can be summarized as follows:

- Maintain a desirable body weight.
- Eat a varied diet—foods not only contain a variety of nutrients with anticarcinogenic properties, such as antioxidants, but they also provide nonnutritive substances such as isoflavones, flavonoids, allylic sulfides (garlic), capsaicin, indoles, and protease inhibitors with anticarcinogenic activity. It is especially important to include a variety of fruits and vegetables daily and to include fiber-containing foods such as whole grains, legumes, fruits, and vegetables.
- Minimize total fat intake.
- Limit intake of alcoholic beverages, if consumed at all.
- Limit consumption of salt-cured, smoked, nitrite-preserved, and charbroiled food.

Once cancer has developed, it can have severe adverse effects on nutritional status. Not only does the cancerous tumor draw nutrients from the host, but also the treatment modalities and the psychologic impact of cancer can interfere with maintenance of adequate nutrition. This chapter focuses on nutritional care of the individual with cancer.

Pathophysiology

Cancerous tumors differ according to their site, size, cellular types, and metabolic effects. Some cancers can have very serious impacts on nutritional status, but these impacts are not strongly correlated with tumor size. **Cancer cachexia** is a severe form of malnutrition associated with a poor prognosis and characterized by anorexia, early satiety, weight loss, anemia, weakness, and muscle wasting. Metabolic alterations, including futile metabolic cycles, insulin resistance causing glucose intolerance, increased lipolysis or fat breakdown, and increased tissue protein turnover, contribute to the nutritional problems of people with cancer. Increased release of tumor necrosis factor and other cytokines may be responsible for these metabolic changes; however, most of the weight loss can be traced to reduced nutrient intake. Appetite may be impaired by altered neurotransmitter (serotonin) levels in the central nervous system or elevated levels of lactate produced by anaerobic metabolism, a method of metabolism favored by tumors. Other factors that can inhibit intake include psychologic stress and *dysgeusia* (distorted taste) or aversions to specific foods. About 70% of individuals with cancer experience food aversions, either because of the effects of the tumor itself or because of the effects of chemotherapy. Mucositis, impaired salivation, nausea, vomiting, loss of the senses of taste and smell, and diarrhea resulting from cancer therapies are all factors in reduced food intake.

Treatment

Surgery, radiation therapy, and chemotherapy are used alone or in combination in cancer treatment. Table 13-1 demonstrates some of the nutritional effects of cancer therapies. Poor nutritional status can interfere with cancer treatment. For example, it may be necessary to reduce the chemotherapy dosages or shorten the radiation therapy schedule for a malnourished person. A poorly nourished surgical patient is more likely to develop pneumonia, *wound dehiscence* (separation of the sides of a wound), or other postoperative complications.

Nutritional Care

The goals of nutritional care are: (1) to identify and prevent or correct nutritional deficiencies resulting from cancer or its therapies, and (2) to maintain or improve functional capacity and quality of life.

Assessment

Assessment is summarized in Table 13-2.

Text continued on p. 289

Table 13-1   Nutritional Effects of Cancer Therapy

Site of Resection	Surgery
	Effect on Nutrition
Tongue, mouth, jaw	Oral intake precluded (temporary)
Esophagus	Oral intake precluded (temporary); gastric stasis and fat malabsorption as a result of vagotomy
Stomach	Dumping syndrome; impaired absorption of vitamin B_{12} and iron
Pancreas (pancreatoduodenectomy)	Diabetes mellitus; impaired absorption of fat and fat-soluble vitamins, calcium, zinc, magnesium, and protein
Small bowel	Depends on extent of resection and portion of bowel involved (see Figure 1-5); lactose intolerance possible; ileal resection: impaired absorption of fat and fat-soluble vitamins, calcium, zinc, magnesium, and vitamin B_{12}; impaired absorption of bile salts with resulting diarrhea and loss of fluid and electrolytes. With massive resection, loss of all nutrients, weight loss, and dehydration occur unless adequate nutritional support is given promptly
Colon	Impaired absorption of water and electrolytes

Radiation Therapy

	Effect on Nutrition	
Site	Acute	Long Term*
Central nervous system	Anorexia, nausea, vomiting (occasionally)	
Head and neck	Xerostomia (dry mouth), mucositis, anorexia, hypogeusia ("mouth blindness")	Xerostomia, bony necrosis, dental caries, altered taste
Esophagus, lung	Dysphagia, sore throat	Esophageal stenosis
Upper abdomen	Anorexia; nausea, vomiting	Gastrointestinal (GI) ulcer
Whole abdomen	Nausea, vomiting; diarrhea; cramping	GI ulcer; diarrhea, malabsorption; chronic enteritis or colitis
Pelvis	Diarrhea	Diarrhea; chronic enteritis or colitis

Chemotherapy

Effect on Nutrition	Chemotherapeutic Agent
Anorexia, nausea, vomiting	BCNU, bleomycin, CCNU, carboplatin, cisplatin, cyclophosphamide, cytarabine (ARA-C), dacarbazine (DTIC), doxorubicin, estramustine phosphate sodium, etoposide (VP-16), floxuridine, fluorouracil, ifosfamide, mechlorethamine, mesna, methotrexate, mitotane, mitoxantrone, octreotide, plicamycin, procarbazine, vinblastine

*Long-term effects may occur within a few months after therapy or may appear years later.

Continued

Table 13-1   Nutritional Effects of Cancer Therapy—cont'd

| | Chemotherapy—cont'd |
Effect on Nutrition	Chemotherapeutic Agent
Mucositis (stomatitis, esophagitis, intestinal ulcerations)	Bleomycin, cytarabine (ARA-C), doxorubicin, floxuridine, fluorouracil, methotrexate, mitoxantrone, plicamycin, vinblastine
Diarrhea	Cytarabine (ARA-C), estramustine phosphate sodium, fluorouracil, mesna, mitotane, mitoxantrone, octreotide, plicamycin, vinblastine
Constipation/paralytic ileus	Vinblastine, vincristine
Hyperglycemia	Asparaginase, streptozocin; glucocorticoids

Table 13-2   Assessment in Cancer

Area of Concern	Significant Findings
Protein-Calorie Malnutrition (PCM)	*History* Poor intake of protein and kcal as a result of food aversions, anorexia, nausea, vomiting, dysgeusia, difficulty chewing or swallowing (especially meats), inadequate financial resources; increased needs as a result of infection, abscess or fistula; glucocorticoid treatment; impaired absorption caused by dumping syndrome, ileal or pancreatic resection, or lactose intolerance; weight loss, especially if >2% in 1 wk, >5% in 1 mo, >7.5% in 3 mo, >10% in 6 mo *Physical Examination* Muscle wasting; edema; delayed wound healing; diarrhea (↓ oncotic pressure in the gut); triceps skinfold or arm muscle circumference <5th percentile; weight <90% standard for height or BMI <18.5, or decline of weight and/or height by one or more percentile change (children) (see Appendix D) *Laboratory Analysis* ↓ Serum albumin, transferrin, or prealbumin; ↓ BUN; ↓ creatinine-height index; ↓ lymphocyte count

Continued

Table 13-2   Assessment in Cancer—cont'd

Area of Concern	Significant Findings
Vitamin Deficiencies	
A	*History*
	Poor intake (same reasons as listed for PCM); steatorrhea; ileal or pancreatic resection
	Physical Examination
	Dry, scaly skin; dry cornea; ↓ night vision
	Laboratory Analysis
	↓ Serum retinol
K	*History*
	Antibiotic usage
	Physical Examination
	Petechiae, ecchymoses
	Laboratory Analysis
	↓ Prothrombin time
C	*History*
	Poor intake of citrus and other fruits as a result of stomatitis, esophagitis, or anorexia
	Physical Examination
	Petechiae, ecchymoses; delayed wound healing
	Laboratory Analysis
	↓ Serum or lymphocyte ascorbic acid

Table 13-2   Assessment in Cancer—cont'd

Area of Concern	Significant Findings
Vitamin Deficiencies—cont'd	
Folic acid	*History*
	Poor intake of fruits, vegetables, and fortified foods caused by anorexia, nausea, vomiting, stomatitis, or esophagitis; methotrexate (a folic acid antagonist) treatment; alcohol abuse
	Physical Examination
	Pallor, glossitis
	Laboratory Analysis
	↓ Hgb, ↑ MCV, ↓ serum folate
Mineral/Electrolyte Deficiencies	
Iron (Fe)	*History*
	Poor intake as a result of aversions to or difficulty chewing/ swallowing meats, poultry, or fish; anorexia; nausea; vomiting; dysgeusia; increased losses from acute or chronic blood loss; decreased absorption caused by gastric resection
	Physical Examination
	Pallor, blue sclerae; koilonychia
	Laboratory Analysis
	↓ Hgb, Hct, MCV, MCH, MCHC; ↓ serum Fe or ferritin; ↑ serum transferrin or TIBC

Continued

Table 13-2   Assessment in Cancer—cont'd

Area of Concern	Significant Findings
Mineral/Electrolyte Deficiencies—cont'd	
Zinc (Zn)	*History*
	Poor intake caused by same factors as listed for Fe; increased losses caused by diarrhea or fistula drainage; impaired absorption as a result of pancreatic or small bowel resection
	Physical Examination
	Dysgeusia, hypogeusia; delayed wound healing; dermatitis
	Laboratory Analysis
	↓ Serum Zn
Calcium (Ca)	*History*
	Poor intake caused by lactose intolerance; decreased absorption caused by steatorrhea, pancreatic or small bowel resection
	Physical Examination
	Tingling of the ends of the fingers; muscle cramps
Potassium (K^+)	*History*
	Increased losses from vomiting or diarrhea
	Physical Examination
	Malaise, weakness
	Laboratory Analysis
	↓ Serum K^+

Table 13-2   Assessment in Cancer—cont'd

Area of Concern	Significant Findings
Mineral/Electrolyte Deficiencies—cont'd	
Magnesium (Mg)	*History*
	Poor intake as a result of alcoholism; increased losses/decreased absorption caused by prolonged vomiting, diarrhea, steatorrhea, fistula drainage, pancreatic or small bowel resection
	Physical Examination
	Tremor, hyperactive deep reflexes; disorientation
	Laboratory Analysis
	↓ Serum Mg

Intervention

Providing adequate nutrients to meet the individual's needs for maintenance and building of tissue

Energy needs

Adults with good nutritional status may need no more than 25 to 30 kcal/kg/day to maintain their weight. Undernourished individuals may need 35 kcal/kg/day or more. Children need adequate kcal to promote continued growth, generally no less than 1000 kcal plus 100 kcal/year of life.

Protein needs

Intake of 1.2 to 2 g/kg/day usually provides adequate amino acids for tissue synthesis, if carbohydrate and fat intake is sufficient so that dietary protein is not needed to meet energy needs.

Iron needs

Iron-deficiency anemia may occur as a result of blood loss or aversions to iron-containing foods. Poultry and fish may be acceptable to the individual with aversion to red meat, and green, leafy vegetables and whole-grain or enriched breads and cereals can provide additional iron. Cast iron cookware can be used to increase the iron content of food. Ferrous sulfate, a commonly used supplement, provides 60 mg of iron in a 300 mg tablet. Depending on the severity of the anemia, two to three doses per day may be needed. Milk, tea, or coffee should not be consumed with the supplement because they decrease iron absorption. Foods containing vitamin C improve iron absorption. Iron supplements often cause some gastrointestinal distress. Taking them with meals or just before bedtime may improve tolerance. If ferrous sulfate is poorly tolerated, then ferrous gluconate or another form of iron may be better accepted. Liquid iron supplements are available for individuals receiving tube feedings or those with difficulty swallowing tablets, but they should be sipped through a straw if taken orally because they are likely to cause dental staining if they have direct contact with the teeth. Supplementation continues until concentrations of serum ferritin, a storage form of iron, rise to normal.

Not all anemia in cancer patients is caused by iron deficiency. **Anemia of chronic disease** occurs in patients with some malignancies, as well as those with renal failure and other chronic illnesses. In this type of anemia, the bone marrow fails to produce adequate red blood cells, but iron stores may be normal. The anemia is often normocytic (normal-sized cells), rather than microcytic, as in iron deficiency (see Chapter 2). Iron therapy does not correct anemia of chronic disease. Serum ferritin levels help to distinguish between anemia of chronic disease and iron-deficiency anemia because serum ferritin is low in iron deficiency but may be high or in the high-normal range in anemia of chronic disease. If ferritin measurements do not provide clearcut separation between the two anemias (e.g., ferritin is low-normal), then measurement of iron stores in a bone marrow aspirate will distinguish between them.

Calcium needs

Lactose intolerance is a common result of the intestinal damage caused by radiation or chemotherapy. Calcium intake may be low when dairy products are avoided. Lactose-intolerant individuals may be able to use yogurt, cheese, cottage cheese, buttermilk, or milk treated with lactase enzyme. Other reliable calcium sources include calcium-fortified juices, tortillas, and foods prepared with milk, such as pancakes (see Figure 3-4). A supplement of 800 mg of calcium per day, e.g., calcium carbonate, calcium citrate, or calcium gluconate, can be used to replace milk products.

Zinc needs

Zinc is found in many of the same foods as iron, and food aversions can limit intake. Zinc needs during healing and *anabolism* (tissue building) are high. A supplement (15-30 mg) may be needed.

Promoting comfort and alleviating nutritional problems associated with cancer therapy

Box 13-1 summarizes problems often encountered during cancer therapy and approaches that may help alleviate them.

Nausea and vomiting are especially common during chemotherapy and can accompany radiation therapy. Medications to relieve nausea and vomiting promote comfort and help make adequate nutritional intake possible if they are given on a regularly scheduled basis or before mealtime.

Mucositis can affect any area of the GI tract, but involvement of the mouth and esophagus is especially troublesome during chemotherapy and radiation of the head and neck. Mouth pain greatly inhibits nutritional intake, and the ulcerations are susceptible to infection. Frequent rinsing of the mouth with saline has been shown to be as effective as antiseptic solutions (dilute hydrogen peroxide) in treating stomatitis. Viscous lidocaine is an effective anesthetic, but the patient must be very careful when using it to avoid inadvertently biting the numbed tissues or burning them with hot food. Magnesium hydroxide (milk of magnesia) rinses are soothing but can dry the mucosa. Other treatments that have been used to promote healing include sucralfate application, hydroxypropyl cellulose films used to form a barrier over lesions, and vitamin E. *Cryotherapy* (holding ice chips in the mouth) at the time of chemotherapy administration to cause vasoconstriction and reduce oral damage has shown promise in small trials. Capsaicin, from chili peppers, has had some success in both relief of pain and stimulation of the regrowth of the oral mucosa.

Food aversions can develop as a conditioned response in individuals suffering from nausea and vomiting caused by radiation or chemotherapy. For example, aversions to red gelatin have occurred in individuals receiving doxorubicin (Adriamycin), a red drug. Individualization of the diet through a process of trial and error appears to be the most successful way of dealing with food aversions.

Box 13-1   Common Nutritional Problems and Dietary
Suggestions for Individuals with Cancer

Nausea and Vomiting

Diet: Liquids and soft foods served cold: juices, carbonated
beverages, gelatin, fruits; dry, bland foods: toast, crackers,
plain bagels; tart foods and fluids: lemonade; serve small
amounts frequently

Supplements:* Glucose oligosaccharides, clear liquids such
as Resource Fruit Drink (Novartis)

Suggestions: Keep environment cool, well ventilated, free of
cooking odors; dry starchy foods (crackers, toast) before
rising can help prevent vomiting; liquids should be sipped
slowly; distraction, imagery, and relaxation techniques
may help; premedicate with antiemetics if appropriate; plan the medication schedule so that drugs with
high emetic potential are not given close to mealtime, if
possible; avoid serving favorite foods during nausea to
reduce the risk of developing aversions to them; avoid
coaxing or pressure to increase intake

Problem foods: Hot foods, fatty foods, foods with strong
odors, spicy foods

Anorexia

Diet: Regular foods served attractively, with variety in
texture and color; small, frequent feedings

Supplements: Glucose oligosaccharides and other modular
products; complete liquid supplements (allow the individual to taste several and select the one[s] preferred);
milk powder added to liquid milk, cereals, mashed
potatoes (if lactose tolerance not a problem); Lipomul
(Upjohn); tube feedings if necessary

Suggestions: Avoid offering beverages until individual has
finished eating, since fluids can be filling; encourage
physical activity; children may eat more if they are
involved in food preparation or if foods are decorated
(e.g., with decorating candies and chocolate chips) or
formed in interesting shapes (e.g., sandwiches cut with
cookie cutters)

Problem foods: Large meals can overwhelm the person and
suppress appetite

---

*See Tables 9-1 and 9-2 for listings of supplements.

Box 13-1   Common Nutritional Problems and Dietary Suggestions for Individuals with Cancer—cont'd

Mucositis (Stomatitis, Esophagitis)

Diet: Nonabrasive, soft foods served cold or at room temperature: sherbet, canned or soft, fresh, low-acid fruits, fruit ices, popsicles, custard, gelatin, ice cream, yogurt, cottage cheese, puddings, canned or cooked vegetables, eggs, sandwiches, cooked cereals (warm, not hot)

Supplements: Glucose oligosaccharides, complete liquid supplements

Suggestions: Rinse mouth often with saline, plain water, sodium bicarbonate solution (1 tsp baking soda/500 ml water), or hydrogen peroxide diluted to ⅙ strength; viscous lidocaine provides topical analgesia; but the patient must be careful in eating after using it because numbed tissues may inadvertently be bitten or burned by hot foods or beverages

Problem foods: Acidic fruits and juices such as citrus (evaluate vitamin C intake when citrus fruits are avoided); salty or spicy foods; hard or abrasive foods such as chips, pretzels, nuts, seeds; foods served hot

Dysphagia

Diet: Emphasize foods that form a semisolid bolus in the mouth (e.g., macaroni and cheese)

Supplements: Carbohydrate or protein modules added to foods, thickened liquid supplements (see Suggestions); pudding-type supplements such as Ensure pudding (Ross) or Sustacal pudding (Mead Johnson)

Suggestions: Thicken liquids with dry infant cereals, mashed potatoes, potato flakes, or cornstarch; use gravies and sauces to moisten meats and vegetables; if dysphagia is severe, consider tube feedings

Problem foods: Thin liquids such as water, tea, coffee; foods that are not uniform in consistency such as stews; dry foods such as overcooked meats, hard rolls, nuts; foods that stick to the palate, such as peanut butter and white bread; slippery foods such as gelatin

Continued

Box 13-1   Common Nutritional Problems and Dietary
Suggestions for Individuals with Cancer—cont'd

Xerostomia (Reduced Saliva Production)

Diet: Regular, moist foods: casseroles, gravies, sauces; encourage fluids, including popsicles, fruit ices, sherbet, gelatin, soups

Suggestions: Use good oral hygiene because dental caries is common when saliva production is insufficient to buffer acids produced by mouth bacteria; rinse mouth often with saline or mouthwash; use sugar-free candies and gum between meals to promote saliva flow; use artificial saliva if problem is severe

Problem foods: Breads, dry foods, sweet sticky foods, sugars in gum or candy

Hypogeusia ("Mouth Blindness")

Diet: Regular foods with strong flavors or seasonings and interesting textures

Supplements: Complete liquid supplements with added flavors if necessary

Problem foods: Bland foods

Dysgeusia (Altered Taste)

Diet: Regular foods; use trial and error to determine the most suitable foods

Supplements: Fruit-flavored supplements, glucose oligosaccharides

Problem foods: Coffee, chocolate, red meats, others (varies with the individual)

Diarrhea

Diet: Low-lactose, low-fat; increase fluids; emphasize starches

Supplements: Glucose oligosaccharides, lactose-free liquid supplements

Problem foods: Milk, cream soups, ice cream, fatty or fried foods

---

Box 13-1   Common Nutritional Problems and Dietary
Suggestions for Individuals with Cancer—cont'd

Constipation
Diet: High-fiber; at least 50 ml fluid per kg/day
Supplements: Bran, 2 tbsp/day

Neutropenia with Potential for Infection
Diet: Regular
Suggestions: Cook eggs, meats, poultry, and fish well; thoroughly wash fruits and vegetables to be eaten raw (after bone marrow transplant and in severe neutropenia, it is sometimes necessary to avoid raw foods altogether); avoid cross-contamination (e.g., carefully clean cutting boards used for trimming raw meat before using them to prepare raw vegetables); refrigerate cooked foods immediately after the meal; discard any leftovers within 3 days†
Supplements: Glucose oligosaccharides, canned supplements
Problem foods: Raw or undercooked eggs, meats, poultry, fish, shellfish (e.g., rare meats, sushi, homemade mayonnaise, raw oysters, key lime pie, and "royal" icing or other decorative icings and glazes unless they are known not to contain raw eggs)

---

†For further food safety information, see Appendix K.

Using appropriate nutrition support methods
Oral feedings

- *Indications:* Method of choice whenever feasible; requires bowel motility (presence of bowel sounds), ability to ingest food orally
- *Example of use:* Mild to moderate anorexia related to any type of tumor
- *Comments:* Supplements (modular components or complete formulas) can be used where regular foods are insufficient. See Tables 9-1 and 9-2 for suitable supplements. Oral intake is often insufficient for children and adults receiving intensive chemotherapy or abdominal radiation.

Enteral tube feedings

Nasogastric (NG), nasoduodenal or nasojejunal (ND/NJ), gastrostomy, or jejunostomy

- *Indications:* Inadequate oral intake, impaired digestion or absorption requiring an elemental diet, ND/NJ feedings are useful if delayed gastric emptying is present; requires adequate bowel motility, unobstructed lower gastrointestinal (GI) tract
- *Example of use:* Severe anorexia, oral or upper GI tumor preventing oral intake, short-bowel syndrome, pancreatic resection
- *Comments:* ND/NJ feedings may be tolerated by the nauseated patient who cannot tolerate feedings into the stomach, but the tubes are unlikely to stay in place during active vomiting

Total parenteral nutrition (TPN)

- *Indications:* GI obstruction preventing tube feeding; severely impaired digestion or absorption that prevents adequate enteral intake or causes dehydration, uncontrollable vomiting; need for "bowel rest" to promote healing or regeneration of the bowel
- *Example of use:* Severe short-bowel syndrome; jejunal or ileal obstruction; enterocutaneous fistula, where bowel rest may promote healing
- *Comments:* TPN is generally reserved for malnourished individuals, or those likely to become malnourished as a result of treatment, for whom an effective cancer therapy is available. Those individuals who are terminally ill and for whom no further treatment is contemplated do not receive much benefit from TPN.

Teaching

Principles of a nutritious diet

Encourage a high-energy, high-protein intake. Protein sources are listed in Table 11-4. Energy intake can be increased by following the suggestions in Box 13-2. Where regular foods are inadequate, commercial supplements may be needed. See Tables 9-1 and 9-2 for examples. Sweets and sugar are often distasteful to the individual with cancer. *Glucose oligosaccharides, glucose polymers,* or *corn syrup solids* are terms that refer to short chains of glucose molecules; they are less sweet than sugar and are not objectionable to most individuals. They can be added to beverages (except carbonated beverages) and foods such as cereals and applesauce to increase the energy content.

Box 13-2   Suggestions for Increasing Energy Intake

Use Fat Liberally Because It Is an Especially Concentrated Source of Energy.*

Salad dressings, cooking oils, mayonnaise, nuts, cream, sour cream, sauces, and gravies are some fat sources.

Butter or margarine provides 35 kcal/tsp. Add them to hot foods such as soup, vegetables, mashed potatoes, cooked cereals, and rice. Serve hot bread because more butter is used when it melts into the bread.

Peanut butter is high in fat, providing 90 kcal/tbsp. It can be served on crackers, apple or pear slices, bananas, or celery.

Serve Small Meals Frequently.
Keep Snacks Available at All Times.

Nuts, dried fruits, bagels or muffins, cookies, crackers and cheese, granola, ice cream or sherbet, yogurt or frozen yogurt, milkshakes made with ice cream, and puddings are good energy sources.

Prepare Foods in a Manner That Will Make Them as Energy-Dense as Possible.

Soups, hot cereals, cocoa from a mix, and instant puddings can be prepared with whole milk or half and half, rather than water.

Sauces can be added to cooked vegetables and pastas. Alfredo sauce, prepared with cream, contains more energy than tomato-based pasta sauces.

Do Not Allow Foods of Low Caloric Density To Displace More Concentrated Energy Sources.

Beverage consumption is best delayed until after, rather than before or during, meals. Low-calorie or no-calorie beverages (artificially sweetened drinks, unsweetened tea or coffee, water) should be avoided as much as possible. Glucose oligosaccharides (also called corn syrup solids and glucose polymers) can be added to tea, coffee, or juices (see Table 9-1).

Raw vegetables and salads should be served only at the end of the meal, or energy-dense foods (cheese, egg, poultry, meat, beans, salad dressing) should be added liberally.

---

*Individuals with malabsorption and steatorrhea may not tolerate increased fat intake. MCT oil (see Chapter 9) is one potential source of energy.

Promoting comfort and relieving side effects of therapy

See Box 13-1 for suggestions for coping with side effects of therapy.

Monitoring the patient's nutritional status regularly

The patient should weigh at least weekly while at home. Progressive weight loss should be reported to the health care team so that appropriate interventions can be planned. The patient or family may need to keep daily records of intake. They can be provided with lists showing the nutritional contributions of common foods to ensure that the daily intake meets the goal.

Home tube feeding or TPN

Many individuals find it impossible to maintain their weight and nutritional status without aggressive nutrition support. Home tube feeding or TPN is often appropriate for those receiving long-term therapy. Chapters 9 and 10 describe procedures for safe delivery of nutrition support.

SELECTED BIBLIOGRAPHY

Ford ES: Body mass index and colon cancer in a national sample of adult US men and women. *Am J Epidemiol* 150:390, 1999.

Holmes S: Nutrition in patients undergoing radiotherapy, *Prof Nurse* 12:789, 1997.

Hunter AN: Nutrition management of patients with neoplastic disease of the head and neck treated with radiation therapy, *Nutr Clin Pract* 11:157, 1996.

Kalman D, Villani LJ: Nutritional aspects of cancer-related fatigue, *J Am Dietet Assoc* 97:650, 1997.

Kennedy L, Diamond J: Assessment and management of chemotherapy-induced mucositis in children, *J Pediatr Oncol Nurs* 14:164, 1997.

Shike M: Nutrition therapy for the cancer patient, *Hematol–Oncol Clin N Am* 10:221, 1996.

Skolin I, et al.: Nutrient intake and weight development in children during chemotherapy for malignant disease, *Oral Oncol* 33:364, 1997.

Van Eys J: Benefits of nutritional intervention on nutritional status, quality of life and survival. *Int J Cancer Suppl* 11:66, 1998.

Weitzman S: Alternative nutritional cancer therapies, *Int J Cancer Suppl* 11:69, 1998.

Wilkes JD: Prevention and treatment of oral mucositis following cancer chemotherapy, *Sem Oncol* 25:538, 1998.

HIV Infection

14

Individuals infected with the human immunodeficiency virus (HIV) display a variety of responses, ranging from asymptomatic infection to acquired immunodeficiency syndrome (AIDS).

Pathophysiology

The retrovirus HIV selectively targets lymphocytes bearing the CD4 cell marker. Using the DNA from the host CD4 cell and the reverse transcriptase enzyme, HIV is able to replicate itself and create an inactive provirus. The provirus is activated by protease in the cell nucleus, and the resulting mature, infectious virus is able to bud from the CD4 cell into the plasma, where it can infect other CD4 cells.

The infected individual is susceptible to opportunistic infections and cancers such as Kaposi's sarcoma and non-Hodgkin's lymphoma. Weight loss and malnutrition are common, even in the early stages of the infection, and 80% or more of individuals with AIDS report unintentional weight loss. Malnutrition can decrease functional capacity, contribute to immune dysfunction, and increase the morbidity associated with the disease. Multiple factors are responsible for the nutritional impairments associated with HIV infection. Respiratory infections, such as *Pneumocystis carinii* pneumonia, cause anorexia, dyspnea, fever, and increased needs for protein, energy, and vitamins. Diarrhea is a common finding, occurring as a result of gastrointestinal (GI) pathogens, including fungi, viruses, bacteria, and protozoans; medications used; or enteropathy caused by HIV itself. Central nervous system (CNS) infections caused by HIV or by opportunistic organisms cause confusion, dementia, and impaired coordination, which interfere with food intake. Medications may impair food intake or absorption, and depression can result in anorexia. Finally, some investigations, but not all, have found resting energy expenditure (and thus caloric needs) to be increased in stable individuals infected with HIV.

Treatment

Three types of antiretroviral agents have been approved by the Food and Drug Administration (FDA) for HIV treatment: (1) nucleoside-analog reverse transcriptase inhibitors (zidovudine [AZT], didanosine, zalcitabine, stavudine, and lamivudine), (2) nonnucleoside reverse transcriptase inhibitors (nevirapine and delavirdine), and (3) protease inhibitors (saquinavir, ritonavir, indinavir, and nelfinavir). Combination therapy is common, making the patient vulnerable to a variety of medication side effects and drug-nutrient or drug-drug interactions. Secondary infections require the use of appropriate antibiotic agents, and, when applicable, patients also receive cancer therapy (see Chapter 13). The side effects of commonly used medications include anorexia, nausea and vomiting, mucosal lesions, and diarrhea (Table 14-1).

Nutritional Care

Nutritional care of the person with HIV infection focuses on identifying and correcting, if possible, nutritional deficits that might weaken the individual, exacerbate immune dysfunctions, or impair quality of life.

Several pharmacologic agents to improve nutritional status are in clinical use or are undergoing experimental evaluation. Dronabinol, a marijuana derivative, and megestrol acetate, a progesterone-like drug, are approved for treatment of anorexia. These agents have been successful in promoting weight gain in some HIV-infected individuals. In some studies, however, it appears that much of the weight gained by adults has been fat rather than lean body tissue. Children have been found to gain weight without growing in height when taking megesterol acetate. Human growth factor, insulin-like growth factor-I, and the anabolic steroid oxandrolone have been used experimentally and have shown promise in increasing lean body mass. The most common endocrine abnormality in HIV infection is low testosterone levels, and supplemental testosterone may also increase lean body mass.

Serum levels of several micronutrients have been reported to be low in individuals with HIV infection. These include zinc,

Table 14-1   Nutritional Impacts of Some Drugs Commonly Prescribed for Persons with HIV Infection

	Side Effect					
Drug	Nausea/ Vomiting	Diarrhea	Abdominal Pain	Sore Mouth/ Throat*	Dry Mouth/ Unpleasant Taste	Anorexia
AIDS Chemotherapeutic Agents						
Didanosine	X	X	X			
Indinavir	X	X	X		X	
Lamivudine		X	X			X
Nelfinavir		X				
Ritonavir	X	X	X		X	
Saquinavir	X	X	X			
Stavudine	X	X				X
Zalcitabine	X			X		
Zidovudine	X					
Antifungal Agents						
Amphotericin B	X	X	X			X
Fluconazole	X	X	X			
Ketoconazole	X					X
Nystatin	X	X				

*Esophagitis, glossitis, or oral mucosal lesions.

Continued

Table 14-1   Nutritional Impacts of Some Drugs Commonly Prescribed for Persons with HIV Infection—cont'd

	Side Effect					
Drug	Nausea/Vomiting	Diarrhea	Abdominal Pain	Sore Mouth/Throat*	Dry Mouth/Unpleasant Taste	Anorexia
Antibacterial and Antiprotozoal Agents						
Atovaquone	X	X	X			
Clindamycin	X	X	X	X		
Pentamidine						
IV or IM	X				X	X
Inhalable	X			X	X	X
Rifabutin	X				X	
Trimethoprim-sulfamethoxazole	X	X	X	X		X
Antiviral and Antitumor Agents						
Acyclovir	X	X	X			
Foscarnet	X	X	X			X
Interferon alfa-2	X	X	X	X	X	X
Valacyclovir	X	X				
Vidarabine	X	X				

*Esophagitis, glossitis, or oral mucosal lesions.

magnesium, total carotenes, folic acid, and vitamins B_{12}, B_6, A, and E. Vitamin A deficiency reportedly increases the likelihood of transmission of HIV from the pregnant woman to her fetus.

Assessment

Nutrition assessment is summarized in Table 14-2.

Intervention

Encouraging adequate intake to meet nutrient requirements

Energy (kcal) needs can be estimated by using Table 11-3 (if indirect calorimetry is not available to measure kcal needs). A high-protein diet (> 1.5 g/kg/day) provides the amino acids needed for tissue synthesis. Diarrhea may improve if a low-fat, high-starch diet is followed. Medium-chain triglycerides may be added to the diet if additional calories are needed. Lactose intolerance is common in individuals with HIV infection. Yogurt and hard cheeses are usually better tolerated than liquid milk in lactose intolerance, and milk treated with lactase enzyme to break down the lactose is available commercially. Lactose-free products should be chosen if oral supplements or enteral tube feedings are used (see Table 9-1).

A daily multivitamin and mineral supplement that supplies 100% of the Daily Value for each nutrient is commonly recommended. Some treatment centers also recommend increased supplementation with vitamins C, B_{12}, B_6, and E, as well as zinc, selenium, and beta carotene. The impact of potential drug-nutrient interactions (see Appendix H) must be considered, especially if the individual is taking several drugs, and supplementation regimens must be adjusted accordingly.

Promoting comfort and coping with complications of the infection and therapy

Many of the disease- and drug-related symptoms (anorexia, nausea and vomiting, stomatitis and esophagitis, dysphagia, neutropenia, diarrhea) are similar to those in the person with cancer. Interventions for these problems are summarized in Box 13-1. Antiretroviral therapies can also cause other potentially serious side effects, and individuals taking these drugs must be closely monitored for complications. Protease inhibitors have been associated with new-onset diabetes. Patients taking protease inhibitors must be regularly screened for hyperglycemia and instructed in diabetic care

Table 14-2   Nutrition Assessment of the HIV-Infected Individual

Area of Concern	Significant Findings
Protein-Calorie Malnutrition (PCM)	*History* Nutrient losses caused by diarrhea, malabsorption (from AIDS enteropathy, GI infections, medications), vomiting; increased needs because of infection and fever; poor intake caused by anorexia (related to respiratory or other infections, depression, medications), oral and esophageal pain (e.g., *Candida* or herpes esophagitis, endotracheal Kaposi's sarcoma), dyspnea, dysphagia, dysgeusia related to medication use or zinc deficiency, dementia, or CNS infections *Physical Examination* Recent weight loss; weight <90% of desirable or BMI <18.5, or decline in percentiles for height or weight on growth chart for children; wasting of muscle and subcutaneous tissue; triceps skinfold or AMC <5th percentile *Laboratory Analysis* ↓ Serum albumin, transferrin, or prealbumin; negative nitrogen balance; ↓ creatinine-height index NOTE: Lymphocyte count is likely to be of little value in nutrition assessment.
Mineral Deficiencies	
Iron (Fe)	*History* Poor intake (same causes as PCM); increased losses or impaired utilization caused by medications such as pentamidine, amphotericin B, foscarnet *Physical Examination* Pallor, koilonychia, fatigue, tachycardia *Laboratory Analysis* ↓ Hct, Hgb, MCV, MCH, MCHC, ferritin

Table 14-2   Nutrition Assessment of the HIV-Infected
Individual—cont'd

Area of Concern	Significant Findings
Mineral Deficiencies—cont'd	
Zinc (Zn)	*History*
	Poor intake (same reasons as PCM); impaired absorption in diarrhea
	Physical Examination
	Hypogeusia, dysgeusia, alopecia, dermatitis, diarrhea
	Laboratory Analysis
	↓ Serum Zn
Selenium (Se)	*History*
	Poor intake of meats, fish, poultry (same reasons as PCM); impaired absorption in diarrhea
	Physical Examination
	Congestive cardiomyopathy, muscle weakness, pallor, fatigue, tachycardia
	Laboratory Analysis
	↓ Serum Se; ↓ Hct, ↑ nucleated RBC, Howell-Jolly bodies, Heinz bodies (hemolytic anemia resulting from fragility of the RBC membrane)
Vitamin Deficiencies	
A	*History*
	Decreased absorption as a result of diarrhea; poor intake because of anorexia, nausea, vomiting
	Physical Examination
	Drying of skin and cornea; papular eruption around hair follicles

Continued

Table 14-2   Nutrition Assessment of the HIV-Infected
Individual—cont'd

Area of Concern	Significant Findings
Vitamin Deficiencies—cont'd	
A—cont'd	*Laboratory Analysis*
	↓ Serum retinol; ↓ retinol-binding protein (indicating PCM, with inadequate protein to manufacture carrier for vitamin A)
B_{12}	*History*
	Poor intake because of poverty, difficulty chewing protein foods, anorexia; impaired absorption in diarrhea
	Physical Examination
	Pallor, glossitis, fatigue, paresthesias
	Laboratory Analysis
	↓ Hct; ↑ MCV; ↓ serum vitamin B_{12}; abnormal Schilling test
Folic Acid	*History*
	Poor intake of fruits and vegetables because of mouth soreness, unconventional diet, poverty, anorexia; impaired absorption because of trimethoprim-sulfamethoxazole or pentamidine use
	Physical Examination
	Pallor, glossitis, fatigue
	Laboratory Analysis
	↓ Hct; ↑ MCV; ↓ serum or RBC folic acid

(see Chapter 18) if this complication occurs. Indinavir increases the risk of *renal lithiasis* (kidney stones). Adults taking this drug must consume at least 1500 ml fluid daily to reduce the risk. Didanosine is available in powdered or tablet form. One single-dose (250 mg) packet supplies 1380 mg sodium, a consideration for the patient needing a sodium-restricted diet. Each 200 mg tablet contains 36.5 mg phenylalanine, which must be considered if the individual has phenylketonuria (PKU).

If appetite stimulants (dronabinol, megestrol acetate, or cyprohepatadine) are used, then the patient should take them about 30 minutes before meals (usually twice daily). Acute episodes of diarrhea may be better controlled if antidiarrheals are administered on a routine schedule rather than after diarrhea occurs. Antiemetic medications (if ordered) should be scheduled to be taken before mealtimes.

In dyspneic individuals (e.g., those with pulmonary infections), small, frequent meals are usually best tolerated, and foods of high caloric density (cheese, meats, biscuits, muffins, etc.) are preferred over foods with low caloric density (green leafy vegetables, no- or low-calorie beverages, etc.). If oxygen is needed, use of a nasal cannula during meals often improves eating ability.

Individuals with dementia or neurologic dysfunction may need to be reminded and encouraged to eat. Occupational therapists can assist in evaluating patients with motor problems and selecting special eating utensils that can improve their ability to feed themselves. Those who cannot feed themselves should be fed in a calm, unhurried manner, with family members or friends being involved whenever possible.

Providing enteral and parenteral feedings in a safe and effective manner

For some patients who cannot consume or absorb enough nutrients administered orally, enteral or parenteral (TPN) feedings will be necessary. The enteral route is preferred whenever possible because it is less likely to be associated with septic complications, more economical, and possibly more effective in maintaining normal GI mucosa, an important barrier to infection. TPN may be necessary if the GI tract is nonfunctional or the caloric requirements are so high that they cannot be met entirely via the enteral route. Careful attention to infection control measures is important during both enteral and parenteral feedings (as is the case in all patients, not just those with HIV infection; see Chapters 9 and 10).

Individuals with malabsorption usually tolerate enteral tube feedings better if they are given continuously or slowly delivered intermittently rather than as bolus feedings. Formulas that are low in total fat or those in which a substantial portion of the fat is in the form of medium-chain triglycerides (MCTs) are likely to be better absorbed than formulas that are rich in long-chain triglycerides (see Table 9-1). Where oral or esophageal infections are present, the patient may be unable to tolerate a nasogastric, nasoduodenal, or nasojejunal tube. Gastrostomy or jejunostomy feedings may be more appropriate.

Teaching

Principles of a good diet

Optimal nutrition will help to maintain functional capacity, improve quality of life, and improve tolerance of treatment. Many individuals infected with HIV are extremely interested in nutrition and its potential benefits in controlling disease, and it is possible to build on this interest in teaching about diet. The Food Group Plan in Chapter 1 can be used as a guide.

With the increased use of multidrug therapy including protease inhibitors, particularly in the early stages of HIV infection, some individuals are experiencing weight gain. Unfortunately, these gains are not in lean body mass but instead are accounted for by fat deposits (lipodystrophy), primarily in the trunk. This creates body image disturbances for some patients and may cause them to discontinue the medication. An increase in the level of physical activity, e.g., aerobic exercise and weight training at least 3 to 5 times per week, can help to control weight gain. Avoiding high-fat foods and high-calorie foods that are low in nutritional value can also help to alleviate the problem. Metabolic changes (hyperglycemia, elevated insulin levels, and high serum triglyceride levels) are associated with the lipodystrophy. Patients with hyperglycemia and hyperinsulinemia may benefit from a diet similar to that recommended in diabetes (see Chapter 18). Measures to reduce hypertriglyceridemia include limiting intake of simple carbohydrates and alcohol (see Chapter 15). Alcohol should preferably be avoided altogether or used only occasionally; in no case should more than two drinks be consumed daily.

Complementary and alternative therapies for HIV

Use of **complementary** and **alternative medical (CAM) therapies** is very common among individuals with HIV. Health care providers need to familiarize themselves with the types of therapies being used in order to evaluate them and give informed advice. Many CAM treatments have not been evaluated in large-scale trials, and therefore their risks and benefits are not fully known. Brief descriptions of some popular CAM therapies follow (Freeman and McIntyre, 1999):

- *Vitamin and/or other micronutrient supplements:* Most studies have been short-term and have shown no effect on lymphocyte markers. Vitamin A and beta carotene supplementation are being studied for their effects on reducing perinatal transmission of HIV. In a group of 281 HIV-infected individuals followed for 8 years, being in the quartile with the highest intakes of B vitamins and carotene was a predictor of survival. Chronic vitamin A intakes >50,000 IU/day can be toxic and should be avoided.
- *Exercise:* Some short-term studies have found a trend toward an increase in natural killer activity and CD4 counts with regular exercise. Exercise may also stabilize or increase lean body mass. Weight training, or a combination of aerobic exercise and weight training, appear to be more effective than aerobics alone.
- *Massage:* In small trials, massage does not appear to have any consistent benefit on markers of disease progression, but it has been effective in stress relief.
- *Chinese herbs and acupuncture:* Several Chinese herbs are used, with or without acupuncture. These therapies have afforded symptom relief to some patients. Indications suggest that ginseng may strengthen the immune system, possibly increasing resistance to infection and reducing the risk of cancer. Ginseng is undergoing further study (Yun and Choi, 1998).
- *Other herbal treatments:* Echinacea (coneflower) is reported to enhance immune function. Thus far it has shown little benefit in prevention of respiratory infections, but further studies continue.

Safe handling practices for food

Infection with foodborne organisms is 20 to 300 times more common in individuals with HIV than in the general public, and these infections are more likely to lead to sepsis and other severe complications in HIV-infected patients. Teach individuals with HIV and their caregivers to choose, prepare, and store foods carefully. Appendix K summarizes important food safety guidelines. Food safety information specifically prepared for the individual with AIDS is also available from the FDA Center for Food Safety and Nutrition website (www.cfsan.fda.gov) and the food information hotline (800-FDA-4010).

SELECTED BIBLIOGRAPHY

Clarick RH, et al.: Megestrol acetate treatment of growth failure in children infected with human immunodeficiency virus, *Pediatrics* 99:354, 1997.

Freeman EM, MacIntyre RC: Evaluating alternative treatments for HIV infection, *Nurs Clin N Am* 34:147, 1999.

Kotler DP: Human immunodeficiency virus-related wasting: malabsorption syndromes, *Sem Oncol* 25 (suppl 6):70, 1998.

Melchart D, et al.: Echinacea root extracts for the prevention of upper respiratory tract infections: a double-blind, placebo-controlled randomized trial, *Arch Fam Med* 7:541, 1998.

Rabeneck L, et al.: A randomized controlled trial evaluating nutrition counseling with or without oral supplementation in malnourished HIV-infected patients, *J Am Dietet Assoc* 98:434, 1998.

Salomon SB, et al.: An elemental diet containing medium-chain triglycerides and enzymatically hydrolyzed protein can improve gastrointestinal tolerance in people infected with HIV, *J Am Dietet Assoc* 98:460, 1998.

Silva M, et al.: The effect of protease inhibitors on weight and body composition in HIV-infected patients, *AIDS* 12:1645, 1998.

Walsek C, Zafonte M, Bowers JM: Nutritional issues and HIV/AIDS: assessment and treatment strategies, *J Assoc Nurs AIDS Care* 8:71, 1997.

Yanovski JA, et al.: Endocrine and metabolic evaluation of human immunodeficiency virus-infected patients with evidence of protease inhibitor-associated lipodystrophy, *J Clin Endocrinol Metab* 84:1925, 1999.

Yun TK, Choi SY: Non-organ specific cancer prevention of ginseng: a prospective study in Korea, *Int J Epidemiol* 27:359, 1998.

Heart Disease

15

Heart disease, the leading cause of death in the United States, encompasses a variety of conditions, including atherosclerosis, hypertension, and congestive heart failure.

Coronary Heart Disease
Pathophysiology

Coronary heart disease (CHD) occurs when plaques containing lipoproteins, cholesterol, tissue debris, and calcium form on the intima, or interior surface of blood vessels. The plaques roughen the intima, and platelets are attracted to the roughened areas, forming clots. When the plaques enlarge sufficiently to occlude the blood flow, tissues distal to the occlusion are deprived of oxygen and nutrients, creating an area of infarct. CHD is manifested when a myocardial infarction (MI) occurs or when myocardial ischemia is present, causing the painful disorder known as angina pectoris.

High serum cholesterol levels are a risk factor for CHD. Serum cholesterol is carried by several **lipoproteins** classified by their density. In order of increasing density, the lipoproteins are **chylomicrons, very low-density lipoproteins (VLDLs), low-density lipoproteins (LDLs),** and **high-density lipoproteins (HDLs).** LDLs carry the most cholesterol and are the most atherogenic. HDLs reduce the risk from CHD by transporting cholesterol from the tissues to the liver, where it is metabolized and excreted. Adults can be classified as at risk for CHD on the basis of serum lipid levels (Table 15-1).

In addition to LDL-cholesterol, other factors increase the risk of CHD: (1) age (>45 years in men and >55 years in women, or premature menopause without estrogen replacement therapy), (2) CHD before age 55 in the father or another first-degree male relative or before age 65 in the mother or another first-degree female relative, (3) smoking, (4) blood pressure >140/90 mmHg or

Table 15-1   Classification of Serum Lipid Levels

Classification	Serum Cholesterol (mg/dl)
Total Cholesterol	
Desirable	<200
Borderline-high risk	200-239
High risk	≥240
LDL-Cholesterol*	
Desirable	<130
Borderline-high risk	130-159
High risk	≥160
HDL-Cholesterol	
Low	<35
Triglycerides	
Normal	<200
Borderline-high	200-400
High	400-1000
Very high	>1000

Adapted from National Cholesterol Education Program: *Second Report of the Expert Panel on Detection, Evaluation, and Treatment of High Blood Cholesterol in Adults (ATP II),* NIH Pub No 93-3095, Washington, DC, 1993, US Department of Health and Human Services.

*Not routinely measured but can be calculated by using the following equation: LDL-cholesterol = total cholesterol − HDL-cholesterol − (triglycerides/5)

need for antihypertensive medication, (5) HDL-cholesterol concentration below 35 mg/dl, and (6) diabetes mellitus. The presence of two or more of these factors places the individual at high risk. An HDL-cholesterol >60 mg/dl, on the other hand, is a "negative risk factor." If high HDL-cholesterol is present, then one risk factor can be deducted from the individual's score.

Prevention and Treatment

It can be difficult to determine which people are at risk for heart disease and which individuals will later develop significant risk factors. Therefore, to reduce the heart risk of the general population, the National Cholesterol Education Program has recommended that all adults in the United States follow a diet that includes no more than 30% of total kcal as fat, 8% to 10% of total kcal from saturated fat, and 300 mg of cholesterol daily.

Nutrition therapy is also appropriate for all individuals with CHD, because changes in nutrient intake can help to control serum lipid levels. Drug therapy may also be required to reach lipid goals, however. Commonly used drugs are the bile acid sequestrants cholestyramine and colestipol; nicotinic acid, which lowers total and LDL-cholesterol, as well as triglycerides; statins that inhibit cholesterol synthesis; fibric acid derivatives such as gemfibrozil and clofibrate, which reduce triglycerides and raise HDL-cholesterol; and probucol, which reduces LDL-cholesterol and HDL-cholesterol.

Nutritional Care

Goals of nutritional care are to reduce the risk of CHD in the general population and especially in individuals with elevated LDL-cholesterol levels by achieving the following:

■ Reduce LDL-cholesterol levels below 130 mg/dl in individuals with definite CHD or two CHD risk factors other than high-risk levels of LDL-cholesterol.
■ Reduce LDL-cholesterol levels below 160 mg/dl in individuals with neither definite CHD nor two risk factors other than high levels of LDL-cholesterol.

Assessment

Assessment is summarized in Table 15-2.

Intervention

Reducing risk factors for CHD

If individuals are found to have elevated LDL-cholesterol or other risk factors for CHD, and they are not already following a dietary plan similar to the **Step-One Diet** (Table 15-3), which is similar to the diet plan recommended by the American Heart Association for all adults, then this diet would be the initial medical nutrition therapy for them.

Step-One reduces the most common and obvious sources of saturated fatty acids and cholesterol in the diet and can be implemented without drastic diet or lifestyle changes for most individuals. Total fat intake is limited, in addition to limitations on saturated fat and cholesterol, to aid in weight reduction. The

Table 15-2   Assessment in Heart Disease

Areas of Concern	Significant Findings
Overweight	*History* Excessive kcal intake; sedentary lifestyle *Physical Examination* Wt >120% of ideal or BMI >25; triceps skinfold >95th percentile for age and sex
Underweight (Seen Primarily in Congestive Heart Failure)	*History* Poor intake because of dyspnea or fatigue; impaired absorption because of inadequate bowel perfusion; increased kcal needs if dyspneic or suffering from concomitant infection *Physical Examination* Wt <90% of ideal or BMI <18.5 or height or weight <5th percentile for age (children); triceps skinfold <5th percentile for age and sex
Elevated Serum Lipid Levels	*History* Daily use of foods high in saturated fat and cholesterol; sedentary lifestyle; family history of hyperlipidemia; cultural food pattern that emphasizes foods high in fat or cholesterol; diabetes *Physical Examination* Xanthomas, or yellowish plaques deposited on the skin (not found in the majority of the individuals) *Laboratory Analysis* ↑ Total serum cholesterol; HDL <35 mg/dl; LDL >130 mg/dl

Table 15-2   Assessment in Heart Disease—cont'd

Areas of Concern	Significant Findings
Elevated Blood Pressure	*History* Daily use of high-sodium foods and salt at the table; psychosocial stress; family history of hypertension; cultural food patterns emphasizing foods high in sodium; obesity; excessive alcohol intake; diabetes *Physical Examination* Edema; elevated blood pressure

Table 15-3   Diet Therapy for High Blood Cholesterol*

Diet Component	Recommended Intake	
	Step-One Diet	Step-Two Diet
Energy	Adequate to achieve or maintain desirable weight	
Protein	Approximately 15%	
Carbohydrate	≥55%	
Total fat	≤30%	
Saturated fat	8-10%	≤7%
Polyunsaturated fat	≤10%	
Monounsaturated fat	Up to 15%	
Cholesterol (mg/day)	300	200

Adapted from National Cholesterol Education Program: *Second Report of the Expert Panel on Detection, Evaluation, and Treatment of High Blood Cholesterol in Adults (ATP II).* NIH Pub No 93-3095, Washington, DC, 1993, US Department of Health and Human Services.
*All values except those for cholesterol are expressed as percentage of total energy intake.

physician and nurse can often provide education regarding the Step-One Diet. The diet instruction should not consist merely of handing out a list of foods allowed and those not allowed, however (see Teaching, below). Referral to a dietitian is helpful for people who have difficulty adhering to the diet or who have a disappointing response to the diet (i.e., no improvement in risk factors for CHD after following the diet for 3 months).

The **Step-Two Diet** (see Table 15-3) is designed for individuals who do not succeed in lowering LDL-cholesterol to the desirable level after adhering to the Step-One Diet for 3 months. Instruction and follow-up by the dietitian are important for those needing the Step-Two Diet.

Facilitating cardiac rest in the individual with an acute myocardial infarction

If the person with CHD experiences an acute MI, then efforts are made to avoid stressing the heart as much as possible during the early recovery period. Common diet modifications include the following:

- A low-kcal (1200 to 1500) diet is used to avoid the metabolic stress caused by larger intakes and to begin promoting weight loss.
- Large meals (more than 600 to 700 kcal) are avoided because they increase heart rate and stroke volume.
- A diet low in saturated fat and cholesterol is used to promote lowering of serum cholesterol and to introduce the individual to appropriate dietary changes.
- A moderate sodium restriction (2 to 3 g) is followed to control any tendency for edema and congestive heart failure to develop.
- Ice water and very cold foods are generally avoided. A subset of individuals have electrocardiographic changes after drinking ice water, although most seem to tolerate it well.

Teaching

Recognizing the need to make permanent diet and lifestyle changes to reduce risk

Necessary changes to reduce LDL-cholesterol and increase HDL-cholesterol include achieving weight control, decreasing dietary fat and cholesterol, increasing physical activity, ceasing smoking (if applicable), and developing constructive ways of coping with stress. Instruction begins with a thorough assessment of the individual's lifestyle, particularly activity and eating patterns. The assessment should reveal information about habitual use of foods high in cholesterol and fat, frequency of eating out and kinds of restaurant meals consumed, and the type, frequency, and amount of physical activity. Teaching includes the rationale for making dietary changes, goal setting, appropriate food choices and preparation methods, tips for eating out, and development of a plan for increasing physical activity. The patient should be actively involved in all planning and goal setting. Changes may be better accepted and less overwhelming if people are counseled to make them gradually. For example, the transition from whole milk to skim milk may be easier if the individual first changes to 2% milk, and later to skim milk. Changes do not have to result in a restrictive or unpalatable diet. Tasty, attractive dishes can be readily prepared within the guidelines (Table 15-4).

Individuals who stop smoking may gain 2.5 to 9 kg (5 to 20 lb), both because cigarettes have appetite-suppressing effects and because people may substitute eating for smoking during the stressful time of giving up cigarettes. Smoking cessation produces more immediate benefits for CHD risk than dietary changes, so it is best to focus first on smoking cessation. If the individual tries to make too many lifestyle alterations at once, he or she may become frustrated and fail at all of them.

Reducing fat and cholesterol intake

Table 15-5 provides specific information about foods to include and to decrease in the meal plan, and additional details are provided as follows.

Meats. Meats can be a significant source of fat and cholesterol.

- Eat no more than 6 oz (the size of two decks of cards) of lean meat, chicken, turkey, and fish daily. Combine small amounts of meat with larger amounts of rice, pasta, or vegetables to make more filling entrees. Replace meat entrees with dried beans and peas or tofu several times per week. Legumes and soy products are low-fat, high-protein, and cholesterol-free.
- Choose lean cuts of meat such as: extra-lean ground beef, sirloin tip, round steak, rump roast, arm roast or center-cut ham, loin chops, and tenderloin.
- Trim away all visible fat before cooking meats, and pour off fat after browning. Remove the skin and underlying fat from poultry before or after cooking.
- Use organ meats, including brains, liver, heart, kidney, and sweet-breads, rarely because they are especially high in cholesterol.

Table 15-4 Dietary Changes to Reduce Risk of Heart Disease

Previous Intake	Revised Intake
Breakfast	**Breakfast**
Doughnut	Shredded wheat (Fi, F)*
Orange juice	Sliced strawberries (Fi)
Coffee	Coffee
Nondairy creamer	Skim milk (F)
Lunch	**Lunch**
Quarter-pound hamburger	Salad of lettuce, spinach, green pepper, and garbanzo beans with low-kcal dressing (F, C, Fi, Na)
French fries, salted	Unsalted whole wheat crackers (Fi, F, Na)
Soft drink	Diet soft drink
Fried fruit pie	Fresh pears (F, Fi, Na)
Dinner	**Dinner**
Prime rib	Curried chicken, without salt (F, Na)
Baked potato with sour cream	Brown rice (F, C)
Green beans cooked with salt	Green beans cooked with thyme (Na)
Lettuce wedge with Thousand Island dressing	Lettuce wedge with low-kcal dressing (F)
Whole milk	Skim milk (F, C)
Chocolate cake with icing	Blueberry-oatmeal crisp (F, Fi)

*Abbreviations refer to reduction in cholesterol (C), fat (F), sodium (Na), and increase in fiber (Fi) intake.

■ Avoid most processed meats, such as regular hot dogs (even if made from turkey), cold cuts, bacon, and sausage, which are high in fat.
■ Eat fish regularly. Some fish (e.g., salmon, mackerel, herring, tuna, and swordfish) are good sources of **omega-3** or **n-3 fatty acids.** Omega-3 fatty acids have been reported to reduce serum

Text continued on p. 322

Table 15-5   Recommended Diet Modifications to Lower Blood Cholesterol: the Step-One Diet

Food Group	Choose	Decrease
Fish, chicken, turkey, and lean meats	Fish, poultry without skin, lean cuts of beef, lamb, pork or veal, shellfish	Fatty cuts of beef, lamb, pork; spare ribs, organ meats, regular cold cuts, sausage, hot dogs, bacon, sardines, roe
Skim and low-fat milk, cheese, yogurt, and dairy substitutes	Skim or 1% fat milk (liquid, powdered, evaporated) Buttermilk	Whole milk (4% fat): regular, evaporated, condensed; cream, half-and-half, 2% milk, imitation milk products, most nondairy creamers, whipped toppings
	Nonfat (0% fat) or low-fat yogurt Low-fat cottage cheese (1% or 2% fat)	Whole-milk yogurt Whole-milk cottage cheese (4% fat)
	Low-fat cheeses, farmer, or pot cheeses (all of these should be labeled no more than 2-6 g fat/oz)	All natural cheeses (e.g., blue, Roquefort, Camembert, Cheddar, Swiss) Low-fat or "light" cream cheese, low-fat or "light" sour cream Cream cheeses, sour cream
	Sherbet, sorbet	Ice cream

Adapted from National Cholesterol Education Program: *Second Report of the Expert Panel on Detection, Evaluation, and Treatment of High Blood Cholesterol in Adults (ATP II).* NIH Pub No 93-3095, Washington, DC, 1993, US Department of Health and Human Services.

Continued

Table 15-5   Recommended Diet Modifications to Lower Blood Cholesterol: the Step-One Diet—cont'd

Food Group	Choose	Decrease
Eggs	Egg whites (2 whites = 1 whole egg in recipes), cholesterol-free egg substitutes	Egg yolks (limit to no more than 4/week on Step-One or 2/week on Step-Two)
Fruits and vegetables	Fresh, frozen, canned, or dried fruits and vegetables	Vegetables prepared in butter, cream, or other sauces
Breads and cereals	Homemade baked goods using unsaturated oils sparingly, angel food cake, low-fat crackers, low-fat cookies	Commercial baked goods: pies, cakes, doughnuts, croissants, pastries, muffins, biscuits, high-fat crackers, high-fat cookies
	Rice, pasta	Egg noodles
	Whole-grain breads and cereals (oatmeal, whole wheat, rye, bran, multigrain, etc.)	Breads in which eggs are major ingredient

Fats and oils		
Limit to no more than 6-8 servings per day from the "Choose" list. 1 serving = 1 teaspoon of most items (see text)	Baking cocoa	Chocolate
	Unsaturated vegetable oils: corn, olive, rapeseed (canola oil), safflower, sesame, soybean, sunflower*	Butter, coconut oil, palm oil, palm kernel oil, lard, bacon fat
	Margarine or shortening made from one of the unsaturated oils listed above†	
	Diet margarine	
	Mayonnaise, salad dressings made with unsaturated oils listed above	Dressings made with egg yolk
	Low-fat dressings	
	Seeds and nuts	Coconut

Adapted from National Cholesterol Education Program: *Second Report of the Expert Panel on Detection, Evaluation, and Treatment of High Blood Cholesterol in Adults (ATP II).* NIH Pub No 93-3095, Washington, DC, 1993, US Department of Health and Human Services.

*Olive, canola, and high oleic forms of safflower and sunflower oils are rich in monounsaturated fat.

†Limit use of hydrogenated and partially hydrogenated fats.

triglycerides and inhibit platelet aggregation and inflammation, which contributes to blockage of the coronary blood vessels. Frequent consumption of fish, whether it is a type that is rich in omega-3 fatty acids or not, is associated with reduced risk of CHD.

Eggs. Yolks are high in fat and cholesterol. Egg whites are free of fat and cholesterol and can be used often.

- Limit yolks to four per week on the Step-One Diet and two per week for the Step-Two Diet.
- Cholesterol-free egg substitutes may be used, but note that some brands are not fat-free.

Fruits and vegetables. Fruits and vegetables provide color, texture, vitamins, minerals, and fiber and should be a part of every meal.

- Use fruits and vegetables liberally. Plant products do not contain cholesterol. In addition, almost all fruits and vegetables are low in fat, with a few exceptions such as avocados, olives, and coconut. Avocados and olives are discussed below under fats and oils.
- Avoid frying or adding butter, cream, or cheese sauces.

Breads and cereals. Grains are good sources of vitamins and minerals, and whole grains provide fiber as well.

- Increase intake as meat intake is reduced, to replace energy and nutrients previously provided by meat.
- Avoid items such as commercial bakery products, cereals (e.g., granola), and quick breads (muffins, banana and other fruit or nut breads, corn bread, pancakes, and waffles) that are high in fat or that contain egg yolk. Homemade products made with egg whites or egg substitutes and the fats and oils allowed are acceptable.

Fats and oils. Limit to 6 to 8 servings/day (approximately 1 tsp/serving) to help control body weight and serum triglyceride levels.

- Avoid coconut, palm, and palm kernel oil (also known as tropical oils), which are cholesterol-free but high in saturated fat. These

oils are used in some bakery products, processed foods, popcorn oils, and nondairy creamers.

- Use liquid or soft (tub) margarine made from unsaturated fats
  (see Table 15-5), which have had little **hydrogenation. Unsaturated fats** are those containing one **(monounsaturated)** or
  more than one **(polyunsaturated)** carbon-carbon double bond.
  Both monounsaturated and polyunsaturated fatty acids have a
  lowering effect on serum cholesterol. Polyunsaturated fatty acids
  are usually limited to no more than 5% to 10% of total kcal
  because excessive amounts may increase the risk of some
  cancers. Many nutritionists advocate a "Mediterranean diet"
  loosely based on traditional food intake patterns in Italy, Greece,
  and other Mediterranean nations where heart disease rates have
  been low. Monounsaturated fats (found in olive and canola oils
  and in high oleic acid forms of safflower and sunflower oils) and
  fiber and other complex carbohydrates are key components in
  that diet plan. Hydrogenated and partially hydrogenated fats
  (margarines and shortening) contain *trans* forms of fatty acids,
  rather than natural *cis* forms. (Molecules of *trans* and *cis* fatty
  acids bend in different ways [Figure 15-1].) Trans fatty acids
  apparently raise LDL cholesterol as much as saturated fats do.

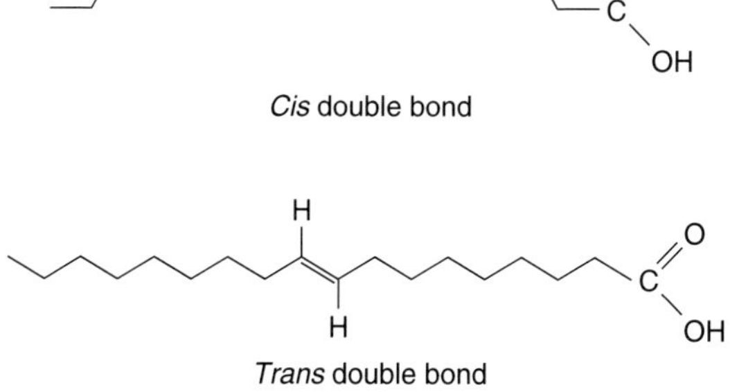

Cis double bond

Trans double bond

Figure 15-1
Structure of *cis* and *trans* fatty acids.

■ Use limited amounts of nuts and seeds. Most contain unsaturated fats, but they are high in kcal. One tbsp of nuts or 2 tsp of peanut butter is equivalent to 1 tsp of fat.
■ Foods equivalent to 1 tsp of fat are regular salad dressings, 1.5 tsp; diet margarine, 2 tsp; olives, 5 large or 10 small; and avocado, one eighth medium.

Preparation methods. Cooking methods that add little or no fat are preferred.

■ Steam, bake, broil, or microwave foods, fry them in a nonstick pan, or stir-fry in a small amount of fat.
■ Prepare soups, stews, and broths in advance so that they can be chilled after cooking and the fat layer that forms on top can be skimmed off.

Snacks and desserts. High-fat chips and crackers are poor choices.

■ Choose low-fat items such as: fruits and fruit ices, melba toast, Ry Krisp, graham crackers, bagels, English muffins, raw vegetables, sherbet, angel food cake, fruit-flavored gelatin, low-fat cookies such as gingersnaps and Newton cookies, and occasionally low-fat frozen yogurt or ice cream.
■ Use cakes, pies, and cookies made with egg whites, egg substitutes, skim milk, and unsaturated oils occasionally, if desired.

Eating out. Individuals should feel free to ask service personnel in restaurants about preparation methods and fat content of foods if this information is not clear from the menu.

■ Avoid fried foods; in fast-food restaurants, choose salads (with as few high-fat ingredients such as meat, cheese, or bacon bits as possible) or grilled items.
■ Order foods without sauces, butter, and sour cream.
■ Ask that salad dressings be served on the side, and use limited amounts.
■ Avoid high-fat toppings such as bacon, chopped eggs, and cheese; eat only small amounts of sunflower seeds and olives.

Convenience foods. Commercial packaged and frozen prepared foods are often high in fat.

■ Prepare casseroles, breads, and desserts with low-fat, low-cholesterol ingredients in advance and freeze them for occasions when preparation time is short.
■ Read labels and choose low-fat, low-kcal frozen entrees and meals.

Controlling hypertriglyceridemia

To control triglyceride levels:

■ Reduce weight, if overweight. The Step-One Diet can be used to reduce fat intake to approximately 30% of kcal, which will aid in weight reduction.
■ Limit intake of simple carbohydrates, e.g., sugars and foods and beverages sweetened with sugars, syrup, pastries, candy, cookies, gelatin, ice cream, and other sweetened desserts.
■ Follow a very low-fat diet (10% to 20% of total kcal) if triglyceride levels are very high (greater than 1000 mg/dl).
■ Increase physical activity.
■ Avoid alcohol, or limit intake to no more than 1 to 2 drinks per day. 1 serving = 12 oz beer, 1 glass (5 oz) of wine, or 1.5 oz (1 jigger) of distilled spirits.
■ Achieve good control of blood glucose if diabetes is present.

Other medical nutrition therapy to reduce the risk of heart disease

A dietary fiber intake of 25 to 30 g/day is recommended. Soluble fibers found in oat bran, barley, legumes, and many fruits and vegetables (see Appendix B) have cholesterol-lowering effects and should be used often.

The combination of soy protein and compounds known as **isoflavones** that are found in soy appear to lower LDL cholesterol. Soy intake can be increased by using tofu to substitute for animal proteins in casseroles, soups, and stir-fried dishes, using soft tofu in place of cottage or cream cheese in some recipes, and by choosing meat substitutes and other products containing "textured vegetable protein."

Increased levels of the amino acid homocysteine increase the risk of CHD. Deficiencies of folic acid and vitamin B_6 increase the levels of homocysteine, and thus a diet adequate in these vitamins is the best protection against hyperhomocysteinemia. Good sources of folic acid include green leafy vegetables, fortified breakfast cereals and other grains, oranges, and legumes. Good sources of vitamin B_6 include whole grains, meat, poultry, fish, and potatoes.

Hypertension

Hypertension is usually defined as a blood pressure of 160/95 or greater. Normotension is a blood pressure less than 140/90. Measurements between these two values reflect borderline hypertension.

Pathophysiology

Increases in blood volume, heart rate, and peripheral vascular resistance can lead to hypertension, but 90% of cases are *essential* hypertension—that is, no cause is known. Obesity, diabetes, and essential hypertension often occur together, which has led to a search for a common causative factor for this so-called **Syndrome X** or metabolic syndrome. Hyperinsulinemia, or increased pancreatic release of insulin, is believed to be the common factor. Hyperinsulinemia is a response to **insulin resistance,** or impaired response of cells (primarily those in the skeletal muscle and adipose tissue) to insulin, and it commonly occurs in obese people and those with type 2 diabetes mellitus. Whatever the cause, hypertension is a risk factor for cerebral vascular accident (CVA or stroke), MI, and renal failure.

Treatment

Drugs used in treatment of hypertension include diuretics, β-adrenergic blocking agents such as propranolol, α-adrenergic blocking agents such as phentolamine, and antihypertensive agents such as methyldopa, calcium channel blockers (e.g., nifedipine), angiotensin converting enzyme (ACE) inhibitors (e.g., captopril), and angiotensin II type 1 receptor blockers (e.g., losartan). Nutrition and lifestyle changes are also important in treatment of hypertension.

Nutritional Care

The goal is to reduce blood pressure to normal if possible. Even if complete normalization is not possible, it is estimated that, for every 2 mmHg reduction in systolic blood pressure, the risk of heart disease is decreased by 5% and the risk of stroke is decreased by 8%.

Assessment

Assessment is summarized in Table 15-2.

Intervention and teaching

Recognizing the need to make diet and lifestyle changes

The individual should participate in assessing personal diet, exercise patterns, weight, and methods for coping with stress and in planning strategies for permanent change. Gradual changes may be more successful than sweeping ones.

Reducing sodium intake

Excessive intake of sodium, in conjunction with chloride, elevates the blood pressure in individuals who are salt-sensitive (approximately 30% to 50% of hypertensive persons). Presently, there is no good method available for determining in the clinical setting which people are salt-sensitive, and therefore, a sodium-restricted diet is recommended for most hypertensive individuals. The level of restriction is usually determined by the severity of hypertension. Box 15-1 describes the levels of sodium restriction. The American Heart Association recommends that the general population consume no more than 6 g sodium chloride (2.4 g sodium) daily in order to reduce the risk of developing hypertension.

The taste preference for salt usually decreases after about 2 to 3 months on a sodium-restricted diet. Commercial salt substitutes contain potassium chloride, rather than sodium chloride. The physician may allow their use if the individual has no renal impairment. Herbs and spices (except high-sodium ones such as celery seeds; parsley flakes; and garlic, onion, or celery salts) and flavorings such as lemon juice can be used to replace salt. Salt-free spice seasoning mixtures are available in supermarkets. Some foods and their suggested low-sodium accompaniments are provided in Table 15-6.

Kosher meats contain two to three times as much sodium as nonkosher. Soaking meats in tap water for 1 hour, then discarding the water and cooking the food is effective in reducing the sodium content while still adhering to the Jewish food laws.

Some drugs, including antibiotics (especially the penicillins),

Box 15-1   Foods To Be Avoided on Sodium-Restricted Diets*

Mild Restriction (2-3 g/day)

Do not use:

Salt at the table (use salt lightly in cooking; 1 tsp salt ≅ 2300 mg sodium)

Smoked, cured, or salt-preserved foods such as salted fish, ham, bacon, sausage, cold cuts, corned beef, kosher meats, sauerkraut, olives

Salted snack foods such as chips, pretzels, popcorn, nuts, crackers

Seasonings such as onion, garlic, and celery salt and monosodium glutamate, bouillon, and meat tenderizers; pickles; condiments such as catsup, prepared mustard, relishes, soy sauce, and Worcestershire sauce

Cheese, peanut butter

Moderate Restriction (1 g/day)

Do not use:

Salt in cooking or at the table

Any food prohibited under Mild Restriction

Canned meat or fish, vegetables, and vegetable juice (except low-sodium)

Frozen fish filets or any frozen vegetables to which salt has been added

More than one serving of any of these in a day: artichoke, beet greens, beets, carrots, celery, dandelion greens, kale, mustard greens, spinach, Swiss chard, turnips

Buttermilk

Regular bread, rolls, crackers

Dry cereals (except puffed wheat, puffed rice, and shredded wheat); instant oatmeal and grits

Shellfish (except oysters)

---

*Low-sodium versions of many of the products are available. These may be included in the diet.

Box 15-1   Foods To Be Avoided on Sodium-Restricted Diets*—cont'd

Moderate Restriction (1 g/day)—cont'd

Do not use:

Salted butter or margarine, commercial salad dressings and mayonnaise

Regular baking powder, baking soda, or any products containing them (e.g., biscuits, corn bread, muffins, cookies, cakes); self-rising flour

Prepared mixes such as breads, muffins, pancakes, entrees, cake, pudding; frozen waffles and French toast

Water treated with a water softener

Bottled water (mineral, sparkling, spring, or other waters), unless information obtained from the bottler indicates it is low in sodium

Regular or diet soft drinks, unless information obtained from the bottler indicates them to be low in sodium

Strict Restriction (0.5 g/day)

Do not use:

Any food listed under Mild or Moderate Restrictions

More than 2 cups milk/day

Commercial foods made with milk, such as ice milk, ice cream, shakes

Artichokes, beet greens, beets, carrots, celery, dandelion greens, kale, mustard greens, spinach, Swiss chard, turnips

Commercial candy, except hard candies, gumdrops, or jelly beans (limit to 10 pieces daily)

*Low-sodium versions of many of the products are available. These may be included in the diet.

Table 15-6   Foods and Suggested Low-Sodium Accompaniments

Foods	Suggested Seasonings
Beef	Horseradish, mustard, cloves, pepper, bay, garlic
Poultry	Curry, sage, coriander, ginger, tarragon
Stews	Bay, garlic, basil, oregano, thyme
Vegetables	Mace, nutmeg, dill, rosemary, savory

sulfonamides, and barbiturates, are high in sodium. Their sodium content should be considered for the individual who is following a sodium-restricted diet. The pharmacist can provide information about the sodium content of these drugs. Individuals should be cautioned about using over-the-counter medications without physician approval. Antacids (except those containing magaldrate), aspirins, cough medicines, and laxatives are often high in sodium.

Other measures

Weight loss, an increase in physical activity, and limiting alcohol intake to no more than two drinks daily help to reduce hypertension. Epidemiologic evidence suggests that a diet rich in potassium, calcium, magnesium, and fiber protects against hypertension. Mineral or fiber supplements, however, have not been effective in controlling hypertension in most studies. A possible explanation is that a combination of all of these nutrients, in proportions similar to those found in a healthful diet, is necessary to reduce the risk of hypertension. Alternatively, it may be that a diet rich in these nutrients is also rich in other nutrients needed to reduce the likelihood of hypertension.

Recently, the prospective Dietary Approaches to Stop Hypertension (DASH) study (Zemel, 1997) has confirmed that a diet containing foods (rather than just supplements) rich in minerals and fiber lowers blood pressure. The DASH diet includes the following numbers of servings daily: grains, 6 to 12; fruits and vegetables, 8 to 12; low-fat milk, yogurt, and cheese, 2 to 4; meat, poultry, or fish, 1 to 2; and oil or other fats, 2 to 4. It also includes 4 to 7 servings per week of nuts, seeds, and beans (which are excellent sources of magnesium, as well as good sources of fiber). Serving sizes are the same as for the Food Guide Pyramid (see Chapter 1); for fats, 1 teaspoon = 1 serving. The number of servings within the suggested range is determined by the individual's energy needs. Another recent study (Joshipura et al., 1999) has determined that an increase in fruit and vegetable intake decreases the risk of stroke. For each increase in fruit and vegetable intake, up to 6 servings daily, the risk of stroke fell by 7% in women and 4% in men. The most effective fruits and vegetables appeared to be the cruciferous vegetables (e.g., broccoli, cabbage, cauliflower, brussels sprouts), green leafy vegetables, and citrus fruits and other vitamin C–containing fruits and vegetables. Because these fruits and vegetables contain a myriad of vitamins and minerals and nonnutritive substances such as fiber and phytochemicals, it is not possible to determine at this time what nutrients or nonnutrients in the fruits and vegetables were responsible for the decrease in risk of stroke.

Congestive Heart Failure
Pathophysiology

Congestive heart failure (CHF), which results from decreased myocardial efficiency, can be caused by MI, disease of the heart valves, hypertension, thiamin deficiency, and many other conditions. Renal blood flow may decrease, with impaired excretion of sodium and water. Peripheral edema, pulmonary edema, and ascites often result.

Treatment

Most of the medications used for treating hypertension are applicable to the treatment of CHF. ACE inhibitors and other vasodilatory agents and diuretics (used to reduce total body water) are often used in the treatment of CHF. Inotropic agents such as digitalis are often given to improve cardiac contractility.

Nutritional Care

The goals of nutritional care are to reduce total body sodium and water to reduce the workload of the heart. Children with CHF often have impaired growth and poor weight gain. This condition may be caused by a combination of factors (see Table 15-2 for a listing). Improvement of growth is a major goal of their nutritional care.

Assessment

Assessment is summarized in Table 15-2.

Intervention and teaching
Decrease workload on the heart

- Achieve weight reduction if overweight.
- Divide daily food intake into five to six small meals. Small meals are often better tolerated by the dyspneic individual than three large meals a day.
- Reduce dietary sodium to decrease fluid retention. The usual sodium allowance is approximately 45 to 70 mg/kg/day in infants and 2 g/day in adults. Box 15-1 provides guidelines for achieving sodium restriction.

■ Control fluid intake to help reduce circulatory volume, if necessary. The fluid allowance commonly ranges from 80 to 160 ml/kg/day in infants to 1.5 to 2 L/day in adults. This includes dietary sources, as well as fluids given with medications. Some foods that are solid at room temperature are liquid at body temperature. Gelatins can be considered to be 100% water, fruit ices 90%, pudding or custard 75%, sherbet 67%, and ice cream 50%. Nutrients must be provided in as small a volume as possible. If the person is tube fed, then a formula providing at least 1.5 to 2 kcal/ml (e.g., Deliver 2.0 [Mead Johnson], TwoCal HN [Ross], Nutren 2.0 [Nestle]) should be used. If parenteral nutrition is necessary, then 20% or 30% fat emulsions (2 or 3 kcal/ml, respectively) can be used as a concentrated kcal source.

Prevent or correct nutritional deficiencies

Increase potassium intake to 4.5 to 7 g/day unless renal impairment is present. Diuretics increase potassium losses, and hypokalemia predisposes to digitalis toxicity. See Appendix A for potassium sources.

If undernutrition is present, increase caloric intake by mouth if possible (see Box 13-2). If oral feedings are not sufficient, malnourished individuals, especially children, have shown improved growth without a worsening of CHF when given continuous tube feedings. Modular ingredients (see Table 9-2) can be used to increase the kcal-density of standard infant formulas to allow provision of adequate kcal within the fluid volume tolerated.

Selected Bibliography

Bostic RM, et al.: Relation of calcium, vitamin D, and dairy food intake to ischemic heart disease mortality among postmenopausal women, *Am J Epidemiol* 149:151, 1999.

Crouse JR III, et al.: A randomized trial comparing the effect of casein with that of soy protein containing varying amounts of isoflavones on plasma concentrations of lipids and lipoproteins, *Arch Intern Med* 159:2070, 1999.

Eckel RH: Obesity and heart disease: a statement for healthcare professionals from the Nutrition Committee, American Heart Association, *Circulation* 96:3248, 1997.

Freeman LM, Roubenoff R: The nutritional implications of cardiac cachexia, *Nutr Rev* 52:340, 1994.

Joshipura KJ, et al.: Fruit and vegetable intake in relation to risk of ischemic stroke, *JAMA* 282:1233, 1999.

Kirchhoff KT, et al.: Electrocardiographic response to ice water ingestion, *Heart Lung* 19:41, 1990.

Kotchen TA, McCarron DA: Dietary electrolytes and blood pressure: a statement for healthcare professionals from the American Heart Association Nutrition Committee, *Circulation* 98:613, 1998.

Mattes RD: The taste for salt in humans, *Am J Clin Nutr* 65(2 Suppl):692S, 1997.

Ornish D, et al.: Intensive lifestyle changes for reversal of coronary heart disease, *JAMA* 280:2001, 1998.

Rimm EB, et al.: Folate and vitamin B_6 from diet and supplements in relation to risk of coronary heart disease among women, *JAMA* 279:359, 1998.

Sidery MB: Meals lie heavy on the heart, *J R Coll Physicians* 28:19, 1994.

Stefanick ML, et al.: Effects of diet and exercise in men and postmenopausal women with low levels of HDL cholesterol and high levels of LDL cholesterol, *N Engl J Med* 339:12, 1998.

Summary of the second report of the National Cholesterol Education Program (NCEP) Expert Panel on Detection, Evaluation, and Treatment of High Blood Cholesterol in Adults (Adult Treatment Panel II), *JAMA* 269:3015, 1993.

Zemel MB: Dietary pattern and hypertension: the DASH study. Dietary Approaches to Stop Hypertension, *Nutr Rev* 55:303, 1997.

Pulmonary Disease

16

Nutrition and acute or chronic respiratory failure interact in a variety of ways. The increased work of breathing in respiratory failure increases energy needs while dyspnea interferes with nutrient intake, and these factors contribute to weight loss and inadequate nutrition status. Malnutrition adversely affects respiratory function by causing (1) wasting of the diaphragm and intercostal muscles, (2) decreased ventilatory response in response to hypoxia, (3) decreased surfactant production, (4) decreased replication of respiratory epithelium with predisposition to infection, (5) decreased cell-mediated immunity with increased susceptibility to pneumonia and other infections, and (6) decreased colloid osmotic pressure with increased likelihood of pulmonary edema. Moreover, phosphate is needed for adequate ATP to allow normal function of muscles, including those of the respiratory system, and for transport of oxygen by the red blood cells. Therefore, hypophosphatemia, which is common during protein-calorie malnutrition and/or the refeeding of malnourished individuals, further impairs respiratory function.

The total energy intake and the proportions of energy nutrients consumed also impact on respiratory function. Respiratory insufficiency is characterized by abnormal gas exchange, in particular the retention of carbon dioxide (CO_2). An excessive energy intake increases the metabolic rate and consequently elevates CO_2 production. Metabolism of carbohydrate yields the most CO_2, approximately 1 mole for every mole of oxygen consumed (or a **respiratory quotient [RQ]** of 1). If excessive carbohydrate is consumed, so that the body makes fat from the carbohydrate, then the RQ is greater than 1. On the other hand, metabolism of fat and protein produces proportionally less CO_2. RQs of these nutrients are approximately 0.7 and 0.8, respectively. Therefore, if the source of most of the energy in the diet is carbohydrate, more CO_2 must be expired than if most of the energy comes from fat.

Chronic Obstructive Pulmonary Disease

Chronic obstructive pulmonary disease (COPD) is a group of diseases that includes asthma, bronchitis, emphysema, and bronchiectasis.

Pathophysiology

The common feature in COPD is chronic obstruction of airflow. Airflow obstruction can result from bronchospasm (asthma); overproduction of mucus in the respiratory system (bronchitis); destruction of elastin, the elastic lung tissue, with air trapping and poor gas exchange (emphysema); or bronchial obstruction caused by a tumor, foreign body, or infection (bronchiectasis).

Treatment

Bronchodilators such as theophylline and aminophylline are often used in treatment of COPD. Antibiotics are prescribed when secondary infections (e.g., pneumonia) occur. Chest percussion and postural drainage may be used in individuals producing large amounts of sputum.

Nutritional Care

Malnutrition is common among individuals with COPD, especially those with emphysema. As many as 70% of people with COPD have lost weight, are underweight, and/or show signs of muscle or fat wasting. Resting energy expenditure is increased in people with moderate to severe COPD because of the increased work of breathing.

Micronutrient levels are also of concern in people with COPD, especially the levels of the **antioxidant** vitamins and minerals. Low blood levels of vitamin A have been reported to be common among people with moderate to severe COPD. Moreover, some individuals with normal blood levels of vitamin A respond to vitamin A supplementation with improvements in respiratory function, indicating that there may be local deficiency of the vitamin in the lung in COPD. Deficiency of vitamin A reduces the replication of epithelial cells and causes degeneration of mucus-secreting cells in the respiratory tract, thus making the person more susceptible to infection. Poor vitamin C status has also been reported to be prevalent among individuals with COPD, which further predisposes them to infection (Gadek, 1999).

Assessment

Assessment is summarized in Table 16-1.

Intervention

Preventing or correcting underweight

- Increase kcal intake through use of kcal-dense foods or supplements; Box 13-2 provides a list of suggestions. Individuals with moderate to severe dyspnea may prefer liquid supplements (shakes, instant breakfast, or commercial nutrient drinks; see Tables 9-1 and 9-2).
- Offer underweight patients with COPD feedings between meals, or save items such as fruit, sherbet, ice cream, or sandwiches for their later consumption if not eaten at mealtimes. Weight gain is usually greater when small, frequent feedings are consumed than when the individual tries to eat three large meals daily, and small feedings minimize the restriction of diaphragmatic movement caused by a full stomach.
- Ensure that patients have sufficient resources to secure an adequate diet. Many individuals with COPD are elderly or retired; they may have a limited income, or they may have a poor diet because of loneliness, apathy about food, or few food preparation skills (especially elderly men). They may need assistance in enrolling in the Food Stamp program, encouragement to eat at a group feeding site for the elderly (usually at senior citizen centers or in apartment houses for the elderly), or, if they are homebound, referral to a program for home-delivered meals.

Improving nutrient intake by promoting comfort

Nutrient intake may be poor because of fatigue or because of the bad taste in the mouth caused by sputum or the aftertaste of bronchodilator medications.

- Provide mouth care often, especially before meals, to clear the palate of the taste of sputum and improve the appetite.
- Schedule treatments and physical activity so that the individual has a chance to rest before meals.

Teaching

Maintaining ideal body weight is a key issue. Underweight individuals have increased morbidity as a result of weakness and

Table 16-1   Assessment in Pulmonary Disease

Areas of Concern	Significant Findings
Protein-Calorie Malnutrition (PCM)	*History* COPD: Poor intake of protein and kcal resulting from breathing difficulty caused by pressure of a full stomach on the diaphragm, unpleasant taste in the mouth from chronic sputum production, gastric irritation from bronchodilator therapy, smoking, inadequate income, loneliness, apathy, inadequate food preparation skills; increased needs because of increased work of breathing, frequent infections Acute respiratory failure: inadequate intake of protein and kcal caused by upper airway intubation, altered state of consciousness, dyspnea; increase in protein and kcal requirements because of increased work of breathing or acute pulmonary infections *Physical Examination* Evidence of weight loss (muscle wasting, lack of fat); weight for height <90% of standard or ideal or BMI <18.5; triceps skinfold or AMC <5th percentile *Laboratory Analysis* ↓ Serum albumin, transferrin, or prealbumin; ↓ lymphocyte count } Uncommon in COPD
Overweight	*History* COPD: decreased kcal needs resulting from decreased basal metabolic rate with aging, decreased activity to compensate for impaired respiratory function *Physical Examination* Weight for height >120% of desirable or ideal or BMI >25; triceps skinfold >95th percentile

Continued

Table 16-1   Assessment in Pulmonary Disease—cont'd

Areas of Concern	Significant Findings
Vitamin Deficiencies	
A	*History*
	Failure to consume at least 1 serving of a food rich in vitamin A or its precursor, carotene. at least every other day
	Physical Examination
	Follicular hyperkeratosis; poor light-dark visual adaptation; dryness of the skin or cornea
	Laboratory Analysis
	↓ Serum retinol
C	*History*
	Failure to consume at least one serving of vitamin C–rich foods per day
	Physical Examination
	Petechiae, ecchymoses; gingivitis
	Laboratory Analysis
	↓ Serum or leukocyte ascorbic acid
Phosphate (P) Deficiency	*History*
	Previous undernutrition; refeeding with high-carbohydrate diet or TPN; use of antacids that bind phosphate
	Physical Examination
	Muscle weakness; acute respiratory failure
	Laboratory Analysis
	↓ Serum P

Table 16-1   Assessment in Pulmonary Disease—cont'd

Areas of Concern	Significant Findings
Magnesium (Mg) Deficiency	*History* Poor food intake, undernutrition *Physical Examination* Diminished ventilation, difficulty weaning from the ventilator (decreased respiratory muscle strength) *Laboratory Analysis* ↓ Serum Mg
Elevated Respiratory Quotient (RQ)	*History* Use of glucose or other carbohydrate to provide most of nonprotein kcal; administration of excess kcal *Physical Examination* Tachypnea (>20 breaths/min in a non–mechanically ventilated adult); shortness of breath *Laboratory Analysis* RQ ≥1; ↑ partial pressure of CO_2 (Pco_2)
Fluid Excess	*History* Administration of more than 35-50 ml fluid/kg/day in an adult, including fluids in IVs, IV medications, tube feedings, TPN, and oral intake; ventilator dependency, which causes ↑ release of antidiuretic hormone (ADH) *Physical Examination* Bounding pulse; sacral or peripheral edema; shortness of breath; pulmonary rales *Laboratory Analysis* ↓ Serum Na

Continued

Table 16-1   Assessment in Pulmonary Disease—cont'd

Areas of Concern	Significant Findings
Excess IV Lipid	*History*
	Rapid administration (over 10 to 12 hours or less) of IV lipid emulsions, especially if >2 g lipid/kg/day is administered
	Laboratory Analysis
	↑ Serum triglycerides; ↓ P_{O_2}, ↑ P_{CO_2}

susceptibility to infection. On the other hand, excess weight increases the work of breathing.

Improving nutrient intake in underweight individuals

Nutrient intake can often be improved by helping the person learn to cope with symptoms that impair food intake. Problems reported by individuals with COPD, along with strategies for dealing with them, are listed as follows:

■ *Early satiety:* Eat high-kcal foods first, then foods of low-kcal density (beverages, raw vegetables) at the end of the meal or between meals. Experiment to see if foods served cold cause fewer problems.
■ *Bloating:* Eat small, frequent meals and avoid hurrying through meals, to reduce air swallowing.
■ *Anorexia:* Eat high-kcal foods first and save lower-kcal ones to eat at the end of the meal; have favorite foods available for snacks; use fat-containing foods, which have higher caloric density.
■ *Dyspnea:* Rest before meals; take bronchodilators before meals; eat slowly; use pursed lip breathing between bites. Avoid excessive protein, which increases ventilatory drive; consume only a moderate (no more than 50% of kcal) carbohydrate diet because excess increases CO_2 production.
■ *Fatigue:* Rest before meals; eat larger meals in the morning or other times when less tired; have easy-to-prepare foods readily available for times when fatigued.

Weight reduction (overweight or obese individuals)

Increase activity within physical limitations. Walking is an example of a good exercise for individuals with COPD. Start with brief periods of light exercise and gradually increase the duration and intensity. Decrease kcal intake by following the guidelines in Chapter 7.

Antioxidant intake

Some evidence suggests that levels of antioxidants (e.g., vitamins A, C, and E and β-carotene) may be low in the respiratory tissues of individuals with COPD. Oxygen therapy increases the need for these nutrients. If dietary intake appears low, counseling should focus on increasing intake of the known antioxidants, and supplements may be needed.

Acute Respiratory Failure

Respiratory failure is one of the leading reasons for admission to intensive care units (ICUs). ICU patients are at increased risk of malnutrition, with more than 40% having signs of malnutrition at the time of admission.

Pathophysiology

Respiratory failure is not a disease but instead is a ventilatory disorder caused by a variety of different conditions. It can result from increased pulmonary capillary pressure or permeability (e.g., pulmonary edema, pneumonia, near drowning), inadequate excretion of carbon dioxide (e.g., chronic bronchitis, emphysema), and depression of the respiratory center or failure of neuromuscular transmission (e.g., drug overdose, spinal cord injury, multiple sclerosis).

Treatment

Treatment of respiratory failure includes administration of oxygen or use of mechanical ventilation to maintain near-normal partial pressures of oxygen and CO_2 in the blood, use of antibiotics if infection is present, and, in some cases, use of corticosteroids to decrease pulmonary edema and stabilize pulmonary membranes.

Nutritional Care

Medical nutrition therapy is aimed at the prevention or correction of nutritional deficiencies or excesses that may worsen respiratory function and predispose the individual to secondary infections. Because individuals with acute respiratory failure tend to have multiple medical problems requiring simultaneous attention, it is easy to neglect nutrition. Persons with acute respiratory failure should be started on nutrition support within the first 3 or 4 days of hospitalization to prevent progression of nutritional deficits. Individuals given nutrition support are more readily weaned from ventilators than those given only intravenous (IV) glucose solutions.

Assessment

Assessment is summarized in Table 16-1.

Intervention

Preventing or correcting protein-calorie malnutrition

Patients able to eat are given a diet of nutrient-dense foods (see Box 13-2). Those unable to eat but who have functioning gastrointestinal (GI) tracts are often given nasogastric (NG) or nasoduodenal/nasojejunal (ND/NJ) feedings. Avoiding pulmonary aspiration of the formula is of key importance in delivering tube feedings in these patients. Measures to avoid pulmonary aspiration include ensuring that the tube is not in the respiratory tract before administering feedings, stopping feedings when the patient must be in Trendelenburg's position (e.g., during postural drainage), and possibly delivering feedings beyond the pyloric sphincter (into the duodenum or jejunum).

Those who are unable to be fully fed by the GI tract may be given total parenteral nutrition (TPN). Excessive amino acid administration should be avoided because it stimulates the ventilatory drive and may increase minute ventilation, fatigue respiratory muscles, and contribute to respiratory arrest.

Providing appropriate amounts of feedings

Avoid either underfeeding or overfeeding. Carefully evaluate energy needs and feed appropriately. Indirect calorimetry is an accurate way of assessing energy needs. This technique requires a metabolic cart and trained staff members. It is not available in all settings, so calculations have been developed to estimate kcal needs in critically ill patients (see Chapter 2).

Overfeeding is particularly likely during nutrition support with enteral tube feedings or TPN because the feedings do not depend on the patient's voluntary food intake. Carbohydrate is the primary energy source in most TPN regimens and in many defined formula diets, making carbohydrate overfeeding a special risk. Indirect calorimetry can detect overfeeding and a high RQ from excessive carbohydrate intake. Where indirect calorimetry is unavailable, physical examination and measurement of arterial blood gases can reveal some of the effects of overfeeding and high RQ. Elevated Pco_2 (partial pressure of CO_2 in the blood), unexpected difficulty in weaning from the ventilator, and tachypnea and shortness of breath (if non–ventilator-dependent) can be associated with overfeeding.

If hypercapnia is present and feedings are high in carbohydrate, then the health care team may consider decreasing the carbohydrate intake to approximately 30% of total kcal and increasing the proportion of the kcal given as fat to as much as 50% to 55%. The response of the patient should be carefully assessed, and the lowest amount of fat and highest amount of carbohydrate tolerated should be provided; however, it is most important that the total energy provided be appropriate to the individual's needs.

Avoiding fluid excess

The fluid required for delivery of tube feedings or TPN, along with medications, to patients with acute respiratory failure puts them at risk for overhydration. Fat is a concentrated source of kcal, and therefore, using fat to supply most of the nonprotein kcal in the diet also helps to control fluid intake. Tube feeding formulas with an increased nutrient density can be used for individuals receiving tube feedings. The formulas designed specifically for respiratory failure (e.g., Pulmocare [Ross], Respalor [Mead Johnson], and Nutrivent [Nestle]) have an increased nutrient density, providing 1.5 kcal/ml. For individuals receiving TPN, 20% or 30% lipid emulsions can be used daily as a kcal source. These emulsions supply 2 or 3 kcal/ml, whereas 10% emulsions provide only 1.1 kcal/ml.

Avoiding lipid excess

Rapid infusion of intravenous lipid emulsions may interfere with pulmonary diffusion capacity in individuals with respiratory impairment. Neonates are at increased risk. Assess the patient's serum triglyceride level after each increase in the infusion rate and at regular intervals thereafter to determine if the lipid infusion rate needs to be reduced. Schedule the delivery of the lipid over 12 to 24 hours each day, which allows the lowest possible infusion rate.

Providing adequate antioxidants

An increase in oxidative stress (e.g., oxygen therapy) increases the needs for antioxidants, including vitamins A, C, and E, β-carotene, and selenium. Supplements of antioxidants should be provided if dietary intake appears to be low.

SELECTED BIBLIOGRAPHY

Baarends EM, et al.: Total free living energy expenditure in patients with severe chronic obstructive pulmonary disease, *Am J Resp Crit Care Med* 155:549, 1997.

Chapman KM, Winter L: COPD: using nutrition to prevent respiratory decline, *Geriatrics* 51:37, 1996.

Cordova FC, Criner GJ: Management of advanced chronic obstructive pulmonary disease, *Comprehensive Therapy* 23:413, 1997.

Dureuil B, Matuszczak Y: Alteration in nutritional status and diaphragm muscle function, *Reprod Nutr Develop* 38:175, 1998.

Gadek JE, et al.: Effect of enteral feeding with eicosapentaenoic acid, gamma-linolenic acid, and antioxidants in patients with acute respiratory distress syndrome. Enteral Nutrition in ARDS Study Group, *Crit Care Med* 27: 1409, 1999.

Mendez C, et al.: Effects of an immune-enhancing diet in critically injured patients, *J Trauma* 42:933, 1997.

Owens MW, Markewitz BA, Payne DK: Outpatient management of chronic obstructive pulmonary disease, *Am J Med Sci* 318: 79, 1999.

Paiva SA, et al.: Assessment of vitamin A status in chronic obstructive pulmonary disease patients and healthy smokers, *Am J Clin Nutr* 64:928, 1996.

Vermeeren MA, Schols AM, Wouters EF: Effects of an acute exacerbation on nutritional and metabolic profile of patients with COPD, *Euro Resp J* 10:2264, 1997.

Renal Disease 17

A variety of diseases can affect the kidneys, including renal failure, **nephrotic syndrome,** and **nephrolithiasis.** The kidneys are responsible for maintaining the optimal chemical composition of all body fluids. When renal failure occurs, there is difficulty in controlling the body content of sodium, potassium, and nitrogenous byproducts of metabolism. In nephrotic syndrome, large amounts of protein are lost in the urine. Nephrolithiasis, or renal calculi formation, refers to the precipitation of stones in the urinary tract.

Acute or Chronic Renal Failure
Pathophysiology

In acute renal failure (ARF), a sudden reduction in glomerular filtration rate occurs, with impairment in excretion of wastes. Causes for this sudden reduction include inadequate renal perfusion (e.g., hemorrhage); acute tubular necrosis following trauma, surgery, or sepsis; nephrotoxic drugs or chemicals; acute glomerulonephritis; and obstruction (e.g., stricture of a ureter). There are two phases, an oliguric phase with urinary output usually less than 400 ml/day (less than 0.5 to 1 ml/kg/hr in children), followed by a diuretic phase when urine output increases. ARF may resolve or it may instead progress to chronic renal failure.

The leading cause of chronic renal failure is diabetes, and good metabolic control of diabetes is the most effective means of prevention. In renal insufficiency or failure, the glomerular filtration rate falls. The kidney is responsible for excretion of urea and creatinine derived from protein metabolism. With impaired renal function, circulating blood urea nitrogen (BUN) and creatinine levels rise, and retention of fluid, potassium, sodium, phosphorus, and other solutes normally excreted by the kidney occurs.

Nutrition-related problems are prevalent in renal failure. Anorexia is common in the presence of high BUN and creatinine levels. In addition, the kidney normally activates **erythropoietin,** which is required for red blood cell formation, and vitamin D, which regulates calcium and phosphorus absorption and bone calcium stores. Anemia, hypocalcemia, bone loss (osteodystrophy), and hyperphosphatemia are common. Retention of sodium and water contributes to hypertension, and potassium retention may lead to cardiac dysrhythmia. Impaired ability to excrete the organic acids produced in metabolic reactions and/or inadequate ability to conserve bicarbonate by the kidney results in metabolic acidosis.

Treatment

Treatment involves removal or, if possible, correction of the cause of renal failure. The major complications during the oliguric phase include acidosis, **hyperkalemia,** infection, hyperphosphatemia, hypertension, and anemia. Alkalinizing agents (e.g., sodium bicarbonate or Shohl's solution), cation-exchange resins to bind potassium, antibiotics, phosphate-binding drugs, antihypertensive agents, and diuretics are the most commonly used treatment measures.

Dialysis or hemofiltration is needed if these measures, combined with dietary restrictions, are insufficient to prevent or control hyperkalemia, fluid overload, symptomatic uremia (drowsiness, nausea, vomiting, and tremors), or rapidly rising BUN and creatinine levels. Different dialysis modalities are available, depending on individual needs. These treatments include hemodialysis, chronic ambulatory peritoneal dialysis (CAPD), or automated peritoneal dialysis (APD). Transplantation is an option for some individuals with end-stage renal disease.

Nutritional Care

The goals of medical nutrition therapy are to reduce the production of wastes that must be excreted by the kidney, avoid excessive fluid and electrolyte intake that will contribute to hypertension, prevent or correct nutritional deficits, prevent or delay development of osteodystrophy, and control hyperlipidemia, which often occurs in these individuals.

Assessment

Assessment is summarized in Table 17-1.

Table 17-1   Assessment in Renal Disease

Areas of Concern	Significant Findings
Protein-Calorie Malnutrition (PCM)	*History* Poor intake of protein-containing and kcal-containing foods as a result of dietary restrictions or anorexia from uremia, abdominal fullness from peritoneal dialysate, zinc deficiency, or depression; losses of amino acids or serum proteins caused by dialysis (hemodialysis losses ≈ 14 g/session, CAPD losses ≈ 5 to 15 g/day), steroid-induced tissue catabolism, and proteinuria; increased needs during infection *Physical Examination* Muscle wasting; thinning of hair; dry weight <90% of ideal for height, BMI <18.5, or decline in growth percentile for height or weight (children) (see Appendix D); triceps skinfold <5th percentile (see Appendix E); NOTE: Loss of weight or decrease in subcutaneous fat may be masked by edema *Laboratory Analysis* ↓ Serum albumin, transferrin, or prealbumin; ↓ lymphocyte count, nitrogen (N_2) losses in urine and dialysate greater than intake (negative N_2 balance)

Continued

Table 17-1   Assessment in Renal Disease—cont'd

Areas of Concern	Significant Findings
Altered Lipid Metabolism	*History* Nephrotic syndrome, excessive consumption of carbohydrates (CHO) caused by dietary emphasis on CHO as a source of kcal or use of glucose as an osmotic agent in dialysis *Laboratory Analysis* ↑ Serum cholesterol, LDL- and VLDL-cholesterol, serum triglycerides
Potential for Fluid Excess	*History* Oliguria or anuria *Physical Examination* Edema; hypertension; acute weight gain (≥1%-2% of body weight) *Laboratory Analysis* ↓ Hct
Potential for Mineral/Electrolyte Imbalance	
Phosphorus (P) excess	*History* Oliguria or anuria *Physical Examination* Tetany *Laboratory Analysis* ↑ Serum P; Ca × P product (Ca in mg/dl × P in mg/dl) >70; renal calcification on radiographs
Calcium (Ca) deficit	*History* Metabolic acidosis (serum pH <7.35, bicarbonate <22 mEq/L); hyperphosphatemia

Table 17-1   Assessment in Renal Disease—cont'd

Areas of Concern	Significant Findings
Potential for Mineral/Electrolyte Imbalance—cont'd	
Calcium (Ca) deficit—cont'd	*Physical Examination*
	Renal osteodystrophy with bone pain and deformities; tetany
	Laboratory Analysis
	↓ Serum Ca (NOTE: ≈45% of Ca is bound to albumin, if the person is hypoalbuminemic, then the Ca level will be misleading; it can be "corrected" by adding 0.8 mg/dl to the total Ca level for each 1 g/dl decrease in albumin below 3.5 g/dl)
Zinc (Zn) deficit	*History*
	↓ Intake caused by restriction of protein-containing foods; loss during dialysis
	Physical Examination
	Hypogeusia, dysgeusia; alopecia; seborrheic dermatitis
	Laboratory Analysis
	↓ Serum Zn
Iron (Fe) deficit	*History*
	Decreased production of erythropoietic factor by diseased kidney; decreased intake as a result of dietary restrictions
	Physical Examination
	Fatigue; pallor
	Laboratory Analysis
	↓ Hct, Hgb, MCV, MCH, MCHC

Continued

Table 17-1   Assessment in Renal Disease—cont'd

Areas of Concern	Significant Findings
Potential for Mineral/Electrolyte Imbalance—cont'd	
Sodium (Na) excess	*History*
	Oliguria or anuria
	Physical Examination
	Edema; hypertension
Potassium (K^+) excess	*History*
	Oliguria or anuria
	Physical Examination
	Weakness, flaccid muscles
	Laboratory Analysis
	↑ Serum K^+; electrocardiogram: elevated T wave, depressed ST segment
Aluminum (Al) excess	*History*
	Use of Al-containing phosphate binders, especially if Al dosages are >30 mg/kg/day
	Physical Examination
	Ataxia, seizures, dementia; renal osteodystrophy with bone pain and deformities
	Laboratory Analysis
	Plasma Al >100 µg/L

Intervention

Modifications of fluid, electrolyte, mineral, and protein intakes are often needed because of the impairment of the kidney's ability to excrete fluid and wastes. Nutrition therapy is designed to reduce edema, hypertension, and uremia. Guidelines for daily nutrient

Table 17-1   Assessment in Renal Disease—cont'd

Areas of Concern	Significant Findings
Potential for Vitamin Imbalance	
A excess	*History*
	Oliguria or anuria
	Physical Examination
	Anorexia, fatigue; alopecia, dry skin; hepatomegaly; irritability (progressing to hydrocephalus and vomiting in infants and children)
	Laboratory Analysis
	↑ Serum retinol
C deficit	*History*
	Losses in dialysis; ↓ intake caused by restriction of K^+-containing fruits and vegetables
	Physical Examination
	Gingivitis; petechiae, ecchymoses
	Laboratory Analysis
	↓ Serum or leukocyte ascorbic acid
B_6 deficit	*History*
	Failure of the diseased kidney to phosphorylate (activate) B_6; loss in dialysis
	Physical Examination
	Dermatitis; ataxia, irritability, seizures
	Laboratory Analysis
	↓ Plasma pyridoxal phosphate (PLP)

Continued

Table 17-1   Assessment in Renal Disease—cont'd

Areas of Concern	Significant Findings
Potential for Vitamin Imbalance—cont'd	
Folic acid	*History*
	Loss of folate during dialysis, $\downarrow$ intake caused by restriction of K^+-containing fruits, vegetables, and meats
	Physical Examination
	Glossitis (inflamed tongue); pallor
	Laboratory Analysis
	$\downarrow$ Hct, $\uparrow$ MCV; $\downarrow$ serum folate
D deficit	*History*
	Failure of the diseased kidney to activate vitamin D, poor intake because of restriction of dairy products
	Physical Examination
	Rickets (children), osteomalacia
	Laboratory Analysis
	$\downarrow$ 1,25-OH$_2$ vitamin D

allowances are given in Table 17-2, but individual needs vary, and continual monitoring and reassessment of the patient is the best guide.

Fluid restrictions

Fluid restriction is necessary when oliguria occurs. For the oliguric person, the daily fluid allowance is approximately 500 ml (to account for insensible losses) plus the volume lost from urine, diarrhea, vomitus and any other sources during the previous 24 hours. Hemodialysis may allow fluid intake to be slightly more liberal. Body weight should be measured daily, with the oral fluid intake adjusted so that gain is no more than 0.45 to 1 kg (1 to 2

Table 17-2   Guidelines for Nutrient Allowances in Renal Failure

Daily Intake	Adults	Children
Kcal/kg	25-35	Pre-adolescent: 100% of RDA for age Adolescent male: 44-55 Adolescent female: 40-50
Protein (g/kg)	UD: 0.6 HD: 1.1-1.2 PD: 1.2-1.3	<3 years: 2.5-3 3 years-puberty: 2-2.5 Puberty: 2 Postpubertal: 1.5
Sodium	1-3 g	50-75 mg/kg
Potassium	UD: often unrestricted until GFR <10 ml/min HD: 1.5-2.5 g PD: 2.5-3+ g	
Phosphorus	UD: <12 mg/kg* HD: <17 mg/kg* PD: <17 mg/kg*	HD: 50 mg/kg PD: 75 mg/kg Maintain serum concentration in normal range

UD, Undialyzed; *HD*, hemodialysis; *PD*, peritoneal dialysis
*Usually totals 550-1100 mg/day.

lb)/day on the days between dialyses. Peritoneal dialysis is very effective at removing fluid, and an oral fluid intake of 2000 ml/day may be tolerated. Acute weight changes are the best guide to fluid deficits and excesses.

Protein modification

For those people with renal impairment who have not yet reached end-stage renal disease, a low-protein diet (<0.6 g/kg/day) has been found to have some benefit in delaying the progression of renal failure; however, there is an increased risk of malnutrition for individuals consuming a low-protein diet, and malnutrition in patients with renal disease is associated with increased morbidity and mortality. Therefore, close monitoring of nutritional status is essential for the person receiving a low-protein diet; the patient should not be allowed to become malnourished simply to delay the time when dialysis must be started.

Table 17-2 provides estimates of protein needs, but the individual's protein catabolic rate (PCR) may also be used to calculate protein needs. (PCR and protein requirements should be equal unless the person is breaking down excessive tissue.)

$$\text{PCR (g/day) m} = 6.25 \times (\text{UNA} + 1.81 + 0.31 \times \text{BW})$$

where *UNA,* or urea nitrogen appearance, is the total urea nitrogen output (measured in the urine and the dialysate fluid) over 24 hours and *BW* is body weight (kg).

The protein in the diet of people with renal disease should be primarily **high biologic value (HBV) protein,** which is rich in essential amino acids (EAAs) in proportions that are favorable for growth and maintenance of human tissues. Good HBV sources are eggs, meat, poultry, fish, soy, and milk products. Supplements of EAAs are sometimes used. The usual dose is 10 to 20 g/day. Intake of other proteins is normally reduced to less than or equal to 0.4 g/kg/day when EAAs are used. EAA preparations are sometimes used temporarily as the sole source of nitrogen in the diet for people with acute renal failure; the usual allowance is 0.4 to 0.5 g/kg/day. EAA formulations are available as tablets, in formulas for oral or tube feeding, and for use in TPN. EAAs have a theoretical advantage in renal failure because the lack of **nonessential amino acids** in the diet should encourage the use of nitrogenous products within the body for synthesis of nonessential amino acids. Nevertheless, balanced amino acid formulations containing both essential and nonessential amino acids are preferred for most individuals with renal failure who can tolerate them. Nonessential amino acids are required for protein formation, and the rate of nonessential amino acid synthesis may not be adequate to meet the body's needs.

Protein and amino acid losses during dialysis can result in protein malnutrition. One approach during peritoneal dialysis is to use a 1.1% amino acid mixture as the primary osmotic agent in one dialysis exchange per day. The amino acids are an effective osmotic agent, and net absorption of amino acids across the peritoneum exceeds the losses of protein and amino acids in the dialysate.

Energy needs

Enough kcal must be consumed to prevent **catabolism** (breakdown of body tissues) because this process not only reduces the amount of functional tissue but also releases nitrogen, which must be excreted by the kidney. In most cases, fat provides about 30% of the calories and carbohydrate provides the remainder of the nonprotein calories (approximately 50% to 60% of total calorie intake). Hypertriglyceridemia affects a significant number of patients, and most carbohydrate should be complex (starches and fiber) to reduce the risk. In addition, alcohol intake should be avoided or severely limited, and saturated fat intake should account for no more than 8% to 10% of total energy intake. If serum triglycerides remain high despite these measures, then the amount of dietary fat can be increased to 40% of calories (with emphasis placed on monounsaturated fats, e.g., canola and olive oil) and the amount of carbohydrate can be correspondingly decreased.

Sugar from peritoneal dialysate must be considered as part of dietary carbohydrate. In peritoneal dialysis, 1.5% to 4.25% glucose solutions (containing 1.5 or 4.25 g glucose/dl) are commonly used as an osmotic agent to remove body fluid. About 70% of the glucose is absorbed by the body. Glucose monohydrate used in the dialysate provides 3.4 kcal/g. Thus the individual receives:

42.5 g/L × 70% × 3.4 kcal/g = 101 kcal/L of 4.25% dialysate

or

15 g/L × 70% × 3.4 kcal/g = 36 kcal/L of 1.5% dialysate

Caloric supplements may be necessary to achieve an adequate energy intake while adhering to the dietary restrictions. These supplements usually contain glucose oligosaccharides or vegetable oils. Some of the more common ones are Moducal, Polycose, and Microlipid.

Electrolyte and mineral restrictions

Sodium and potassium. The kidney is responsible for excretion of electrolytes, and thus their levels may become excessive in renal failure. Some degree of restriction is usually necessary in renal failure, although potassium restriction may not be necessary until the glomerular filtration rate falls to 10 ml/hr. Peritoneal dialysis is very effective in removing sodium and potassium, and thus people receiving peritoneal dialysis can usually have more liberal electrolyte allowances than those receiving hemodialysis.

Box 15-1 lists major dietary sodium sources. Some medications, including antibiotics (especially penicillins), sulfonamides, and barbiturates, are significant sources of sodium. The sodium supplied by any medications must be deducted from the dietary sodium allowance. Consult a pharmacist for the sodium content of drugs. The richest potassium sources are fruits and vegetables, meats, and dairy products.

Phosphorus. Progression of renal insufficiency is delayed in adults consuming diets containing less than 600 mg of phosphorus per day. By reducing milk intake to no more than 1 cup per day, omitting soft drinks and beer, and reducing the intake of meats, poultry, fish, eggs, cereals, and breads (especially whole grains) sufficiently to comply with protein restrictions, it is usually possible to achieve this level of intake. In the past, aluminum hydroxide antacids were used as phosphate binders, to reduce the absorption of phosphate, but their long-term use has resulted in aluminum toxicity, with ataxia, dementia, and worsening of renal osteodystrophy. Consequently, they are no longer used unless other therapy is ineffective in reducing phosphorus levels. Calcium carbonate or calcium acetate antacids are sometimes used as phosphate binders, but there are risks in the use of large doses of calcium. These risks include potential hypercalcemia, gastrointestinal discomfort, and the possibility that the combination of high levels of calcium and phosphorus will cause calcification of the soft tissues. Sevelamer hydrochloride (Renagel) is a relatively new phosphate binder that contains neither calcium nor aluminum.

Calcium. Calcium is needed to prevent or delay the progression of renal osteodystrophy, or loss of minerals from the bones, resulting from chronic acidosis (from inability to excrete acids produced in metabolism) and impaired vitamin D metabolism.

The preferred intake is 1 to 1.5 g daily for adults and adolescents, and young children should consume the Dietary Reference Intake. Restriction of dairy products may be necessary to reduce phosphorus and protein intake, so a supplement (e.g., calcium carbonate or citrate) may be needed.

Vitamin-mineral supplementation

Water-soluble vitamins, iron, and zinc are often prescribed at the level of the Recommended Dietary Allowance (RDA) because the renal diet tends to be low in these. Additional supplements of vitamin B_6 (5 to 10 mg/day), vitamin C (70 to 100 mg/day), and folic acid (0.8 to 1 mg/day) are needed to replace losses in dialysis. Vitamin A levels are usually high in renal failure, and supplements are avoided.

Iron, folic acid, and vitamin B_{12} intake must be adequate in the person receiving recombinant human erythropoietin to allow for adequate red blood cell formation. If dietary intake is inadequate, then supplements should be used. Calcitriol, a synthetic form of 1,25-dihydroxyvitamin D_3, is often prescribed to prevent renal osteodystrophy in individuals undergoing dialysis. Calcium intake must be at least 800 to 1200 mg/day for calcitriol to be effective (see Figure 3-4 for food sources of calcium).

Nutrition support

Anorexia resulting from uremia, medications, or depression; the restrictions of the renal diet; abdominal fullness from the peritoneal dialysis; infections or inflammation; metabolic acidosis that stimulates protein degradation; and electrolyte imbalances or circulatory instability associated with renal failure or dialysis are all factors that can interact to impair nutritional status. When oral intake is inadequate, nutrition support measures may be needed. Enteral tube feeding is preferred if the enteral route is available. Specialized formulas for renal failure, with low protein, phosphorus, and electrolyte content, are available if needed by the undialyzed patient (see Table 9-1). Usually, the dialyzed patient tolerates a formula designed for general use. Some general-use formulas are available in concentrated forms (2 kcal/ml) for individuals needing fluid restriction.

Individuals who do not tolerate enteral feedings may require total parenteral nutrition (TPN). Specialized amino acid mixtures for renal failure are available; however, the dialyzed patient usually tolerates a balanced amino acid solution containing both essential and nonessential amino acids. Intradialytic TPN (TPN administered during hemodialysis, usually three times weekly) is given to some patients. The advantages are that the patient receives supplemental nutrition, and **ultrafiltration** during dialysis prevents any fluid overload from the TPN; however, these short infusions provide insufficient energy to meet daily needs, and the expense of these treatments is likely to be high in comparison to their benefit.

Impaired growth is very common among children with renal failure. Intensive dietary counseling, oral supplements, enteral tube feeding, and TPN are used as needed to maximize nutrient intake. In addition, growth hormone is approved for use in children with short stature associated with renal failure.

Emotional support

Renal failure and subsequent dependence on dialysis create severe emotional demands on the individual. Furthermore, the diet includes many restrictions to which the individual must adjust. Health care professionals must provide reinforcement and encouragement. Some techniques that have been successful in encouraging patients to follow the diet restrictions include the following:

■ *Self-monitoring:* The health care professional provides feedback regarding diet records kept by the individual; the diet records can also be used to individualize teaching regarding needed diet changes.
■ *Modeling:* Providing the patient samples of low-protein food products and recipes for their use is especially effective.
■ *Anticipatory guidance:* Discussing or role-playing strategies for incorporating diet modifications into social situations and holiday meals is one way the health care professional can help the patient. It is also beneficial to work with the patient in preventing relapse into old dietary habits.

Teaching

Dietary restrictions and their rationale

The renal diet is complex, and the dietitian is the professional best prepared to plan the diet and perform initial teaching. Individualization of the diet as much as possible (to incorporate favorite foods and respond to the demands of the individual's lifestyle) improves quality of life and compliance with the diet.

Fluid

- Measure body weight and check for edema daily.
- Include foods that are liquids at room temperature in the fluid allowance. Water content of some common foods is as follows: gelatins, 100% water; fruit ices, 90%; pudding or custard, 75%; sherbet, 67%; and ice cream, 50%.

Protein

- At least half of dietary protein should be HBV. Approximately 7 g of HBV protein is contained in 1 oz of meat, fish, poultry; ¼ cup cooked soybeans or ¼-⅓ cup soy product such as tofu, tempeh, or miso; 1 egg; or 7 fluid oz of whole, low-fat, or skim milk.
- Half or less of the protein should be low biologic value (LBV). Cereals, breads, vegetables, and legumes are the primary sources of LBV protein. An individual who is allotted 28 g of HBV protein and 18 g LBV protein daily can consume the equivalent of 4 oz of meat, 6 slices of bread (2 g protein/slice), 3 servings of vegetables (1 g/serving), 3 servings of fruits (0.5 g/serving), and 5 servings of carbohydrate supplements such as Polycose or Moducal (0.1 g protein/3 tbsp serving).
- Low-protein pasta and bread products, available via mail order, some pharmacies, and some larger grocery chains, are a source of complex carbohydrate for the person on a very limited protein diet.

Kilocalories

- Fats are valuable energy sources, but saturated fats raise serum cholesterol levels and should be restricted as in the Step One Diet described in Chapter 15. Individuals with hypercholesterolemia should use oils and margarine high in monounsaturated and polyunsaturated fats (those containing primarily liquid canola [rapeseed], olive, safflower, sunflower, corn, soybean, or cotton-seed oils); lean meats, fish, or skinned poultry; and skim milk products. If hyperlipidemia does not respond to these changes, then more extensive dietary modifications to control heart disease are needed (Step Two Diet; see Chapter 15). Unfortunately, hypercholesterolemia often continues even after renal transplant. Dietary problems in the posttransplant patient are discussed in Chapter 11.

■ Simple carbohydrates, such as sugar, jam, syrup, hard candy, gumdrops, jelly beans, and popsicles, are widely used as calorie sources because they contribute little or no sodium, potassium, and protein.

■ Reduce intake of simple carbohydrates if hypertriglyceridemia occurs. To compensate, substitute complex carbohydrates (breads, cereals, and vegetables) up to the amount allowed by the protein restriction. Monounsaturated fatty acids are also a useful energy source for the person with hypertriglyceridemia.

■ Limit alcohol intake (preferably to none or only an occasional drink, but in no case more than a maximum of 1 to 2 drinks a day) if hypertriglyceridemia occurs.

Sodium

■ Limit intake of sodium in foods; see the list in Box 15-1. This will reduce fluid retention, edema, and hypertension. Note that this restriction is unnecessary for many individuals during peritoneal dialysis or after renal transplants.

■ Salt substitutes are not usually used because they are high in potassium.

■ Avoid over-the-counter drugs unless approved by the physician or responsible care provider. Many drugs, including antacids (except magaldrate), aspirin, cough medicines, and laxatives, are high in sodium.

Potassium

■ The kidney is the primary route of excretion, and toxic levels of potassium can occur in renal failure.

■ The richest sources of potassium are meats, milk products, fruits, and vegetables.

■ Choose canned, drained fruits or vegetables (processed without salt), rather than fresh or frozen.

■ Decrease potassium in fresh vegetables and fruits by cutting them into small pieces and soaking or cooking them in a large amount of water, then discarding the water.

Example. An example of an individualized diet plan is shown in Table 17-3. The diet order in this case is for 45 g protein (34 g HBV), 1000 mg sodium, 1650 mg potassium, 2650 kcal or more, and 720 ml fluid per day.

Preventing constipation

■ Increase fiber intake to 25 to 30 g/day (see Appendix B).
■ Exercise regularly.
■ Restrict phosphorus intake so that use of phosphate binders can be decreased. Constipation often occurs with regular use of phosphate binders.

Nephrotic Syndrome
Pathophysiology

Nephrotic syndrome results from an increase in permeability of the glomerular capillary membrane. It is associated with proteinuria (2 g/day or more), hypoalbuminemia, edema, and hyperlipidemia. It may be idiopathic or may result from conditions such as glomerulonephritis, diabetes mellitus, collagen vascular diseases, or sickle cell anemia. The disorder can resolve spontaneously or follow a pattern of remissions and relapses.

Treatment

Drug therapy includes corticosteroids, which help lessen protein-uria, and diuretics. If hypercholesterolemia or hypertriglyceridemia is severe, bile acid–binding resins, nicotinic acid, and inhibitors of cholesterol synthesis (statins) may be used to help control the hyperlipidemia.

Nutritional Care

Medical nutrition therapy in nephrotic syndrome is designed to maintain adequate nutritional status and to help control edema and hyperlipidemia.

Assessment

Assessment is summarized in Table 17-1.

Table 17-3 Meal Plan of Man with Chronic Renal Failure (CRF)

Menu	Pro (g)	Na (mg)	K (mg)	Kcal
Breakfast				
Shredded wheat, ½ cup	2	1	38	70
Frozen strawberries, ½ cup	0.5	1.5	115	80
Sugar, 1 tsp	—	—	—	16
Half and half, ½ cup	4	60	170	160
Cinnamon toast:				
Low-protein bread, 1 slice	0.1	9	9	100
Margarine, 2 tsp	—	100	2	90
Sugar, 2 tsp	—	—	—	32
Snack				
Jelly beans, 1 oz	0.1	9	9	100
Lunch				
Shrimp salad:				
Shrimp, 2 oz	13.8	60	190	150
Mayonnaise, 3 tsp	—	150	3	135
Lettuce, ¼ cup shredded	0.5	4.5	57	13
Matzo, 1 piece	2	1	38	70
Margarine, 2 tsp	—	100	2	95

	Pro	Na	K	Cal
Cranberry juice, 1 cup	0.1	9	9	100
With Polycose powder, 1 tbsp	—	6	—	31
Tangerine, 1 medium	0.5	1.5	115	40
Snack				
Hard candy, 1 oz	0.1	9	9	100
Dinner				
Grilled chicken, 2 oz	13.8	60	190	75
Rigatoni, low protein, 1/2 cup	0.1	9	9	100
With margarine, 2 tsp	—	100	2	90
Stirfry				
Mushrooms, 1/2 cup	1	9	113	25
Zucchini 1/2 cup	1	9	113	25
Oil, 3 tsp	—	—	—	115
Hi-C, 1 cup	0.1	6	9	100
With Polycose powder, 1 tbsp	—	—	—	31
Peaches, 1/2 cup, canned, drained	0.7	3.5	215	75
Sugar mints, 37	0.1	9	9	100

Continued

Pro, Protein; Na, sodium; K, potassium.

Table 17-3   Meal Plan of Man with Chronic Renal Failure (CRF)—cont'd

Menu	Pro (g)	Na (mg)	K (mg)	Kcal
Snack				
Low-protein toast, 2 slices	0.2	18	18	200
Margarine, 3 tsp	—	150	3	135
Honey, 1 tbsp	0.1	9	9	100
Milk, whole, ½ cup	4	60	184	80
With Polycose powder, 1 tbsp	—	6	—	31
TOTALS	44.8	979	1640	2664

HBV protein = 35.6 g   Fluid = 720 ml

Intervention and teaching
Low-sodium diet

A diet restricted in sodium is the most effective way to reduce the edema. The sodium allowance is usually 1 to 2 g (40 to 90 mEq)/day until the edema is reduced. See Box 15-1 for this level of restriction. If the edema resolves, then the sodium restriction can be removed.

Protein intake

Increasing protein intake to replace urinary losses is ineffective and results in increased proteinuria. A diet providing approximately the RDA for protein (0.8 g/kg/day for adults) usually supplies adequate protein.

Dietary control of hyperlipidemia

A diet that is low in saturated fat and cholesterol (see Chapter 15) will help to reduce serum cholesterol. Lean meat, fish, and skinned poultry should be used, and low-fat dairy products should be used. A moderate intake of fat (30% of kcal) is recommended because diets extremely low in fat (and consequently high in carbohydrates) could worsen hypertriglyceridemia. Monounsaturated and polyunsaturated fats should supply most of the fat kcal. Weight reduction usually helps reduce serum lipid levels if the individual is overweight. Alcohol intake should be avoided if possible, but if this is unacceptable to the patient, then intake should not exceed 1 to 2 drinks daily.

Hyperglycemia related to corticosteroid use

Reduce intake of simple carbohydrates such as desserts, soft drinks, and pastries. Increase intake of fiber and other complex carbohydrates such as whole-grain breads, cereals, legumes, and starchy vegetables.

Renal Calculi, or Nephrolithiasis
Pathophysiology

Calculi, or stones, can precipitate in any part of the urinary tract when the urine becomes supersaturated with the solute. The most important solutes, in terms of nephrolithiasis, are calcium, oxalate, and uric acid. Approximately 70% to 88% of all stones contain calcium, and 36% to 70% of stones are composed of calcium oxalate. Normal urine contains inhibitors of stone formation, and some people with stones have been found to have abnormalities of inhibitor production. In other individuals with stones, however, no abnormalities were found. Risk factors for stone formation include recurrent urinary tract infections, hyperparathyroidism, prolonged immobilization, ileostomy, Crohn's disease, laxative abuse, gout (excessive uric acid production), paraplegia, and milk-alkali syndrome (excessive intake of milk or other dietary calcium sources and antacids).

Treatment

Many calculi pass through the urinary tract spontaneously, and therapy consists of analgesics to relieve the pain associated with calculi and treatment of any underlying causative factors such as urinary tract infection, obstruction, or gout. Some stones that do not pass spontaneously can be fragmented through lithotripsy, to make it possible for the smaller fragments to be excreted. Calculi that are very large, too hard to be fragmented, or in an inappropriate location for lithotripsy can be removed either endoscopically or surgically.

Nutritional Care

Nutrition therapy can reduce the risk of recurrence of stones in some individuals. The most important aspect of nutritional care is maintaining an adequate fluid intake.

Assessment

Assess the quantity of fluids usually consumed, and determine whether there is a history of previous stone formation. The composition of any stones excreted should be determined, if possible.

Intervention and teaching

Adequate fluid intake

Fluid intake should be sufficient to produce at least 2 liters of dilute urine (specific gravity <1.010) daily, which reduces the risk of precipitation of calculi. Water should be encouraged, but juices, herbal teas, and soft drinks can provide some of the liquid. It is especially important to consume fluids at bedtime because the urine tends to become concentrated during the night. People who are unconscious, unaware of thirst, or unable to drink fluids need to receive sufficient fluid via a feeding tube or intravenous infusions to produce dilute urine.

Dietary substrates contributing to calculi formation

Calcium-containing stones. In the past, it was common to use calcium-restricted diets in an effort to reduce the recurrence of calculi in people who formed calcium-containing stones. It is now recognized that hypercalciuria (excessive calcium excretion in the urine) is common among individuals with a history of stone formation, but only a subset of individuals benefit from calcium restriction. This subset includes people with absorptive hypercalciuria type II, who have normal urinary calcium levels even when receiving a calcium-restricted diet. For these individuals, dietary calcium may need to be restricted to approximately 400 mg/day. This can be accomplished by limiting milk products and deep green leafy vegetables to about one serving each per day. A high-fiber diet has also been suggested as a way to reduce calcium absorption.

Excessive intakes of protein and sodium increase urinary calcium losses and may contribute to stone formation. Limiting protein intake to no more than the RDA and sodium intake to no more than 2 to 3 g/day may reduce the risk of recurrence of stone formation.

Oxalate-containing stones. Many foods contain oxalates, but only a few have been proven to increase urinary excretion of oxalate significantly. These foods include spinach, beets, rhubarb, chocolate, peanuts and peanut butter, strawberries, black or green tea, and wheat bran, and these items should be avoided by people who form oxalate stones. At present, it is not clear whether it is safe to consume other foods rich in oxalates such as plums, berries other than strawberries, tomatoes, celery, beans (dried, baked, green, and wax), deep green leafy vegetables (spinach, kale, and collards), tofu and other soy products, almonds, and cashews.

Vitamin C yields oxalate when it is metabolized. It has not been proven that vitamin C promotes stone formation, but the safest course is for people who form oxalate stones to avoid megadoses (1 g or more/day) of vitamin C.

If hypercalciuria is not present, then a high-calcium intake may be beneficial. Calcium decreases oxalate absorption in the intestine. If the person has fat malabsorption, then a low-fat diet or reduction of long-chain triglycerides in the diet and supplementation with medium-chain triglycerides may be effective. Excessive calcium is lost in the feces during fat malabsorption because calcium undergoes soap formation with fat that is not absorbed.

"Ash" from diets. Foods are metabolized in the body to yield acid or alkaline "ash," or end products. The original pH of the food has no relationship to the acidity or alkalinity of its end products. Acid-ash diets are sometimes used to help acidify the urine and prevent precipitation of calcium stones. Acid urine also reduces the growth of bacteria in the bladder, and prevention of urinary tract infections decreases the risk of stone formation. On the other hand, alkaline-ash diets are sometimes used to prevent recurrence of uric acid and cystine stones. Individuals on these diets make most of their food choices from the acid- or alkaline-ash food groups, as appropriate. Medications are often used to change urine pH, but acid- or alkaline-ash diets are prescribed occasionally.

- Acid-ash foods: meat, whole grains, eggs, cheese, cranberries, prunes, and plums.
- Alkaline-ash foods: milk; vegetables; fruits except cranberries, prunes, and plums.

Physical activity

Whenever possible, individuals should have daily weight-bearing exercise. The stress of this type of exercise helps prevent hypercalciuria caused by the release of calcium from the bone. It is especially important that caregivers in long-term care and rehabilitation facilities be aware of this problem and make every attempt to assist patients to obtain exercise.

SELECTED BIBLIOGRAPHY

Brewer ED: Pediatric experience with intradialytic parenteral nutrition and supplemental tube feeding, *Am J Kidney Dis* 33:205, 1999.

Foulks CJ: An evidence-based evaluation of intradialytic parenteral nutrition, *Am J Kidney Dis* 33:186, 1999.

Klahr S: Prevention of progression of nephropathy, *Nephrology, Dialysis, Transplantation* 12 (Suppl 2):63, 1997.

Kopple JD: The nutrition management of the patient with acute renal failure, *J Parent Ent Nutr* 20:3, 1996.

Kopple JD: Therapeutic approaches to malnutrition in chronic dialysis patients: the different modalities of nutritional support, *Am J Kidney Dis* 33:180, 1999.

Mitch WE, Maroni BJ: Factors causing malnutrition in patients with chronic uremia, *Am J Kidney Dis* 33:176, 1999.

Modification of Diet in Renal Disease Study Group (prepared by Kopple JD et al.): Effect of dietary protein restriction on nutritional status in the Modification of Diet in Renal Disease Study, *Kidney Int* 52:778, 1997.

Parivar F, Low RK, Stoller ML: The influence of diet on urinary stone disease, *J Urology* 155:432, 1996.

Sedman A, et al.: Nutritional management of the child with mild to moderate chronic renal failure, *J Pediatr* 129:s13, 1996.

Wolfson M: Nutritional management of the continuous ambulatory peritoneal dialysis patient, *Am J Kidney Dis* 27:744, 1996.

Wolfson M, Jones M: Intraperitoneal nutrition, *Am J Kidney Dis* 33:203, 1999.

Diabetes Mellitus 18

Diabetes mellitus is a disorder characterized by impaired carbohydrate, fat, and protein metabolism. Hyperglycemia and glucosuria commonly occur in untreated diabetes (Box 18-1).

Pathophysiology

The following terms are used in classifying diabetes:

Type 1 diabetes (previously known as insulin-dependent) is characterized by insulin deficiency that results from destruction of the beta cells of the pancreas, usually by an autoimmune process. Most individuals with type 1 diabetes are normal weight or underweight at the time of diagnosis. Classic symptoms of untreated type 1 diabetes include polyuria, polydipsia (increased fluid intake), polyphagia (increased food intake), and weight loss.

Type 2 diabetes (previously known as non–insulin-dependent) is characterized by insulin resistance, or decreased tissue uptake of glucose in response to insulin. Individuals with type 2 diabetes also have an insulin secretory defect that makes it impossible for them to release enough insulin to compensate for the insulin resistance. Type 2 diabetes is much more common than type 1 diabetes, and most individuals with type 2 diabetes are overweight or obese. Individuals with type 2 diabetes can survive without insulin injections at least initially and sometimes throughout their lives.

Gestational diabetes mellitus is the term given to any glucose intolerance that first occurs or is recognized during pregnancy.

Impaired glucose tolerance (IGT) and *impaired fasting glucose (IFG)* are not considered to be overt forms of diabetes, but they are risk factors for later development of diabetes and cardiovascular disease. IGT is defined as a glucose concentration ≥140

Box 18-1   Criteria for Diagnosis of Diabetes Mellitus in Adults

---

Two of these findings, on different days (either two different tests, or two abnormal findings with the same test) are required for the diagnosis of diabetes:

■ Casual (any time of day without regard to time since the last meal) plasma glucose level ≥200 mg/dl (11.1 mM) plus symptoms of diabetes such as excessive thirst and urination and unplanned weight loss

OR

■ Fasting plasma glucose level ≥126 mg/dl (7.0 mM). "Fasting" means no energy intake for at least 8 hours.

OR

■ Plasma glucose level ≥200 mg/dl (11.1 mM) 2 hours after consuming a 75 g glucose load*

From report of the expert committee on the diagnosis and classification of diabetes mellitus, *Diabetes Care* 22(suppl 1):S5, 1999.

*Oral glucose tolerance test; this is not recommended for routine clinical use.

mg/dl (7.8 mmol/l) and <200 mg/dl (11.1 mmol/l) 2 hours after ingestion of a 75 g glucose load. IFG is present when fasting (no food intake for at least 8 hours) plasma glucose is ≥110 mg/dl (6.1 mmol/l) and <126 mg/dl (7.0 mmol/l).

Diabetes is associated with many complications. The major chronic ones are accelerated coronary heart disease, peripheral vascular disease, cerebrovascular disease, retinopathy, nephropathy, and neuropathy. Gastrointestinal (GI) motility disorders occur in 20% to 76% of people with diabetes, with **gastroparesis** or delayed gastric emptying being the most common of these disorders. Symptoms include early satiety, abdominal discomfort and/or distension, bloating, nausea, vomiting, anorexia, and unexplained hypoglycemia. The cause of these motility disorders is not fully understood, although neuropathy probably plays a role, at least in some individuals.

Acute complications of type 1 diabetes include diabetic ketoacidosis (DKA) and hypoglycemia, and those of type 2 diabetes include hyperglycemic hyperosmolar nonketotic syndrome (HHNS) and infections such as pneumonia, cellulitis, bacteriuria, and vulvovaginitis. DKA results from insulin deficiency—too small a dosage, omission of a dose or doses, increased need for insulin, or elevation of the insulin-antagonizing counterregulatory hormones (glucagon, catecholamines, cortisol, and growth hormone), such as occurs during infection or trauma. In response to the insulin deficiency, hyperglycemia and glucosuria occur. Glucosuria leads to an osmotic diuresis with resulting dehydration and loss of electrolytes. The insulin deficit also allows increased lipolysis, or release of fatty acids from storage sites. Accelerated synthesis of ketones from the fatty acids results in ketosis (increased blood ketone levels because of increased production of ketones from fatty acids), and acidosis (because ketones are acidic). HHNS, on the other hand, is almost always precipitated by some stressor that increases blood glucose levels (surgery, trauma, burns, chronic disease, infection, drugs such as corticosteroids or diuretics, dialysis). Insulin levels are high, although they are not high enough to normalize the blood glucose. HHNS results in marked hyperglycemia (often greater than 1000 mg/dl), elevation of serum osmolality, glucosuria, and dehydration. Ketosis is absent or only very mild.

Treatment

Treatment of diabetes hinges on an appropriate plan for meals and physical activity, as well as medications if necessary. The Diabetes Control and Complications Trial showed that intensive management of diabetes to maintain blood glucose levels as near normal as possible reduces retinopathy, nephropathy, and neuropathy in type 1 diabetes (American Diabetes Assoc, 2000). Furthermore, data from the United Kingdom Prospective Diabetes Study (the largest and longest study ever performed on patients with type 2 diabetes) demonstrate that reduction of the occurrence of retinopathy, nephropathy, and possibly neuropathy in this form of diabetes is possible with intensive treatment to achieve near-normal blood glucose concentrations (UKPDS Group, 1998a and b). Diabetic care is a team effort that usually involves several health professionals—one or more physicians, dietitians, nurses, and other professionals such as a podiatrist and optometrist or opthalmologist—as well as the patient and family members. Certified diabetes educators (CDEs) are physicians, nurses, or dietitians who have received extensive education in diabetes care and have passed a certification examination to show that they have special qualifications for patient teaching related to diabetes.

Nutrition Therapy

Medical nutrition therapy is an essential component of the care of all people with diabetes. A registered dietitian (RD) who is knowledgeable in diabetes care is the best person to carry out nutrition planning and teaching. All health professionals on the team should be familiar with the principles of nutrition care in diabetes so that they can reinforce the instruction provided by the dietitian, however.

Medications

Insulin or oral hypoglycemic agents may be needed to help control hyperglycemia and excessive hepatic glucose production. Current practice is to recommend intensive therapy for all people with diabetes who are able to manage it. The goal of intensive therapy is to reduce long-term complications by maintaining glucose at normal or near-normal levels almost all the time. For intensive therapy of type 1 diabetes, several insulin injections are usually needed daily. Insulin is available in four forms: (1) ultra-short-, (2) short-, (3) intermediate-, or (4) long-acting (Table 18-1). Injections of ultra-short- or short-acting insulin are taken before each meal, often combined with one or two daily injections of long- or intermediate-acting insulin. Alternatively, motivated individuals may use continuous subcutaneous insulin infusion (CSII), or insulin pump therapy, which delivers short-acting insulin continuously to provide basal levels and allows the patient to administer boluses as needed with meals or snacks. Hypoglycemia is more prevalent with intensive therapy than with less intensive therapy. Also, the individual is more likely to become overweight with intensive therapy than with traditional therapy. With their diabetes under better control, patients lose less glucose in the urine, and insulin stimulates storage of glucose as fat.

Intensive management is not recommended for patients who are unwilling to participate actively in their care. The risk of hypoglycemia is heightened with intensive therapy. Thus, intensive management is also not recommended for children <2 years of age and only with caution for those 2 to 7 years old because hypoglycemia may impair normal brain development. Hypoglycemia may precipitate strokes or heart attacks if atherosclerosis is

Table 18-1   Insulin Activity*

Insulin	Approximate Number of Hours After Injection		
	Onset	Peak	Duration
Ultra-Short Acting			
Lispro	0.25-0.33	0.5-1.5	3-4
Short Acting			
Regular	0.5-1	2-5	6-8
Intermediate Acting			
NPH	1.5-5	4-12	14-24
Lente	2.5-5	4-12	18-24
Long Acting			
Ultralente	6-10	10-30	24-36

*The times of onset, peak activity, and duration may vary widely from individual to individual and at different times in the same individual. Therefore these times are guidelines only.

present, and thus older adults or others with significant atherosclerosis need to be especially careful if they choose to use intensive therapy.

Oral hypoglycemic agents, including metformin, repaglinide, and the sulfonylureas (tolbutamide, chlorpropamide, tolazamide, glipizide, and glyburide), are used in treatment of some individuals with type 2 diabetes. Metformin acts primarily by making the tissues more sensitive to insulin, whereas the major role of repaglinide and the sulfonylureas is to stimulate insulin release from the pancreas. Acarbose is a medication that delays the digestion of starches and other complex carbohydrates, thus reducing the peak postprandial blood glucose concentrations. Some individuals with type 2 diabetes require daily insulin injections to maintain good control of blood glucose.

Monitoring Blood Glucose

The American Diabetes Association (2000) has suggested goals for glycemic control as follows:

1. Average preprandial glucose (in capillary blood), 80-120 mg/dl (4.4-6.1 mmol/l)

2. Average bedtime glucose, 100-140 mg/dl (5.6-7.8 mmol/l)
3. **Glycosylated hemoglobin** (HbA_{1c}), <7% (HBA_{1c} reflects the blood glucose levels over the two- to three-month period before the test was performed.)

Self-monitoring of blood glucose (SMBG) is an important tool for achieving these goals. When intensive therapy is used in type 1 diabetes, SMBG is done at least 3 to 4 times daily to achieve the goals of preventing complications while maintaining patient safety. Daily monitoring is necessary in patients with type 2 diabetes who are treated with insulin or sulfonylureas, in order to detect asymptomatic hypoglycemia. The frequency of monitoring is less clearcut in individuals with type 2 diabetes than those with type 1 diabetes, however. It is not known whether stable patients who can control their glucose levels with dietary modifications alone require routine SMBG.

Nutritional Care
Assessment

A diet history to determine the usual intake and activity level is an essential part of planning nutritional care for the individual with either type 1 diabetes or type 2 diabetes. Other aspects of assessment are summarized in Table 18-2.

Intervention and Teaching

The goals of intervention and teaching are for the person to:

■ Improve metabolic control and, more specifically, to keep blood glucose as near normal as possible by balancing food intake with insulin or oral hypoglycemic therapy and physical activity levels.
■ Achieve optimal serum lipid levels.
■ Consume adequate energy to maintain or attain reasonable weights for adults, normal growth and development in children and adolescents, increased metabolic needs during pregnancy and lactation, or recovery from catabolic illnesses.
■ Prevent and treat short- and long-term complications.
■ Improve overall health through optimal nutrition.

Nutrition guidelines in type 1 diabetes

Planning of care begins with a diet history to determine the person's usual pattern of food intake and physical activity, which is used to

Table 18-2   Assessment in Diabetes Mellitus

Area of Concern	Significant Findings
Overweight	*History*
	Type 2 diabetes; sedentary lifestyle; excessive insulin or kcal intake
	Physical Examination
	Weight >120% of desirable or BMI >25; triceps skinfold >95th percentile
Underweight	*History*
	Type 1 diabetes
	Physical Examination
	Weight <90% of desirable or BMI <18.5; triceps skinfold <5th percentile; failure of children to follow established growth patterns (see Appendix D)
Glucose Tolerance	
Hyperglycemia	*History*
	Type 1 and 2 diabetes with inadequate treatment (too low a drug dosage or too great a kcal intake), noncompliance to the treatment regimen, or stress such as infection or surgery
	Physical Examination
	Flushed skin, thirst, polyuria, poor skin turgor; drowsiness, dizziness, weakness; pain in abdomen; nausea, vomiting
	Laboratory Analysis
	↑ Blood glucose; urine positive for glucose; urine positive for ketones (in ketoacidosis); ↑ serum osmolality (in nonketotic hyperosmolar coma); Hb A_{1c} >6% (hyperglycemia over a period of several weeks)

Table 18-2   Assessment in Diabetes Mellitus—cont'd

Area of Concern	Significant Findings
Glucose Tolerance—cont'd	
Hypoglycemia	*History*
	Excessive intake of insulin; unusual exertion without increased food intake; omission of scheduled meal or snack; gastroenteritis or other illness with vomiting; excessive alcohol use; use of drugs that reduce blood glucose (e.g., salicylates, chloramphenicol)
	Physical Examination
	Hunger, headache, trembling, excessive perspiration, faintness, double vision
	Laboratory Analysis
	↓ Blood glucose
Adequacy of Mineral Nutriture	
Zinc (Zn)	*History*
	↑ Excretion
	Physical Examination
	Anorexia; hypogeusia; poor wound healing; diarrhea; dermatitis
	Laboratory Analysis
	↓ Serum Zn
Magnesium (Mg)	*History*
	↑ Excretion, especially in ketoacidosis
	Physical Examination
	Weakness, muscle pain, disorientation
	Laboratory Analysis
	↓ Serum Mg

Continued

Table 18-2   Assessment in Diabetes Mellitus—cont'd

Area of Concern	Significant Findings
Adequacy of Mineral Nutriture—cont'd	
Chromium (Cr)	*History*
	Inadequate intake, especially a diet with many refined foods
	Laboratory Analysis
	↑ Blood glucose

develop an individualized meal plan and schedule of insulin therapy. All individuals taking insulin must perform daily SMBG so that hypoglycemia and hyperglycemia are detected early and insulin dosages can be adjusted as needed. For most individuals, eating at regular times every day and synchronizing food intake with the time of action of the insulin used (see Table 18-1) is recommended. For example, if a dose of NPH insulin is taken at 6:00 AM, then breakfast should be eaten by 7:30 AM, when the onset of insulin activity could occur. Both lunch and an afternoon snack are needed because the peak insulin activity will occur between noon and late afternoon; and a bedtime snack is needed because insulin activity can last 24 hours. For people who are willing to participate in intensive therapy, with multiple daily insulin injections or CSII, there is more flexibility in the timing and composition of meals and snacks. Insulin dosages and administration times can be adjusted to compensate for changes in the meal plan. Ultra-short-acting insulin, taken at the time of a meal or snack, allows for quick changes in plans.

Nutrition guidelines in type 2 diabetes

Nutritional care in type 2 diabetes is aimed at controlling blood glucose and lipids and blood pressure. Most individuals with type 2 diabetes are overweight or obese, and weight loss improves metabolic control, but efforts to achieve and maintain an ideal body weight are often unsuccessful. A nutritionally adequate, reduced-fat meal plan providing 250 to 500 kcal less than the average daily intake should be recommended, along with an increase in physical activity. A weight loss of only 5 to 9 kg (10 to 20 lb), regardless of the starting weight, usually reduces blood glucose levels, dyslipidemia, and blood pressure.

Nutrition guidelines in pregnancy

The infant of a diabetic woman in poor control at the time of conception is at risk for fetal malformations or death, prematurity, respiratory distress syndrome, and macrosomia (excessive body size). Very good control of blood glucose during pregnancy reduces the risk of complications in the infant. Thus, SMBG and intensive therapy to maintain near-normal blood glucose levels are preferred during pregnancy. To prevent congenital anomalies, it is best if intensive therapy begins before conception because most organ formation occurs very early in pregnancy.

Gestational diabetes mellitus (GDM) increases the risk of fetal macrosomia, maternal hypertensive disorders, and need for Caesarean delivery, as well as complications in the neonatal period, including hypoglycemia, hypocalcemia, and polycythemia (excessive red blood cell concentration). Good metabolic control reduces these risks. The goal is to maintain fasting blood glucose levels at 95 mg/dl (5.3 mmol/l) or less and two-hour postprandial levels at 120 mg/dl (6.7 mmol/l) or less. A bedtime snack is usually advisable to reduce the risk of hypoglycemia during the night. Ideally, women with GDM will be counseled by a registered dietitian to adhere to a meal plan that provides adequate calories and nutrients to promote normal growth of the fetus. Weight gain goals during pregnancy are provided in Chapter 3. Obese women (BMI >30) have had improved glucose and triglyceride levels when following a moderately energy-restricted diet (approximately 1800 kcal/day). Physical activity should also be encouraged as a means of improving control of blood glucose. Women with GDM need thorough instruction in self-monitoring. Daily SMBG is an important part of diabetic care in pregnancy. When insulin is used, postprandial glucose levels appear to be more useful than preprandial levels. Some evidence suggests that excessive ketone levels may have adverse effects on the fetus, and therefore, urine monitoring of ketones may be of benefit in determining the adequacy of energy intake and/or insulin dosages.

Components of the diet in diabetes

Protein

Adults with diabetes and normal renal function are believed to have protein needs similar to those of the general population, and a protein intake providing 10% to 20% of caloric intake is usually considered appropriate. If nephropathy develops but the glomerular filtration rate (GFR) is still normal, then the diabetes care team may consider limiting protein intake to no more than 0.8 g/kg/day (the adult RDA, and approximately 10% of caloric intake). Once the GFR begins to fall, restricting protein intake to no more than 0.6 g/kg/day may slow the progression of the nephropathy in some patients.

Fat

Diabetes is a risk factor for dyslipidemias and coronary heart disease, and overweight and obesity are very common among people with diabetes. To help control these problems, fat should provide no more than 30% of the total kcal in the diet. Saturated and polyunsaturated fats should each provide less than 10% of the total kcal, leaving monounsaturated fats to provide as much as 10% to 15% of total kcal. Cholesterol intake should be limited to 300 mg/day (see Chapter 15). If low-density lipoprotein (LDL) cholesterol is not reduced with these measures, then saturated fat intake can be further reduced to no more than 7% of total kcal and cholesterol intake can be restricted to <200 mg/day. If serum triglyceride levels are elevated, then an increase in monounsaturated fats and a decrease in carbohydrate intake may help to reduce them. In severe hypertriglyceridemia (>1000 mg/dl or 11.3 mmol/l), however, it is usually necessary to restrict fat to <10% of kcal to reduce the risk of pancreatitis.

Carbohydrate

Carbohydrate usually accounts for 50% or more of the kcal consumed. Even when insulin is not used, carbohydrate (and other energy nutrients) should be spread as evenly as possible among the meals, and meals should be far enough apart (4 to 5 hours) to allow blood glucose to return to basal concentrations before each meal. Although most of the carbohydrate should come from nutritious foods within the meal plan, sucrose can be substituted for other carbohydrate foods without impairing metabolic control. Soluble fiber from oats, legumes, fruits, and vegetables can help to reduce serum lipid levels. Diabetic individuals should consume at least 25 to 30 g of fiber daily, as should the general population.

Some foods have been identified as having a low **glycemic index**—that is, they cause less change in the blood glucose than some reference carbohydrate (usually white bread or glucose). Rice is a food of relatively high glycemic index, and legumes are low, for example; however, the speed of digestion is a major determinant of how much blood glucose changes, and many factors affect the speed of digestion, including preparation method, the presence of fat in the meal or snack, and the ripeness of fruits or vegetables. Some individuals may wish to plan their diets with a focus on foods of low glycemic index, but many others find it more practical to control total carbohydrate intake than to try to control the glycemic index. See Foster-Powell and Miller (1995) for a compilation of glycemic index data for various foods.

Nonnutritive sweeteners (those containing negligible or no calories) include aspartame, acesulfame K, sucralose, and saccharin. These sweeteners can be consumed in moderation by people with diabetes. Individuals with phenylketonuria should not use aspartame (Nutrasweet). Nutritive sugar substitutes such as sugar alcohols (e.g., sorbitol) are sometimes used in products marketed to people with diabetes. They provide about half the kcal per gram as sugars do, but their kcal contribution must be considered as part of the meal plan. Excessive amounts may cause diarrhea.

Alcohol

Limited amounts of alcohol can be included in the meal plans of most diabetic individuals if they so desire. Alcohol is not metabolized to glucose, and it inhibits gluconeogenesis (formation of glucose from noncarbohydrates, i.e., amino acids and glycerol). Therefore, people taking insulin or oral hypoglycemic agents might become hypoglycemic if they consume alcohol without food. The recommendation in diabetes is the same as for the general population—no more than 2 drinks (1 drink = 12 oz beer, 5 oz wine, or 1.5 oz distilled spirits) daily. Normally, these drinks are consumed in addition to the usual meal plan because they do not elevate blood glucose. For overweight or obese individuals, however, each serving of alcohol should be substituted for fat in the diet (1 alcohol serving = 2 fat exchanges). Pregnant women and people with a history of alcohol abuse should not consume alcohol, and those with pancreatitis, hypertriglyceridemia, or neuropathy should consume very little, if any.

Vitamins and minerals

No sound evidence suggests that individuals with diabetes have an increased need for vitamins, compared with nondiabetic adults. Deficiencies of two minerals, chromium and magnesium, are associated with resistance to the effects of insulin and glucose intolerance. Supplements may improve glucose tolerance if the individual is deficient in these nutrients, but there is no benefit from supplementation if stores are adequate. Apparently, most people with diabetes are not deficient in chromium or magnesium.

Sodium

Recommendations for sodium intake for nonhypertensive people with diabetes are the same as for the general population—no more than 2400 to 3000 mg/day. If mild to moderate hypertension is present, limiting daily sodium intake to 2400 mg or less may be beneficial. For the person with hypertension and nephropathy, an intake of 2000 mg/day or less is reasonable. Box 15-1 provides guidelines for these levels of sodium restriction.

Tools for meal planning

The American Diabetes Association and American Dietetic Association have jointly developed *Exchange Lists for Meal Planning* (1995), in which foods are grouped according to similarities in their carbohydrate, protein, and fat content. In working with the person with diabetes to develop a meal plan, the dietitian considers the person's optimal energy intake (Table 18-3), as well as the desirable proportions of carbohydrate, protein, and fat in the diet (see previous discussion). Once these parameters are established, the number of exchanges (servings) from each group can be identified, and the exchanges can be assigned to specific meals and snacks so that the carbohydrate is spread evenly throughout the day. Starch, milk, and fruit exchanges contain approximately the same amount of carbohydrate (12 to 15 g/exchange) and can be substituted for one another.

Carbohydrate counting is a technique that focuses on the carbohydrate content of foods consumed. Protein and fat content of the diet must be considered, along with carbohydrate, because otherwise excessive weight gain may occur. The emphasis on carbohydrate is justified, however, by the fact that carbohydrate is the main component of the diet that affects postprandial blood glucose levels and insulin requirements. The Exchange Lists and Nutrition Facts on food labels can be used to identify the carbohydrate content of foods. Depending on the skills and interest of the diabetic individual, carbohydrate counting can be a very simple or very complex technique. At its simplest, the dietitian teaches the person with diabetes to identify sources of carbohydrate

Table 18-3   Estimating Daily Energy Needs

Adults*

Basal calories	20-25 kcal/kg desirable body wt	
Add calories for activity	If sedentary	30% more calories
	If moderately active	50% more calories
	If strenuously active	100% more calories
Adjustments†	Add 300 kcal/day during pregnancy	
	Add 500 kcal/day during lactation	
	Add 500 kcal/day to gain 1 lb/wk	
	Subtract 500 kcal/day to lose 1 lb/wk	

Infants and Children‡

	Age (yr)	Calories/kg	Calories/day
Infants	0-0.5	108	650
	0.5-1.0	98	850
Children	1-3	102	1,300
	4-6	90	1,800
	7-10	70	2,000
Males	11-14	55	2,500
	15-18	45	3,000
	19-24	40	2,900
Females	11-14	47	2,200
	15-18	40	2,200
	19-24	38	2,200

From *Medical management of type 1 diabetes,* ed 3. Alexandria, VA: American Diabetes Association, 1998. Used with permission.

Note: From birth to age 10, no distinction between sexes is made regarding energy requirements. Separate allowances are recommended for boys and girls older than age 10 because of differences in the age and onset of puberty and patterns of physical activity. Considerable variability is seen in the timing and magnitude of the adolescent growth spurt and in activity patterns. Consequently, the range of the recommendation for children older than age 20 is wider, and energy allowances should be adjusted individually to take into account body weight, physical activity, and rate of growth.

*Adapted from Joyce M: Issues in prescribing calories. In Powers M: *Handbook of diabetes medical nutrition therapy,* Gaithersburg, MD, 1996, Aspen Publishers (p. 368).

†Adjustments are approximate: weight changes should be monitored and compared with caloric intake.

‡Adapted from National Academy of Sciences: *Recommended Dietary Allowances.* 10th ed. Washington, DC, National Academy Press, 1989.

in the diet, and they work together to make carbohydrate intake at a meal consistent from day to day. Keeping food records is encouraged, to help the person recognize the relationship between carbohydrate intake and blood glucose levels. At an intermediate level, the person further develops record-keeping skills, comparing blood glucose records with food intake records. The person learns to recognize patterns in blood glucose readings and to understand how they relate to food intake, physical activity, and diabetes medications. At its most complex level, carbohydrate counting is appropriate for people with type 1 diabetes who are receiving intensive insulin therapy. At this level, the person with diabetes matches insulin dosages precisely with carbohydrate intake, decreasing or increasing the insulin dosage to allow consumption of less or more carbohydrate than usual.

Exercise

Regular exercise (continuous activity lasting at least 20 to 30 minutes and performed at least 3 to 4 days a week) can promote weight control, reduce the risk of heart disease, help relieve psychologic stress, and increase the sensitivity of the tissues to insulin. The guidelines in Chapter 6, for becoming and remaining physically fit, are appropriate for individuals with diabetes, but these individuals should undertake an exercise program only under a physician's supervision. If neuropathy is present in the feet, then exercise that causes impact on the feet (e.g., jogging, treadmill running) should be avoided, and swimming, cycling, rowing, or other low-impact activities should be chosen.

Individuals with type 1 diabetes should monitor their blood glucose before and after exercise to determine whether insulin or food intake needs to be adjusted. The person should not exercise if the blood glucose is >250 mg/dl (13.9 mmol/l) and ketosis is present and use caution if the blood glucose is >300 mg/dl (16.6 mmol/l) whether or not ketosis is present (American Diabetes Association, 2000). If the preexercise blood glucose concentration is less than 100 mg/dl (5.6 mM), then the individual needs to consume a carbohydrate-containing snack before exercise. Snacks may be needed every 30 to 60 minutes to prevent hypoglycemia during exercise lasting more than 30 minutes. Appropriate snacks provide approximately 10 to 15 g of rapidly absorbed carbohydrate. Examples include 1 small apple or banana, 1/2 cup regular soft drink, 1/2 bagel, or 4 to 6 oz fruit juice. Some individuals become hypoglycemic several hours after exercise ends, and they need a snack or meal after exercise. Strenuous activity lasting 45 minutes or longer may result in a need to decrease the insulin dosage.

Coping with acute illness

Individuals with diabetes must be taught to cope with sick days (e.g., acute viral illnesses) before they occur. They must learn to do the following:

- Check blood glucose and urine ketones frequently, often every 2 to 4 hours.
- Consume approximately 10 to 15 g carbohydrate every 1 to 2 hours (Box 18-2). When vomiting, diarrhea, or fever is present, small amounts of liquids every 15 to 30 minutes help to prevent dehydration, replace electrolyte losses, and provide energy.
- Notify the health care provider if it is impossible to take and retain carbohydrate-containing foods and fluids for 4 hours or more, blood glucose is difficult to control or ketonuria is present, persistent diarrhea occurs, severe abdominal pain is present, or the illness lasts more than 24 hours.

Minimizing acute complications

Hypoglycemia

Hypoglycemia is most common in people treated with insulin but can also occur with oral hypoglycemic therapy. Instruction should be planned to help the person (and significant others, as appropriate):

- Be aware of and avoid precipitating factors: failing to eat scheduled meals and snacks, eating meals or snacks late, vomiting or poor food intake during acute illness, prolonged or intense physical activity without a compensatory increase in carbohydrate intake or decrease in insulin dosage, alcohol intake, and impaired mentation and self-care skills, resulting from alcohol intoxication or illicit drug use.
- Recognize signs and symptoms of hypoglycemia: hunger, irritability, headache, shakiness, sweating, and altered neurologic status ranging from drowsiness to unconsciousness and convulsions. Repeated episodes of hypoglycemia can cause symptom unawareness, e.g., if hypoglycemia occurs one day, then the person with diabetes may be unaware of symptoms if an episode of hypoglycemia occurs the following day.

Box 18-2   Foods and Fluids for Sick Days*

½ cup (120 ml) regular gelatin dessert
½ cup (120 ml) fat-free, light, or regular ice cream
½ cup (120 ml) sherbet or sorbet
1 frozen fruit juice bar
6 saltine crackers
4 slices melba toast
1 cup (240 ml) tomato, vegetable, chicken noodle, or
    cream soup
½ cup (120 ml) sugar-free (or ¼ cup regular) pudding
¾ cup (180 ml) regular ginger ale
½ cup (120 ml) regular cola or lemon-lime soda
½ cup (120 ml) orange juice

---

*Each serving provides approximately 15 g carbohydrate.

- Test blood glucose regularly and any time signs of hypoglycemia appear.
- Correct hypoglycemia (blood glucose <70 mg/dl [3.8 mmol/l]) if it occurs. The diabetic individual should have a carbohydrate source, such as glucose in tablet or liquid form, granulated sugar, or hard candy, always available for use if symptoms occur. One guideline is to consume 15 g carbohydrate (e.g., 2 tbsp raisins, 1/2 cup orange or apple juice, 1/2 cup regular soft drink, 5 LifeSavers) if blood glucose falls below 70 mg/dl and to retest the blood glucose in 15 minutes and eat another 15 g carbohydrate if still hypoglycemic. Following the initial carbohydrate feeding with a more substantial snack or meal containing protein, fat, and carbohydrate helps to reduce the risk of recurrence of the hypoglycemia.
- Wear a Medic-Alert bracelet so that treatment can be given if the individual becomes confused or unconscious.

Diabetic ketoacidosis

This complication occurs primarily in individuals with type 1 diabetes. Instruction should help the person (and significant others, as appropriate) with the following goals:

- Be aware of precipitating factors, such as acute infectious illnesses or failure to take the prescribed dosage of insulin or oral hypoglycemic agents.

■ Recognize the signs and symptoms such as elevated blood glucose, thirst, warm dry skin, nausea and vomiting, "fruity"-smelling breath, pain in abdomen, drowsiness, and polyuria.

■ Check blood glucose if the symptoms occur, and obtain medical treatment if blood glucose is excessively elevated.

Hyperglycemic hyperosmolar nonketotic syndrome

This complication is more common in the individual with type 2 diabetes. Instruction should help the individual (and significant others, as appropriate) with the following goals:

■ Be aware of precipitating factors, such as infections or other stress.

■ Recognize the symptoms such as excessive thirst, polyuria, dehydration, shallow respirations, and altered sensorium.

■ Check blood glucose if symptoms occur, and obtain medical attention if the blood glucose level is high.

Coping with diabetic gastroparesis

Prokinetic agents, including metoclopramide, erythromycin, and the investigational drug domperidone, can be effective in stimulating GI motility in some instances. Correcting hyperglycemia can help relieve symptoms because hyperglycemia has an inhibitory effect on gastric emptying. People with gastroparesis should be encouraged to keep detailed food intake, blood glucose, and symptom records so that insulin administration can be fitted to peak absorption times. Use of short- and ultra-short-acting insulins increases flexibility in coping with the problem (e.g., a dose of insulin lispro can be injected postprandially if SMBG reveals that blood glucose is excessively high).

Medical nutrition therapy in gastroparesis includes counseling to reduce fat intake because fat tends to delay gastric emptying. People with gastroparesis are at risk for formation of gastric bezoars (hardened gastrointestinal contents, often containing food fibers), and decreasing the intake of high-fiber foods (see Appendix B) may decrease this risk. Small, frequent meals may be better tolerated than large meals if early satiety is a problem. Food should be chewed thoroughly. Maintaining an upright posture for at least 30 to 60 minutes after a meal allows gravity to facilitate gastric emptying.

SELECTED BIBLIOGRAPHY

American Diabetes Association, American Dietetic Association: *Exchange lists for meal planning,* Alexandria, Va, and Chicago, 1995, The Associations.

American Diabetes Association: Clinical practice recommendations 2000, *Diabetes Care* 23 (suppl 1): S1-S116, 2000.

Anderson RA: Nutritional factors influencing the glucose/insulin system: chromium, *J Am Coll Nutr* 16:404, 1997.

Foster-Powell K, Miller JB: International tables of glycemic index, *Am J Clin Nutr* 62 (suppl):871S, 1995.

Gillespie SJ, Kulkarni KD, Daly AE: Using carbohydrate counting in diabetes clinical practice, *J Am Dietet Assoc* 98:897, 1998.

Jones MW, Stone LC: Management of the woman with gestational diabetes mellitus, *J Perinatal Neonatal Nurs* 11:13, 1998.

UK Prospective Diabetes Study (UKPDS) Group: Intensive blood-glucose control with sulphonylureas or insulin compared with conventional treatment and risk of complications in patients with type 2 diabetes (UKPDS 33), *Lancet* 352:837, 1998a.

UK Prospective Diabetes Study (UKPDS) Group: Effect of intensive blood-glucose control with metformin on complications in overweight patients with type 2 diabetes (UKPDS 34), *Lancet* 352:854, 1998b.

Valmadrid CT et al.: Alcohol intake and the risk of coronary heart disease mortality in persons with older-onset diabetes mellitus, *JAMA* 282:239, 1999.

Valentine V, Barone JA, Hill JVC: Gastropathy in patients with diabetes: current concepts and treatment recommendations, *Diabetes Spectrum* 11:248, 1998.

Williams KV, et al.: Improved glycemic control reduces the impact of weight gain on cardiovascular risk factors in type 1 diabetes. The Epidemiology of Diabetes Complications Study, *Diabetes Care* 22:1084, 1999.

Alcohol-Related, Mental, and Neurologic Disorders

19

Alcohol Abuse and Alcoholism
Pathophysiology

Alcohol abuse can be defined as heavy drinking with an increasing tolerance for ethanol but no withdrawal symptoms when drinking stops. **Alcoholism** refers to a strong craving for ethanol, associated with increasing tolerance to alcohol's intoxicating effects and symptoms of withdrawal when drinking is discontinued. Approximately two thirds of adults in the United States drink alcohol, but heavy drinkers (about 10% of those who drink or 7% of the total adult population) account for most of the social and physical problems associated with alcoholism and alcohol abuse. Both genetic and environmental factors appear to contribute to development of alcoholism and alcohol abuse.

Alcoholism and alcohol abuse are found in all socioeconomic classes and cultural groups. The rates of alcohol-related problems tend to be lower in Japanese and some other Asian groups, however, because there is a very high (~50%) prevalence of acetaldehyde dehydrogenase deficiency in these groups. This enzyme is a part of the pathway for metabolism of alcohol, and a deficiency allows the accumulation of acetaldehyde following alcohol ingestion. High levels of acetaldehyde can cause many unpleasant symptoms, including nausea, vomiting, hypotension, faintness, respiratory difficulties, throbbing head, and chest pain, and these symptoms deter most affected individuals from heavy drinking.

Heavy alcohol use has adverse effects on nutrition both because it displaces other, more nutritious, foods in the diet and because chronic use impairs absorption and metabolism of many nutrients. Ethanol provides approximately 7 kcal/g, and alcoholics often obtain as much as 50% of their energy intake from ethanol (Table 19-1). The most common nutritional problems in heavy drinkers include deficiencies of protein, thiamin, folate, vitamin B_6

Table 19-1   Approximate Alcohol and Kilocalorie Content of Some Common Alcohol Beverages

Beverage and Serving Size	Alcohol (g/Serving)	Kcal/ Serving
Beer, Ale, and Malt Liquor		
Beer, 12 fl oz	13	150
Beer, light, 12 fl oz	11	100
Beer, low alcohol, 12 fl oz	6.5	75
Malt liquor or ale, 12 fl oz	15	150
Cocktails*		
Bloody Mary, 5 fl oz	14	120
Gin & tonic, 7.5 fl oz	16	170
Martini, 2.5 fl oz	22	160
Piña colada, 4.5 fl oz	20	260
Distilled Spirits (Gin, Rum, Vodka, Whiskey), 1.5 fl oz Jigger		
80 proof	14	97
90 proof	16	110
100 proof	18	124
Wines		
Dessert, 2 fl oz	9	75
Table, 3.5 fl oz	9.6	75

Abbreviation: fl oz, fluid ounce (approximately 30 ml).
*Components: Bloody Mary = tomato juice, vodka, and lemon juice; gin & tonic = tonic water, gin, and lime juice; martini = gin and vermouth; piña colada = pineapple juice, rum, sugar, and coconut cream.

(pyridoxine), niacin, riboflavin, magnesium, zinc, and calcium. The protein deficiency, along with generalized nutritional deficits, contributes to the development of fatty liver. Fatty liver occurs when inadequate protein is available to form lipoproteins for the transport of lipids out of the liver, causing the lipids synthesized in the liver to be stored there.

In addition to the nutritional deficiencies associated with alcohol abuse, the metabolism of alcohol can result in metabolic complications such as hypoglycemia, lactic acidosis, hyperuricemia (contributing to gout), hypertriglyceridemia, and ketoacidosis. Both underweight (because of poor food intake) and overweight are problems among alcoholics. Overweight is a problem especially in middle- and upper-income alcoholics because of the significant amount of energy provided by alcohol. A variety of other medical problems are associated with heavy alcohol use, including cirrhosis of the liver, hepatic encephalopathy, pancreatitis, gastritis, cerebral atrophy, hypertension, osteopenia (thinning of the bones), and neuropathy associated with demyelination of the nerves. **Wernicke-Korsakoff syndrome** is a serious disorder of the central nervous system that can occur in alcoholism. Symptoms are mental confusion, memory loss, confabulation, ataxia, abnormal ocular motility (ophthalmoplegia and nystagmus), and peripheral neuropathy. The cause of Wernicke-Korsakoff syndrome appears to be multifactorial, but both genetic susceptibility and thiamin deficiency play roles in its development.

Treatment

Alcoholics tend to deny that they have a problem. Effective therapy for alcoholism comes only after the individual has acknowledged the illness. Comprehensive therapy includes individual or group counseling, usually involving family members and/or close friends, and a nutritious diet. Prolonged follow-up (e.g., through participation in a group such as Alcoholics Anonymous) is necessary for most recovering alcoholics. Pharmacologic agents are often used early in treatment of alcoholism. Antianxiety agents such as diazepam may be used to reduce anxiety during alcohol withdrawal. Disulfiram (Antabuse), which interferes with the metabolism of alcohol, is sometimes administered for several weeks or months to help the individual resist the compulsion to drink. When alcohol is ingested by the person taking disulfiram, acetaldehyde levels in the blood rise, causing many unpleasant symptoms (see previous Pathophysiology discussion).

Nutritional Care

Most forms of alcohol are low in micronutrients (vitamins and minerals). Chronic alcohol abuse can cause low hepatic stores of folic acid, niacin, and vitamins B_6 (pyridoxine) and B_{12}, as well as impaired utilization of folic acid and vitamins B_1 (thiamin) and B_6. In addition, zinc and magnesium levels may be low as a result of increased urinary excretion of these minerals during heavy drinking. Bone loss may occur because of increased calcium loss in the urine. Organ damage associated with alcohol abuse, including hepatitis, hepatic cirrhosis, and pancreatitis, interferes with absorption of fat, fat-soluble vitamins, and minerals. Gastritis related to alcohol abuse may result in iron-deficiency anemia from blood loss.

Goals of medical nutrition therapy are to support the individual in avoiding alcohol and to correct nutritional deficits.

Assessment

Assessment is summarized in Table 19-2.

Intervention and teaching

Promoting hepatic regeneration and correcting nutritional deficits

The most important dietary change is abstinence from alcohol to allow the liver to heal. People who abuse alcohol are likely to have a variety of nutritional deficits, as described previously. A nutritious diet adequate in energy, protein, and micronutrients can promote hepatic regeneration. If esophageal varices are present, bland foods and foods that are soft in texture (see Appendix J) reduce the risk of bleeding varices. Medical nutrition therapy of hepatitis, hepatic encephalopathy, and steatorrhea related to alcohol abuse are described in Chapter 12. If ascites (excessive accumulation of serous fluid within the peritoneum) are present, then a sodium restriction (usually 1 g/day) is commonly used (see Box 15-1).

In the severely malnourished alcoholic, especially if Wernicke-Korsakoff syndrome is suspected, thiamin 100 mg/day is given parenterally for three days because absorption is likely to be impaired. After the initial three days of treatment, oral thiamin 50 mg/day is recommended for at least 6 weeks and 50 mg weekly thereafter. The other B vitamins, particularly folate and vitamin B_6, zinc, and magnesium, are often administered orally at dosages two

Table 19-2   Assessment in Alcoholism and Disruptions
of Mental Health

Area of Concern	Significant Findings
Protein-Calorie Malnutrition (PCM)	*History* Chronic alcohol or other drug abuse (inadequate intake of nutritious foods or impaired absorption of nutrients); paranoia, delusions (e.g., fear that food is poisoned); confusion, disorientation, inability to care for self (e.g., schizophrenia, Alzheimer's disease) *Physical Examination* Hepatomegaly (can be from both malnutrition and toxic effects of alcohol); ascites, edema; muscle wasting; triceps skinfold or AMC <5th percentile; weight <90% of standard or BMI <18.5 ($\downarrow$ body weight may be masked by presence of ascites and edema) *Laboratory Analysis* $\downarrow$ Serum albumin, transferrin, or prealbumin ($\downarrow$ levels may indicate liver failure instead of or in addition to malnutrition); $\downarrow$ lymphocyte count
Overweight/Obesity	*History* Excessive intake of kcal (sometimes occurs in depression or alcoholism) *Physical Examination* Weight >120% of standard or BMI >25; triceps skinfold >95th percentile

Continued

Table 19-2   Assessment in Alcoholism and Disruptions of Mental Health—cont'd

Area of Concern	Significant Findings
Vitamin Deficiencies	
B complex, especially B_1, B_6, folic acid	*History* Alcohol abuse; high ethanol or carbohydrate intake without adequate vitamins; severely restricted diet (e.g., canned soups, soft drinks, candy, snack foods) *Physical Examination* Peripheral neuropathy; dermatitis; glossitis, cheilosis; edema, congestive heart failure; confusion, memory loss *Laboratory Analysis* ↓ Hct, ↑ MCV, ↓ serum or RBC folic acid; NOTE: Laboratory assessment of vitamins B_1 and B_6 is rarely done; these vitamins have low toxicity; large doses are given and response is evaluated clinically
Mineral Deficiencies	
Zinc (Zn)	*History* Alcohol abuse, with poor intake and ↑ excretion of Zn *Physical Examination* Hypogeusia, dysgeusia; diarrhea; dermatitis *Laboratory Analysis* ↓ Serum Zn

Table 19-2   Assessment in Alcoholism and Disruptions
of Mental Health—cont'd

Area of Concern	Significant Findings
Mineral Deficiencies—cont'd	
Magnesium (Mg)	*History*
	Alcohol abuse, with poor intake and ↑ excretion of Mg
	Physical Examination
	Tremor, ataxia; mental disorientation
	Laboratory Analysis
	↓ Serum Mg
Calcium (Ca)	*History*
	Alcohol abuse, with poor intake and ↑ excretion of Ca
	Laboratory Analysis
	Osteopenia on radiograph

to three times the Dietary Reference Intake (DRI) for several weeks, to replenish the tissue stores of these nutrients. A daily oral multivitamin-multimineral supplement providing the DRI is usually recommended for several months thereafter.

Recovered alcoholics need continued help, particularly advice for coping with social events and holidays when alcohol is usually served. Role-playing before these occasions can be helpful. The likelihood of success is increased by involvement of family and friends. Organizations such as Al-Anon can be of great benefit in providing support to family and friends and in helping them to learn how to help the recovering alcoholic.

Disorders of Mental Health
Pathophysiology

Mental illnesses have a variety of diverse origins too extensive to describe here. It is important to note that most mental illnesses have no nutritional cause. "Orthomolecular psychiatry," a treatment approach using vitamin supplements containing 10 to 500 times the recommended intakes, is not supported by scientific evidence or recognized as acceptable therapy by the American Psychiatric Association. There is also no reason to believe, as some individuals do, that many cases of mental illness arise from allergies or hypersensitivity to common foods. In most cases, nutritional care is primarily a supportive measure during the treatment of mental health disorders.

Treatment

A variety of treatment modalities may be used in mental disorders, including psychoanalysis, behavioral therapy, and family therapy. Some of the medications used are major and minor tranquilizers and lithium. Appendix H lists effects of these drugs on appetite and nutrient needs.

Nutritional Care

The goal of care is for the person to be able to cope with nutrition-related symptoms often seen in disruptions of mental health.

Assessment

Table 19-2 describes assessment in mental disorders.

Intervention

A variety of nutrition-related symptoms are found among individuals with disruptions of mental health. Most of these conditions are corrected when the individual receives adequate treatment for the underlying disorder; however, Table 19-3 summarizes approaches that can be used until the person has responded to treatment.

Neurologic Disorders

Convulsive (Seizure) Disorders

Pathophysiology

Numerous types of convulsive disorders (generally referred to as epilepsy) occur. Partial seizures affect only one cerebral hemisphere so that consciousness is maintained but some cognitive functions such as speech are transiently lost. Generalized seizures affect the brain as a whole, and consciousness is lost, but the loss

Table 19-3 Intervention in Mental Disorders

Symptoms	Example of Mental Disorder	Suggested Interventions
Anorexia/apathy about food	Depression	Provide small, frequent feedings of foods high in kcal; determine likes and dislikes, and try to accommodate these; serve foods in an attractive manner; use nutritional supplements (see Tables 9-1 and 9-2) as needed
Constipation	Depression	Encourage high-fiber foods and liberal fluid intake
Overeating	Depression	Make low-kcal foods available, but avoid emphasizing weight control until mental condition stabilizes
Confusion/disorientation	Schizophrenia, organic brain syndrome, Alzheimer's disease (AD, or senile dementia)	Remind individual to eat, if necessary; may need to direct him to take each bite; feed in an unhurried manner if self-feeding is not possible

Continued

Table 19-3   Intervention in Mental Disorders—cont'd

Symptoms	Example of Mental Disorder	Suggested Interventions
Excessive activity with "no time to eat"	Manic behavior	Provide high-kcal foods that can be carried with the person who is too active to sit for a meal: sandwiches; muffins; sliced cheese; fruit, custard, or pudding served in unbreakable containers; liquid nutritional supplements (see Table 9-1) in plastic glasses
Delusions (e.g., fear that food is poisoned or, conversely, belief that certain foods have magical powers)	Schizophrenia	Allow individual to choose foods and beverages until delusions have responded to treatment; try to avoid tube feeding of persons with paranoia because this may increase the feeling of persecution

of consciousness may be so brief that it is barely noticeable. Signs of convulsive disorders range from subtle (a blank stare or a brief twitching of the mouth or eyelids) to severe (tonic-clonic seizures, with alternate sustained contraction and relaxation of the muscles). Convulsive disorders may occur as a result of hypoxia or central nervous system trauma, malformations, neoplasms, or infections. A variety of metabolic disorders (hypoglycemia, hypocalcemia, hypomagnesemia, water intoxication, lead poisoning, medication side effects) can cause seizures; in these cases, correcting the underlying disorder is the primary treatment. A significant percentage of convulsive disorders are idiopathic (have no known cause).

Treatment

Anticonvulsant medications are the primary means of treatment. Anticonvulsants used include carbamazepine, hydantoins (phenytoin and ethotoin), ethosuximide, valproic acid, and phenobarbital.

Nutritional care

Long-term use of anticonvulsant medications increases the risk of drug-nutrient interactions and may impair nutritional status. In some instances, medications are unsuccessful in controlling seizures. Ketosis (an elevated level of ketones in the blood), achieved with a "ketogenic" high-fat diet, has been found to improve control in some individuals with seizures that respond poorly to medication.

Assessment

Nutritional assessment is summarized in Table 19-4.

Intervention and teaching

Anticonvulsant medications. Many commonly used anticonvulsants, including phenytoin, phenobarbital, and primidone, accelerate the turnover of vitamin D and can contribute to poor bone mineralization (osteomalacia). Intake of the anticonvulsants and calcium at the same time impairs the absorption of both the drug and the nutrient. Vitamin D and calcium supplements may be needed by people who take these medications, but they should not be taken at the same time as the medications.

Ketogenic diet. High levels of blood ketones produced from the metabolism of fat appear to decrease seizure activity. A diet that

Table 19-4   Assessment in Neurologic Disorders

Area of Concern	Significant Findings
Protein-Calorie Malnutrition (PCM)	*History*
	Restricted protein intake (e.g., ketogenic diet in seizure disorder, low-fat diet in multiple sclerosis); unpalatable diet (e.g., ketogenic diet); feeding/swallowing difficulties such as dribbling of food and beverages from the mouth, dysphagia, weakness of muscles required for chewing, incoordination or spasticity interfering with chewing and swallowing; dementia or memory loss (refusing or forgetting to eat); use of corticosteroids
	Physical Examination
	Muscle wasting; triceps skinfold or AMC <5th percentile; weight <90% of standard or BMI <18.5; or weight-for-height or weight-for-age <5th percentile (children); edema, ascites
	Laboratory Analysis
	↓ Serum albumin, transferrin, or prealbumin; ↓ lymphocyte count
Overweight/Obesity	*History*
	↓ Kcal needs resulting from inactivity; reliance on soft or pureed foods, which are often more dense in kcal than higher fiber foods
	Physical Examination
	Triceps skinfold >95th percentile; weight >120% of standard or BMI >25 or weight-for-height or weight-for-age >95th percentile (children)

Table 19-4   Assessment in Neurologic Disorders—cont'd

Area of Concern	Significant Findings
Vitamin and Mineral Deficiencies	
Folic acid	*History*
	Phenytoin use
	Physical Examination
	Pallor; glossitis
	Laboratory Analysis
	↓ Hct, ↑ MCV; ↓ serum folic acid
D	*History*
	Use of phenobarbital, primidone, or phenytoin, especially when combined with ketogenic diet; lack of sun exposure (e.g., institutionalization)
	Physical Examination
	Rickets; osteomalacia
	Laboratory Analysis
	↓ Serum 1,25-dihydroxyvitamin D; ↓ serum Ca (uncommon); ↑ alkaline phosphatase
Iron (Fe)	*History*
	Inadequate intake (ketogenic diet used in seizure disorders, low-fat diet used in MS, difficulty chewing meats)
	Physical Examination
	Pallor, blue sclerae; koilonychia
	Laboratory Analysis
	↓ Hct, Hgb, MCV, MCH, MCHC; ↓ serum Fe; ↑ serum transferrin or TIBC

Continued

Table 19-4 Assessment in Neurologic Disorders—cont'd

Area of Concern	Significant Findings
Vitamin and Mineral Deficiencies—cont'd	
Zinc (Zn)	*History*
	Inadequate intake (ketogenic diet, low-fat diet, difficulty chewing meats)
	Physical Examination
	Diarrhea; dermatitis; hypogeusia, dysgeusia
	Laboratory Analysis
	↓ Serum Zn
Calcium (Ca)	*History*
	Phenytoin use (↓ Ca absorption) or corticosteroid use with increased losses; inadequate intake (ketogenic diet, low-fat diet used in MS, lactose intolerance)
	Physical Examination
	Rickets; osteomalacia
	Laboratory Analysis
	↓ Serum Ca (uncommon); ↑ serum alkaline phosphatase
Fluid Deficiencies	*History*
	Poor intake caused by difficulty swallowing fluids (as in CP or ALS) or inability to express thirst
	Physical Examination
	Poor skin turgor; ↓ urinary output; dry, sticky mucous membranes
	Laboratory Analysis
	↑ Serum Na, serum osmolality, BUN, Hct, urine specific gravity

stimulates ketone production (a **ketogenic diet**) is recommended for selected individuals who exhibit a poor response to anticonvulsant medications. The diet is effective only if adherence is rigid because a small excess of carbohydrate will inhibit ketosis. Adherence becomes much more difficult as children age, unless they are severely retarded. The high fat intake is unpalatable to many individuals, and the strict diet can be a burden. Potential side effects include nephrolithiasis (kidney stones) and hypocalcemia. These side effects probably occur because the diet is so high in fat that some is not absorbed, and calcium is trapped in the fat in the feces. Calcium in the intestine reduces the absorption of oxalate, whereas loss of calcium in the stools allows increased absorption of oxalate. Oxalate is a component of many kidney stones. The diet may also result in an acidic urine that promotes formation of uric acid stones. Drugs that make the urine alkaline inhibit uric acid stone formation.

To accelerate development of ketosis, the diet is usually initiated after a 36- to 48-hour period of fasting, or a period of partial fasting (50 kcal/kg/day for young children). The diet is introduced over a period of 3 to 4 days to reduce the likelihood of nausea and vomiting. There are two forms of ketogenic diets: the classic form and the medium-chain triglyceride (MCT) or partial MCT diet. In the classic diet, the ratio of dietary fat to the combined carbohydrate and protein intake is between 3:1 and 4:1 (3 to 4 g fat for every gram of carbohydrate plus protein). The diet usually includes the following protein allowances (per kg of desirable body weight per day): 1.2 g for children <2 years of age, 1 g for children between 2 and 19 years, and 0.75 g for people over 19 years. To promote ketosis, energy intake is limited to approximately 75 kcal/kg/day for children ages 1 to 3, 68 kcal/kg/day for children ages 4 to 6, and 60 kcal/kg/day for children ages 7 to 10. Exchange lists (Walser M, et al, 1984) are available to assist in planning daily food intake.

Soft (tub or squeeze bottle) margarine and polyunsaturated and monounsaturated oils such as corn, soybean, safflower, sunflower, canola, and olive oil are preferred over butter and cream to avoid increasing serum lipid levels unnecessarily. Hyperlipidemia is common, but it apparently resolves once the diet is discontinued.

Fluids are restricted to approximately 600 to 1200 ml/day, with no more than 120 ml taken in a two-hour period, to prevent expansion of plasma volume with dilution of the ketones. Urine specific gravity must be maintained between 1.020 and 1.025.

Caffeine and aspartame (Nutrasweet) are avoided because they might inhibit ketosis.

Some clinicians prefer the use of MCTs to long-chain triglycerides (LCTs). MCTs appear to be more ketogenic than the LCTs found in most common foods, which allows the combined carbohydrate and protein content of the diet to be increased to 20% to 40% of the total energy intake and the energy and fluid allowances to be more liberal. Results are still better if moderate energy and fluid restrictions are practiced, however. There are disadvantages to the MCT diet. MCTs are more expensive than LCTs, and excessive intakes of MCTs can result in abdominal cramping and diarrhea. Incorporating MCTs into the diet can be accomplished by blending them into skim milk, using them in place of other cooking oils, making salad dressing from them, or mixing them into unsweetened applesauce, scrambled eggs, meat or pasta salads, or casseroles. Gastrointestinal side effects are lessened and seizure control is improved if small amounts are served throughout the day, rather than larger amounts once or twice daily. A modification of the MCT diet supplies approximately 30% of the kcal as MCT and 41% as LCT, with the remainder of the kcal from protein and carbohydrate.

The ketogenic diet may be low in vitamins C, A, and B complex and in iron, zinc, and calcium. A daily supplement providing the DRI for the person's age is advisable.

Cerebral Palsy

Pathophysiology

Cerebral palsy (CP) is usually the result of hypoxia during the perinatal period. Motor centers of the brain are affected, with resulting incoordination, physical disabilities, and sometimes impairments of speech, sight, and hearing. There are several types of CP: spastic paralysis, with hyperactivity of the extensor muscles; choreoathetosis, with involuntary muscle movements; ataxia, or incoordination; and flaccidity, or decreased muscle tone.

Treatment

Physical therapy and judicious use of devices, such as computers that make communication by nonverbal individuals possible, can help people with CP achieve their maximum potential. Orthopedic surgery is sometimes used to correct deformities.

Nutritional care

Goals of care are to maintain adequate intake of nutrients and to prevent obesity, which further impairs mobility in individuals with CP.

Assessment

Assessment is summarized in Table 19-4.

Intervention and teaching

Chewing and swallowing problems. Provision of adequate nutrients may be difficult because of neuromuscular impairments and persistence of primitive reflexes. To minimize these problems:

- Foods offered should be tailored to the needs of the individual. Beverages often leak out of the mouth. Leakage can be decreased by thickening fluids with infant cereals or yogurt, or liquids can be offered in the form of gelatin, fruit ices, ice cream, or sherbet.
- Individuals with CP should be placed in good anatomic position for feeding. Those with spastic CP are especially likely to hyperextend their necks, which makes swallowing difficult. Positioning them with back straight and hips and knees flexed reduces hyperextension. Separating the legs promotes stability.
- Underweight is a common problem, largely because of difficulty ingesting food. Parents and caregivers of some children with CP spend between 3 and 7 hours daily feeding the children. Because of the prolonged mealtimes, provision of snacks is often not effective in increasing intake. Thus, increasing the kcal content of foods eaten at mealtimes is the best alternative. Skim milk powder, margarine, oils, or modular ingredients (see Table 9-2) can be added to foods to increase kcal density. Gastrostomy feedings have been beneficial for many children who cannot eat enough to maintain their nutritional status and obtain adequate nutrients to support growth.

Promoting self-feeding. To make it easier for people with CP to feed themselves:

- Utilize plates with rims to allow food to be scooped up by pushing it against the rim.
- Use specially made silverware with thick handles or insert the

spoon or fork handle into a rolled washcloth to make it easier to grip.
- Prevent scooting of plates or bowls by putting suction cups, such as those used for soap holders, under them.

Preventing or correcting obesity. Individuals who are very inactive, such as those with severe motor impairments who are confined to a wheelchair, may become overweight or obese. To prevent or alleviate this problem:

- Reduce fat in the diet. Choose lean meat and skinless poultry; use skim or low-fat milk and dairy products made with skim or low-fat milk; limit intake of fried or fatty foods; serve pastries, doughnuts, and high-fat cookies and cakes rarely; use butter or margarine sparingly; use low-fat or fat-free salad dressings.
- Serve unsweetened beverages or those sweetened with sugar substitutes often. Beverages consumed before or with meals help the person feel full faster.
- Increase intake of fibers and starches. Whole grains and fresh fruits and vegetables are bulky and help the individual to feel full more quickly.
- See Chapter 7 for further suggestions.

Preventing or correcting constipation

- Good sources of fiber such as whole grains, legumes, fruits, and vegetables should be served daily. Bran (2 tablespoons) can also be added to food daily.
- Liberal fluid intake helps produce soft, bulky stools.
- Increase activity as tolerated to stimulate gastrointestinal motility.

Amyotrophic Lateral Sclerosis
Pathophysiology

Amyotrophic lateral sclerosis (ALS) is a progressive degenerative neurologic disease that results in atrophy of the muscles. Eventually, it affects most of the body, including the muscles involved in chewing and swallowing.

Treatment

There is no specific therapy and no cure for ALS. Physical therapy can help maintain as much muscle mass as possible.

Nutritional care

Goals of care are to prevent nutritional deficits and maintain feeding safety (i.e., prevent choking or aspiration of foods and beverages into the lungs).

Assessment

Assessment is summarized in Table 19-4. Weight loss is inevitable because of muscle wasting. Nutritional deficits, however, accelerate loss. When weight loss in 6 months is greater than 10% of the usual body weight, energy deficits should be suspected. Chair or bed scales are often necessary to obtain weights.

Intervention and teaching

Preventing nutritional deficits

- Encourage small, frequent feedings to maintain optimal intake. Box 13-2 offers suggestions for increasing kcal intake. Supplements in the form of puddings or thick liquids may be the easiest to consume.
- Try utensils with loops to fit over the hands to help prevent dropping of utensils and improve grip.
- Protein foods may be difficult to chew, especially if dry. Good protein sources are tender, chopped meats and poultry; moist casseroles made with meat, fish, or poultry; cheese and cottage cheese; yogurt; and poached, soft-cooked, or scrambled eggs. Gravies and sauces served with meats make chewing and swallowing easier.
- Commercial supplements (high-protein puddings and beverages or protein powders to be added to other foods; see Tables 9-1 and 9-2) are available, but home-prepared products are often tastier.
- Vitamins and minerals may be lacking because of impaired intake. A daily multivitamin-multimineral supplement can be recommended if assessment indicates a need.
- Fluids are among the most difficult foods to swallow. Plain water is especially likely to cause choking. Semisolid sources of fluid (e.g., sherbet, sorbet, fruit ices, and gelatin) can be used to promote adequate intake. Fluids can also be thickened with baby cereal to make swallowing them easier.

Reducing dysphagia and potential for pulmonary aspiration

- Serve soft, moist foods such as casseroles, meats and vegetables with gravies and sauces, applesauce, mashed potatoes, and cooked cereals.

- Do not rush the individual while eating. Serving foods in insulated dishes or on a warming tray can help maintain their temperature during prolonged mealtimes.
- Suggest that the person try turning the head to the side while swallowing or swallowing twice after each bite. Speech or physical therapists may help the individual in dealing with dysphagia.
- If excessive mucus is a problem, reduce intake of milk, which is thought to increase mucus production. Calcium can be obtained from cheese or calcium supplements.
- Keep suction equipment available.
- Gastrostomy feedings are sometimes instituted where dysphagia is severe and the risk of aspiration is high. Blended foods or commercial formulas may be used. Fluoroscopic examination while the individual is swallowing foods and liquids containing small amounts of barium has been used to evaluate the likelihood of aspiration and to determine when gastrostomy is necessary.

Preventing constipation. Inactivity and muscle weakness contribute to decreased bowel motility and constipation. To help alleviate this problem:

- Increase fiber intake with daily servings of bran, cooked legumes, whole grains, fruits, and vegetables.
- Prunes and prune juice contain a natural laxative and can be used regularly if acceptable to the individual.
- If tube feedings are used, choose a blended formula made of regular foods or a commercial formula containing added fiber (see Chapter 9).

Multiple Sclerosis

Pathophysiology

Multiple sclerosis (MS), a disease of the central nervous system, affects the myelinated nerve fibers and the muscles they innervate. Patches of the myelin surrounding the nerves degenerate, and the myelin is replaced by scars. MS tends to follow a pattern of exacerbations and remissions.

It appears that the disease is autoimmune, with cell-mediated and humoral responses being generated against myelin proteins. The cause of MS is unknown, but evidence suggests that some individuals have a genetic susceptibility that makes them vulnerable to MS when exposed to certain environmental influences. Viruses or toxic substances have been proposed as possible environmental triggers for the disease. Some epidemiologic evidence indicates that a diet rich in plant foods (grains, fruits, and vegetables) is associated with a reduced risk for development of MS.

Treatment

Although there is no cure for MS, a variety of medications are used for palliation of symptoms associated with MS. Muscle spasms are a common problem that is often alleviated by baclofen (a drug that mimics a neurotransmitter). Diazepam may be used as an adjunct to potentiate the effects of baclofen. Dantrolene is an alternative antispastic drug. Clonazepam can be used if intention tremor is a problem. Urinary retention, which contributes to urinary tract infections, is another frequently encountered symptom, which can be treated with anticholinergic agents such as oxybutynin or propantheline. Nonsteroidal antiinflammatory drugs (NSAIDs, e.g., ibuprofen) relieve muscle and joint pain, and antidepressants such as amitriptyline may be effective in controlling emotional lability. Steroids are sometimes used for their antiinflammatory properties in acute exacerbation of the disease. Immune modifiers such as type I interferons, methotrexate, cyclosporine, cyclophosphamide, and azathioprine have been used in an effort to slow the progression of the disease, but at present their use remains largely experimental.

Even small increases in environmental temperature may worsen symptoms, and thus cool showers or air conditioning may be effective in promoting comfort. It is suggested that avoidance of physical and psychologic stress helps prevent relapses.

Nutritional care

Assessment

Assessment is summarized in Table 19-4.

Intervention and teaching

There is no proof that a special diet is effective in alleviating the effects of MS; however, long-term use of a low-fat diet, especially one low in saturated fat, is postulated to reduce the number of acute exacerbations and slow the progress of the disease. Although firm evidence for the efficacy of this diet is lacking, it should not be harmful if individuals are carefully instructed so that the diet is nutritionally adequate.

Low-fat diet. The low-fat diet should consist of protein, 60 to 70 g/day; total fat, 50 to 60 g/day; and carbohydrates sufficient to provide the balance of needed kcal. Saturated fat is restricted to 10 g/day. Meat, fish, and poultry intake must be reduced to about 2 oz/day, and dairy products must be prepared from skim milk. Fish oil, 1 tsp/day (equivalent to 4.5 g fat), is recommended. Other unsaturated fats include safflower, sunflower, corn, soybean, olive, and cottonseed oils.

Intake of calcium, iron, and zinc should be evaluated. Supplements are often needed because of the restriction of animal products.

Constipation. Constipation is reported by more than 40% of people with multiple sclerosis. Generalized muscle weakness, immobility, and constipating medications probably are etiologic factors. To help prevent or correct constipation:

■ Increase intake of fiber-containing foods (whole grains, legumes, fruits, and vegetables; see Appendix B).
■ Consume prunes or prune juice regularly (if acceptable to the individual).
■ Maintain a liberal fluid intake to encourage formation of soft, bulky stools.
■ Increase physical activity as tolerated to increase gastrointestinal motility.

Parkinsonism (Parkinson's Disease)

Pathophysiology

Parkinsonism is a progressive neuromuscular disorder characterized by a low content of dopamine in the basal ganglia of the central nervous system. This results in tremor, rigidity, a characteristic "pill rolling" movement of the fingers, and hypoactivity. The cause is not known, but it has been speculated that oxidative damage from free radicals in the central nervous system may be involved. Two genes have been linked to Parkinsonism, and it has been suggested that there is a genetic-environmental cause for this disorder, i.e., a genetic susceptibility to develop the disease upon exposure to environmental factors, which might include toxins, smoking, or head trauma.

Treatment

Levodopa, a precursor of dopamine, or a combination of levodopa and carbidopa is used to treat Parkinsonism.

Nutritional care

People with Parkinson's disease may experience weight loss because the tremors and involuntary movements increase energy expenditure and may make it difficult for them to feed themselves adequately. Parkinson's disease may also impair the ability to swallow, interfering with intake of foods and beverages. In addition, levodopa has significant drug-nutrient interactions that must be understood in order to maximize the benefits of the medication.

Assessment

Assessment is summarized in Table 19-4.

Intervention and teaching

Preventing or correcting weight loss

■ Monitor weight regularly.
■ Encourage the individual to consume energy sufficient to reach the upper limit of the recommendation for age and sex (usually approximately 25 to 30 kcal/kg).
■ Choose foods that are easy to get to the mouth (sandwiches and other foods eaten with the hands, or foods that can be impaled with a fork such as chunks of fruit or vegetables), rather than soups or other foods that must be balanced on a utensil.

Optimizing drug therapy. Avoid antagonists of levodopa, which include alcohol and excessive amounts of vitamin B_6 (pyridoxine). Use vitamin supplements that provide no more than the DRI of vitamin B_6.

After several years of levodopa therapy, individuals may become less responsive to the drug. If this occurs, the first steps should be to ensure that:

■ Levodopa is taken at least 30 minutes before eating. Protein in meals and snacks may interfere with the drug action.
■ Protein intake does not exceed the RDA. The "typical" North American diet often includes twice the RDA of protein.

Individuals who do not respond to the aforementioned changes in medication schedules and protein intake sometimes benefit from the following:

■ Limit protein intake from morning through afternoon to ≤7 g (approximately three servings of grain products or starchy

vegetables). Fruits, green leafy vegetables, juices, candies, and small amounts of bread, cereal, or starchy vegetables can be consumed.
- Consume legumes, meats, and dairy products at dinner because control of Parkinsonism symptoms is less important during the night.
- Monitor weight and evaluate intake of protein, calcium, iron, riboflavin, and niacin on this diet. Calcium or other supplements may be needed.

Preventing constipation

- Increase intake of bran, whole grains, legumes, and fresh fruits and vegetables to provide fiber.
- Consume prunes or prune juice regularly (if acceptable to the individual).
- Increase activity as tolerated.

Coping with feeding difficulties

- Increase intake of semisolids such as gelatin, sherbet, ice cream, or fruit ices if swallowing is a problem. Thin liquids, especially plain water, are often harder to swallow.
- Keep foods warm and palatable for slow eaters by using insulated dishes or a warming tray.
- Avoid interruptions (e.g., medication administration) during meals and snacks. Any distraction can cause the elderly person with Parkinsonism to lose focus on eating and have difficulty starting again.
- Plate guards (a high rim around the plate) may be needed to help affected people scoop up food and bring it to their mouths.
- Avoid soups or other foods that may be especially difficult to convey to the mouth when a tremor is present.
- Avoid especially tough, hard, and chewy foods.

Cerebrovascular Accident (Stroke)

Pathophysiology

Cerebrovascular accident (CVA), or stroke, refers to neurologic symptoms resulting from the interruption of blood flow to the brain. Stroke can result from ischemia (diminished blood flow usually related to blood vessel occlusion) or hemorrhage (subarachnoid or intracerebral). Symptoms vary, depending on the extent and location of the CVA. Some individuals experience hemiplegia, or paralysis of one side of the body; visual field defects (e.g., hemianopia, or failure to see half of the visual field); apraxia (inability to perform a known task in response to verbal instructions); and dysphagia. Cerebral edema, increasing the intracranial pressure and damage to the brain, occurs in about 10% to 20% of individuals with ischemic stroke. Vasospasm, or narrowing of the cerebral arteries, is common following hemorrhagic stroke.

Treatment

Pharmacologic therapy is aimed at decreasing or preventing extension of the damage. Anticoagulants are used in selected individuals, especially those with emboli arising from the heart, to reduce the formation of a clot. Antifibrinolytic agents such as aminocaproic acid are often used to prevent recurrence of bleeding in some individuals with stroke resulting from a ruptured aneurysm. Early use of antithrombolytic agents such as recombinant tissue plasminogen activator (t-PA) has been effective in improving the status of some people with ischemic stroke. Steroids or osmotic agents such as mannitol may be used to reduce cerebral edema. Calcium channel blockers (nimodipine) are used to decrease cerebral vasospasm. Surgery (thrombectomy or embolectomy) is sometimes required to reestablish cerebral perfusion.

Nutritional care

The extent and location of the CVA will determine the severity and exact type of problems experienced. Thorough assessment to provide the basis for an individualized plan of care is thus essential.

Assessment

Assessment is summarized in Table 19-4.

Intervention and teaching

Prevention of stroke. High blood levels of the amino acid homocysteine have been found to be predictors of cardiovascular diseases, including stroke, and adequate dietary folate is an important factor in maintaining low levels of homocysteine. Moreover, epidemiologic evidence indicates that the risk of stroke, particularly in people with hypertension, is lessened by a diet rich in potassium, magnesium, calcium, and fiber. It is not clear that potassium, magnesium, calcium, and fiber by themselves (i.e., taken in the form of a supplement) would be effective in prevention of strokes. It may be that they are simply markers of a nutritious diet and a healthful lifestyle. It appears, however, that a diet rich in fruits and vegetables (5 or more servings a day) and grain products, which would provide good sources of fiber, minerals, and folate, might reduce the likelihood of stroke.

Coping with feeding difficulties after stroke

Hemiplegia. Self-feeding will be more difficult if the dominant hand is affected.

- Provide unobtrusive help in opening packages of utensils or condiments, cutting or buttering foods, or feeding the person, if necessary.
- Check for "pocketing" of food in the cheek on the affected side during meals, which occurs because the individual cannot sense that the food is there.
- Provide good mouth care after meals. Teach the patient or home caregivers to do this before discharge.

Visual field defects. The individual may fail to eat half the food on the tray because he or she does not see it.

- Teach the individual to compensate by scanning, or routinely turning the head and moving the eyes toward the affected side.

Dysphagia. Muscle weakness or incoordination, impaired gag or swallowing reflexes, and impaired cough contribute to dysphagia. Dysphagia, in turn, reduces the adequacy of nutrient intake and increases the likelihood of pulmonary aspiration.

- Position the individual upright, if possible, during and for at least 30 minutes after a meal.
- Try thick liquids such as shakes or beverages thickened with infant cereals, cornstarch, instant potatoes, or mashed potatoes, which may be easier to swallow than thin liquids such as water or tea.
- Avoid slick foods (e.g., gelatin, pasta salad).

■ Use foods served at temperature extremes, either chilled or hot, and foods with interesting textures, which may stimulate the swallowing reflex.
■ Do not leave the individual alone during meals, and ensure that suction is available. Enteral tube feedings may be necessary if the problem is severe.

Correcting constipation. Immobility and altered muscle function often lead to constipation. To help prevent or correct constipation:

■ Obtain adequate fiber by increasing intake of whole grains, fruits, and vegetables (see Appendix B), and use bran (2 tbsp) daily.
■ Use prunes or prune juice regularly, if acceptable to the individual.
■ Increase physical activity as tolerated.

Alzheimer's Disease and Dementia
Pathophysiology

Alzheimer's disease (AD) is the most common cause of dementia, or progressive loss of mental function because of an organic cause. The cause is not definitely known, but the most common findings in the brains of individuals with AD are cerebral atrophy, senile plaques, and neurofibrillary tangles, as well as low levels of the neurotransmitter acetylcholine. Genetic factors are believed to be involved in 25% to 40% of cases of AD. Oxidative damage to the neurons has also been suggested as a likely cause. Affected people experience memory loss, shortened attention span, expressive and receptive language disorders, apraxia (inability to perform a task in response to verbal commands), loss of reasoning skills, and intolerance of frustration.

Treatment

A cure for AD is unavailable at this time, but some medications can improve symptoms. The cholinesterase inhibitors (agents that reduce the rate of degradation of acetylcholine) tacrine and donepezil are approved for use in AD. Estrogen, NSAIDs, and antioxidants (e.g., vitamins E and C, β-carotene) have all improved symptoms in some patients. Gingko biloba, an extract derived from the gingko tree, has antioxidant and anticholinesterase properties and has improved memory in some patients with early AD.

Antipsychotropic medications may be needed to control the agitation experienced by some individuals with more advanced AD.

Nutritional care

Progressive loss of self-care skills affects food intake and nutritional status. Weight loss and underweight are common in individuals with Alzheimer's disease, and some investigators have suggested that the metabolic rate and kcal needs may be increased in this condition.

Assessment

Assessment is summarized in Table 19-4.

Intervention

Nutrition interventions are designed to encourage an adequate intake in order to maintain weight and strength, lessen morbidity (e.g., decubitus ulcers and pneumonia), and optimize comfort.

Encouraging adequate intake. The following list summarizes nutritional management of some of the more common problems experienced by the individual with AD.

- *Memory loss.* The individual may forget to eat or to finish a meal. Provide verbal and nonverbal cues that it is mealtime (e.g., announce the meal to the person; put utensils in his or her hand). Eating in a group setting may improve intake because the individual observes models of eating behavior.
- *Poor swallowing.* Swallowing difficulties increase the risk of pulmonary aspiration. Food consistency may have to be altered to cope with swallowing difficulties (see discussion on Intervention and Teaching for Cerebrovascular Accident). Position the person upright to reduce dribbling of food from the mouth, coughing, and choking. Keeping the chin slightly downward reduces the possibility of aspiration.
- *Poor intake.* Inadequate consumption is common even in the individual with no swallowing problems. Provide adequate time for the individual to eat, and avoid distractions during mealtimes. Many affected people experience "sundowning," or restlessness and agitation in the evening, and food intake is poor at this time. For these individuals, maximize intake at the noon and morning meals when cognitive abilities are better. The affected person

may need to be fed. When feeding a person with AD, try alternating bites of sweetened with unsweetened foods to see if this improves intake. Sweet items may be preferred to other foods. Use diversions (singing, cheerful conversation, touching, holding hands) to redirect behavior if the person is combative or resistive when being fed.

SELECTED BIBLIOGRAPHY

Bostom AG, et al.: Nonfasting plasma total homocysteine levels and stroke incidence in elderly persons: the Framingham Study, *Ann Intern Med* 131:352, 1999.

Elmst~ahl S, et al.: Treatment of dysphagia improves nutritional conditions in stroke patients, *Dysphagia* 14:61, 1999.

Finley B: Nutritional needs of the person with Alzheimer's disease: practical approaches to quality care, *J Am Dietet Assoc* 97(10 Suppl 2):S177, 1997.

Folstein M: Nutrition and Alzheimer's disease, *Nutr Rev* 55(1 Pt 1):23, 1997.

Freeman JM, et al.: The efficacy of the ketogenic diet—1998: a prospective evaluation of intervention in 150 children, *Pediatrics* 102:1358, 1998.

Gloria L, et al.: Nutritional deficiencies in chronic alcoholics: relation to dietary intake and alcohol consumption, *Am J Gastroenterol* 92:485, 1997.

Gorelick PB, et al.: Prevention of a first stroke: a review of guidelines and a multidisciplinary consensus statement from the National Stroke Association, *JAMA* 281:1112, 1999.

Henderson RC: Vitamin D levels in noninstitutionalized children with cerebral palsy, *J Child Neurol* 12:443, 1997.

Lauer K: Diet and multiple sclerosis, *Neurology* 49(2 Suppl 2): S55, 1997.

Pandarinath G, Lenhart A: Nutrition and Parkinson's disease, *N Carolina Med J* 58:186, 1997.

Phelps SJ, et al.: The ketogenic diet in pediatric epilepsy, *Nutr Clin Pract* 13:267, 1998.

Sarin SK, et al.: Dietary and nutritional abnormalities in alcoholic liver disease: a comparison with chronic alcoholics without liver disease, *Am J Gastroenterol* 92:777, 1997.

Stallings VA, et al.: Energy expenditure of children and adolescents with severe disabilities: a cerebral palsy model, *Am J Clin Nutr* 64:627, 1996.

Suresh-Babu MV, Thomas AG: Nutrition in children with cerebral palsy, *J Pediatr Gastroenterol Nutr* 26:484, 1998.

Suter PM: The effects of potassium, magnesium, calcium, and fiber on risk of stroke, *Nutr Rev* 57:84, 1999.

Walser M, et al.: *Nutritional management: The Johns Hopkins Handbook,* Philadelphia, 1984, WB Saunders.

Low Birth Weight Infants

20

Low birth weight (LBW) infants are those with birth weights less than 2500 g. They are premature and/or **small-for-gestational age (SGA)**. Preterm or premature infants are those born before 37 weeks of gestation. **Very low birth weight (VLBW)** infants have birth weights less than 1500 g, and **extremely low birth weight (ELBW)** infants weigh less than 1000 g at birth.

Pathophysiology

The smaller and the more premature the infant, the greater the nutritional risk. The following list provides some of the factors contributing to nutritional problems:

- *Decreased nutrient stores:* Most fat, glycogen, and minerals, such as iron, calcium, phosphorus, and zinc, are deposited during the last 8 weeks of pregnancy. Thus, preterm infants have increased potential for hypoglycemia, rickets, and anemia.
- *Increased kcal and nutrient needs for growth:* The LBW infant requires approximately 120 kcal/kg/day, compared with the term neonate's 108 kcal/kg/day. Needs for protein and other nutrients are also increased (Table 20-1).
- *Immature mechanical function of the gastrointestinal (GI) tract:* A coordinated suck-and-swallow function, which is necessary for nipple-feeding an infant, does not develop until 32 to 34 weeks of gestation. Delayed gastric emptying and poor intestinal motility are common in preterm infants.
- *Reduced digestive capability:* Preterm infants have a smaller pool of bile salts, which are required for fat digestion and absorption, than do term infants. Production of pancreatic amylase and

Table 20-1   Nutritional Requirements for Premature Infants
Weighing Fewer Than 1000 g

Ingredient (Unit/Day)	Enteral	Parenteral
Water (ml/kg)	150-200	120-150
Energy (kcal/kg)*	110-130	90-100
Protein (g/kg)†	3-3.8	2.5-3.5
Carbohydrates (g/kg)	8-12	10-15
Fat (g/kg)	3-4	2-3.5
Sodium (mEq/kg)	2-4	2-3.5
Chloride (mEq/kg)	2-4	2-3.5
Potassium (mEq/kg)	2-3	2-3
Calcium (mg/kg)‡	120-230	60-90
Phosphorus (mg/kg)‡	60-140	40-70
Magnesium (mg/kg)	8-15	5-7
Iron (mg/kg)§	2-4	0.1-0.2
Vitamin A (U)‖	700-1500	700-1500
Vitamin D (U)	400	40-160
Vitamin E (U)¶	6-12	2-4
Vitamin K (µg)	7-9	6-10
Vitamin C (mg)	20-60	35-50
Vitamin B_1 (mg)	0.2-0.7	0.3-0.8
Vitamin B_2 (mg)	0.3-0.8	0.4-0.9
Vitamin B_6 (mg)	0.3-0.7	0.3-0.7
Vitamin B_{12} (µg)	0.3-0.7	0.3-0.7
Niacin (mg)	5-12	5-12
Folate (µg)	50	40-90
Biotin (µg)	6-20	6-13
Zinc (µg/kg)	800-1000	400
Copper (µg/kg)	100-150	20
Selenium (µg/kg)	1.3-3	1.5-2
Chromium (µg/kg)	0.7-7.5	0.2
Manganese (µg/kg)	10-20	1
Molybdenum (µg/kg)	0.3	0.25
Iodine (µg/kg)	30-60	1

From Pereira GR: Nutritional care of the extremely premature infant, *Clin Perinatol* 22:62, 1995.

*Adjust according to weight gain and stress factors.

†Requirements increase with increasing degree of prematurity.

‡Inadequate amount in total parenteral nutrition solutions because of risk of precipitation.

§Initiate at 2 weeks of age. Higher values recommended for erythropoietin therapy.

‖Supplementation might reduce incidence of bronchopulmonary dysplasia.

¶Supplementation might reduce severity of retinopathy of prematurity.

lipase, enzymes involved in carbohydrate and fat digestion, is also reduced. Lactase (the enzyme required for milk sugar digestion) levels are low until about 34 weeks of gestation.

■ *Immature lungs with increased work of breathing and increased kcal needs:* Respiratory problems also interfere with enteral feedings. A tachypneic infant, with a respiratory rate greater than 60 breaths/min, cannot be safely nipple-fed, nor can an infant requiring mechanical ventilation.

■ *Potential for heat loss:* Preterm infants have a large body surface area in relation to body weight, as well as little subcutaneous fat to provide insulation. Loss of heat increases energy needs.

■ *Susceptibility to* **necrotizing enterocolitis (NEC):** NEC is a serious disease of the GI tract that can result in intestinal perforation and even death. The risk of developing NEC is increased by prematurity, birth asphyxia (as indicated by low Apgar scores), catheterization of the umbilical arteries (used for arterial blood gases), formula feedings, and hyperosmolar enteral intake (e.g., vitamin supplements, medications given as oral elixirs, and oral calcium or potassium supplements).

Treatment

Immaturity of the lungs (particularly inadequate surfactant production, resulting in respiratory distress syndrome or RDS) is the primary problem for many preterm infants. Surfactant replacement, oxygen therapy, and mechanical ventilation are often needed until respiratory function improves. Oxygen therapy is an essential part of the care of many LBW infants, yet oxygen is toxic to the tissues, particularly the retina and lung. Retinopathy of prematurity and **bronchopulmonary dysplasia (BPD)** are two of the long-term consequences of oxygen administration. The use of mechanical ventilation in combination with supplemental oxygen increases the risk of BPD, a lung injury characterized by a persistent oxygen requirement beyond 36 weeks gestational age. Right-sided heart failure is common in BPD, as are hypoxia, hypercarbia, and oxygen dependency. Severe BPD is associated with pulmonary fibrosis, bronchoconstriction, emphysematous changes, and a mismatch between ventilation and perfusion. Treatment includes diuretics, bronchodilators, steroids, and gradual weaning from oxygen.

Nutritional Care

Ideally, caregivers would deliver adequate nutrients so that the infant could grow as rapidly as he or she would have in the uterus. Unfortunately, this goal is elusive in many sick, stressed, or extremely premature infants.

Assessment

Assessment is summarized in Table 20-2.

Intervention

Commonly used feeding methods

Total parenteral nutrition (TPN)

TPN is used in a variety of conditions, including severe RDS, congenital bowel anomalies (e.g., intestinal atresia, where some portion of the lumen of the bowel fails to form), NEC, or intolerance of enteral feedings. It may be delivered through an umbilical artery catheter, a central venous catheter inserted into the subclavian vein, or a peripheral vein. Peripherally inserted central catheters (PICCs) are increasingly popular routes of TPN delivery.

TPN is composed of solutions of glucose, amino acids, vitamins, and minerals. Lipid emulsions (2 to 4 g/kg/day, or 10 to 20 ml/kg/day of 20% lipid emulsion) are often given to provide part of the needed kcal. Lipid administration may be delayed in jaundiced infants until the indirect (unconjugated) bilirubin is low enough that phototherapy is not needed. High levels of indirect bilirubin are toxic to the central nervous system (CNS), and indirect bilirubin is transported by albumin in the blood. Free fatty acids in the blood can displace bilirubin from its binding sites on serum albumin, and displacement of the indirect bilirubin from albumin increases the likelihood of CNS damage. Blood levels of free fatty acid levels are increased by lipid infusions.

Complications of long-term TPN include osteopenia (inadequate calcification of the bones) and cholestasis (poor flow of bile, which can cause liver damage). Several factors may contribute to osteopenia in LBW infants, including difficulty in providing adequate calcium and phosphorus in TPN because of problems related to insolubility, metabolic acidosis often present in very immature infants, and potential for impaired vitamin D metabolism.

Table 20-2   Assessment in Low Birth Weight Infants

Area of Concern	Significant Findings
Protein-Calorie Malnutrition	*History* Increased kcal needs for growth and physiologic stress—cold, infection, respiratory disease; poor kcal reserves; poor enteral feeding tolerance caused by immature GI function; impaired digestive ability; limited fluid tolerance, which limits the amount of nutrients delivered (excess fluid contributes to patent ductus arteriosus, which worsens cardiorespiratory function) *Physical Examination* Poor weight gain (gain should average 20-30 g/day once LBW infants are stable) *Laboratory Analysis* Serum albumin <3 g/dl or pre-albumin <11 mg/dl
Vitamin Deficiencies A	*History* Poor stores; oxygen therapy, with ↑ need for antioxidants such as vitamin A *Physical Examination* Poor growth *Laboratory Analysis* Serum retinol <20 µg/dl

Table 20-2   Assessment in Low Birth Weight Infants—cont'd

Area of Concern	Significant Findings
Vitamin Deficiencies—cont'd	
E	*History*
	Poor stores; use of oxygen and IV lipid emulsions, with ↑ need for antioxidants such as vitamin E
	Physical Examination
	Pallor, tachycardia, mild generalized edema
	Laboratory Analysis
	↓ Serum tocopherol, Hct, Hgb (hemolytic anemia)
Electrolyte/Mineral Deficiencies	
Sodium (Na)	*History*
	Poor renal conservation caused by immaturity; increased Na needs for growth; use of diuretics in infants with cardiorespiratory disease
	Laboratory Analysis
	↓ Serum Na
Iron (Fe)	*History*
	Poor stores; iatrogenic blood loss—frequent laboratory testing
	Physical Examination
	Pallor; tachycardia
	Laboratory Analysis
	↓ Hct, Hgb, MCV, MCH, MCHC

Continued

Table 20-2   Assessment in Low Birth Weight Infants—cont'd

Area of Concern	Significant Findings
Electrolyte/Mineral Deficiencies—cont'd	
Calcium (Ca)	*History*
	Decreased reserves with great needs for bone mineralization; limited amount of Ca soluble in formulas or IV fluids
	Laboratory Analysis
	↓ Serum Ca; ↑ alkaline phosphatase; radiographic evidence of poor mineralization or fractures
Phosphorus(P)	*History*
	Decreased reserves with great needs for bone mineralization; limited amount of P soluble in formulas or IV fluids
	Laboratory Analysis
	↓ Serum P; ↑ alkaline phosphatase; radiographic evidence of poor mineralization
Zinc (Zn)	*History*
	Poor stores; great needs for tissue anabolism during rapid growth; use of Fe supplements, which compete with Zn for absorption
	Physical Examination
	Delayed growth; diarrhea; seborrheic dermatitis
	Laboratory Analysis
	↓ Serum Zn

Small amounts of enteral feedings seem to "prime" the GI tract by stimulating the development of the GI mucosa, GI motility, and gut hormone release. Therefore "minimal" feedings of formula or human milk delivered at 0.1 to 20 ml/kg/day are often begun when TPN is still needed.

Enteral tube feedings

Enteral tube feedings can be used when there are GI motility (active bowel sounds or passage of stools); no excessive abdominal distention; soft, nontender abdomen (indicating no signs of peritonitis); no bilious nasogastric drainage, which would indicate abnormal bowel motility; no evidence of GI bleeding; and no signs of intestinal obstruction.

Nonnutritive feeding, or sucking a pacifier, during tube feedings may calm the infant and improve oxygenation, and some researchers have reported that it speeds the transition to nipple feedings, improves growth, and shortens hospitalization.

Routes and types of tube feedings include:

■ Intermittent oral-gastric or nasogastric (OG or NG) feedings
   Uses: Intermittent (gavage) feedings every 1 to 3 hours are often used for infants receiving routine feedings.
   Advantages: This is the most physiologic schedule for feeding because intermittent feedings stimulate GI and pancreatic hormone secretion in a cyclic manner.
   Shortcomings: There is a potential for pulmonary aspiration. Bolus feedings are not tolerated well by infants with delayed gastric emptying and in some infants recovering from severe RDS, who have decreased arterial oxygen tension and lung volumes with bolus feedings. Nasogastric feeding tubes increase upper airway resistance and may compromise gas exchange in infants.

■ Continuous OG or NG feedings
   Uses: Often used for infants recovering from severe RDS or those with diminished absorptive capacity (such as short-bowel syndrome) or gastroesophageal reflux.
   Advantages: These methods are slightly more energy efficient (fewer kcal are used for absorption and metabolism of nutrients) than intermittent feedings and may allow intake of slightly greater volumes.

Shortcomings: There is a potential for pulmonary aspiration. Nasogastric feeding tubes increase upper airway resistance and may compromise gas exchange in infants. The cream may separate if human milk is fed continuously, and the infant may not receive all of the fat (and much of the kcal) of the feeding.

■ Continuous transpyloric (nasoduodenal) feedings

Uses: Often used in cases of delayed gastric emptying, severe gastroesophageal reflux and aspiration, and use of continuous positive airway pressure (CPAP) in which the stomach may be distended with air.

Shortcomings: This method has no advantage over oral-gastric feedings in promotion of kcal intake or weight gain. It bypasses the stomach, where lingual (from the mouth) and gastric lipases perform a significant amount of fat digestion in the infant and thus can cause malabsorption of fat. Other potential problems are bacterial overgrowth of the upper intestine, potential for intestinal perforation, and difficulty positioning the tube tip beyond the pylorus. The cream may separate if human milk is fed continuously, and the infant may not receive all of the fat (and much of the kcal) of the feeding.

Nipple feedings

Nipple feedings are used in infants with a normal respiratory rate (<60 breaths/min) and the ability to coordinate breathing, sucking, and swallowing. Usually, these infants are at least 33 to 34 weeks gestational age (either born after that period of gestation, or the combined prenatal and postnatal ages are equivalent to that period).

Milk and formulas

Milk from mothers of preterm infants (preterm milk) has higher levels of minerals and protein than milk of mothers delivering at term (term milk). Nevertheless, levels of calcium, phosphorus, calories, zinc, and sodium in preterm milk are probably too low for rapidly growing premature infants. Fortifiers containing protein, carbohydrates, lipid, minerals, and vitamins are available for addition to human milk. Infants who receive fortified human milk have a reduced incidence of necrotizing enterocolitis and sepsis, compared with infants receiving a formula designed for preterm infants (described as follows). The rate of growth in length and weight is lower in infants fed fortified human milk, but the reduction in the rate of infection by human milk tends to outweigh this disadvantage. Thus, mothers of LBW infants should be encouraged to breastfeed. Providing breast milk for the baby gives her an important role in his or her care and can strengthen the bond between the mother and her hospitalized infant. Most mothers of LBW infants will need to pump or hand-express milk for some period of time after birth until the infant is well and strong enough to suckle.

Specially prepared formulas with greater protein, mineral, vitamin, and kcal content than formulas for term infants are available for preterm infants. They are usually used until the infant's weight is about 1800 g (approximately 4 lb). Characteristics of these formulas are as follows:

- Carbohydrate calories are provided by corn syrup solids or glucose oligosaccharides in addition to lactose because lactose digestion is not mature.
- Fat includes medium-chain triglycerides (MCTs) in addition to long-chain triglycerides (LCTs). MCTs require fewer bile salts for absorption.
- Calories are concentrated into a smaller volume than in formulas for term infants (24 kcal/oz rather than 20 kcal/oz).
- Levels of minerals and protein are increased in comparison to formulas for term infants to promote growth.
- Taurine, an amino acid needed for retinal and brain development and for conjugation of bile salts, is included. Taurine-conjugated bile salts are better emulsifiers of fat than glycine-conjugated bile salts. (Glycine is usually substituted for taurine during bile salt formation when insufficient taurine is available.)
- Very long-chain polyunsaturated fatty acids are included. These fatty acids (arachidonic acid and docosahexaenoic acid) are normally transferred to the fetus via the placenta during gestation and are found in human milk, but are not abundant in cow's milk, which is used to make many infant formulas. These fatty acids are believed to be important in development of the central nervous system.

Safe delivery of nutrition support

LBW infants are especially vulnerable to mechanical and infectious complications of nutrient delivery. To prevent these complications, nutrition support must be carefully administered and monitored (see Chapters 9 and 10).

TPN

- Measure weight daily, and measure head circumference and length regularly.
- Monitor state of hydration continually. Fluid overload increases the workload on the heart and can interfere with closure of the ductus arteriosus. On the other hand, phototherapy and the use of radiant warmers increase fluid requirements.
- Check blood glucose every 4 to 8 hours or as ordered until stable. LBW infants often have poor glucose tolerance and a low renal glucose threshold. Thus, they can experience hyperglycemia and glucosuria, with loss of energy and excessive fluid in the urine, on relatively low doses of glucose.
- Note serum triglyceride levels in infants receiving lipid infusions, especially in infants with respiratory compromise and those with sepsis. Excessive lipid doses may decrease the partial pressure of oxygen in the blood Po_2, and septic infants may have impaired ability to metabolize lipids.

Enteral feedings

- Include all assessment measures listed above for infants receiving TPN.
- Measure abdominal girth (usually just above the umbilicus) every 2 to 8 hours or as ordered. Girth should not increase more than 2 cm after feedings. Report increases greater than this to the physician.
- Evaluate the color of the gastric residual before each intermittent feeding or every 2 to 3 hours during continuous feedings. Bile-stained (green or yellow) fluid usually indicates reduced GI motility and should be reported to the physician. Feedings may need to be decreased or stopped until the problem resolves.
- Position the infant on the right side after feedings, if possible, to promote gastric emptying.
- Note infant's color, respiratory effort, oxygen saturation, and any increase in prevalence of apnea and bradycardia in assessing response to feedings.
- Check stools for occult blood, which may signal NEC. Check for an anal fissure if blood is present in stools.
- Check stools for reducing substances with Clinitest tablets (not with urine test strips); presence of reducing substances indicates lactose malabsorption.
- Check the pH of the urine regularly. Immature infants have a low

renal capacity for acid excretion, and many infant formulas result in a large renal acid load. (Human milk contains a low renal acid load.) The blood pH may be normal, even when the renal acid load is excessive, because of compensatory mechanisms maintaining acid-base balance; however, a persistently acid urine may indicate a need for alkali therapy or use of a formula with a reduced renal acid load.

■ Weigh the breastfed infant on an electronic scale before and after breastfeeding if there is concern about whether intake is adequate. The number of grams gained is approximately equal to the milliliters of milk consumed. Mechanical scales are not usually sufficiently accurate to measure the small weight change resulting from feeding.

Supplementation

Common supplements are 5 to 25 IU of vitamin E and 400 IU of vitamin D per day. If receiving human milk, the infant may be prescribed 2 to 3 mg/kg/day of elemental iron as ferrous sulfate drops. Iron-fortified formula usually provides enough iron to meet needs.

Bronchopulmonary dysplasia (BPD)

BPD increases the work of breathing and thus increases energy needs. Infants with BPD often exhibit delayed growth. It is common practice to supplement the formula or human milk fed to infants with BPD with an energy source (e.g., carbohydrate); however, recent work has shown that "catch-up" growth in infants with BPD is more rapid when feedings are supplemented with more protein, zinc, calcium, and phosphorus than are available in standard infant formulas (Brunton, 1998).

SELECTED BIBLIOGRAPHY

Battaglia FC, Thureen PJ: Nutrition of the fetus and the premature infant, *Diabetes Care* 21 Suppl 2:B70, 1998.

Brunton JA, Saigal S, Atkinson SA: Growth and body composition in infants with bronchopulmonary dysplasia up to 3 months corrected age: a randomized trial of high-energy nutrient-enriched formula fed after hospital discharge, *J Pediatr* 133:340, 1998.

Crawford MA, et al.: Are deficits of arachidonic and docosahexaenoic acids responsible for the neural and vascular complications of preterm babies? *Am J Clin Nutr* 66 (4 Suppl):1032S, 1997.

Darby MK, Loughead JL: Neonatal nutritional requirements and formula composition: a review, *JOGNN* 25:209, 1996.

Ehrenkranz RA, et al.: Longitudinal growth of hospitalized very low birth weight infants. *Pediatrics* 104:280, 1999.

Gordon N: Nutrition and cognitive function, *Brain & Development* 19:165, 1997.

Hay WW Jr: Assessing the effect of disease on nutrition of the preterm infant, *Clin Biochem* 29:399, 1996.

Manz F, Kalhoff H, Remer T: Renal acid excretion in early infancy, *Pediatr Nephrol* 11:231, 1997.

Neu J, Weiss MD: Necrotizing enterocolitis: pathophysiology and prevention, *J Parent Ent Nutr* 23:S13, 1999.

Schanler RJ, Shulman RJ, Lau C: Feeding strategies for premature infants: beneficial outcomes of feeding fortified human milk versus preterm formula, *Pediatrics* 103:1150, 1999.

APPENDIXES

Appendix A
Functions and Dietary Sources of Some Important Nutrients

Appendix A   Functions and Dietary Sources of Some Important Nutrients

Function	Signs and Symptoms of Deficiencies/ Individuals at Increased Risk of Deficiencies (if applicable)	Food Sources
Water		
Solvent for many chemical reactions in metabolism, participant in some chemical reactions (e.g., sugar digestion), temperature regulation, removal of wastes, lubrication and cushioning, transport of nutrients throughout the body	Dehydration, or fluid volume deficit: thirst, flushed skin, sense of apprehension, nausea, heat exhaustion, increased pulse rate and temperature, mental confusion, cyanosis, poor skin turgor, loss of body weight *At risk:* Infants and young children with diarrhea or vomiting, elderly	Water and other beverages; water contained in foods (esp. fruits, vegetables); metabolic water released from the oxidation of nutrients in the body
Carbohydrates		
Glucose and carbohydrates that yield glucose: Energy (4 kcal/g carbohydrate from food, 3.4 kcal/g IV glucose), protein sparing*	Ketosis (excessive production of ketones from incomplete metabolism of fat): increased urination and thirst, dehydration (see above), flushed dry skin, rapid shallow respirations, fruity odor of breath *At risk:* Individuals with diabetes	Grain products, vegetables, fruits, milk, yogurt, ice cream, sugar, honey, syrup, jelly, jam, candy, other sweets

Fiber, insoluble†: Improve elimination by increasing fecal mass	Constipation, diverticula (herniations that protrude through the musculature of the large intestine and can become inflamed), hemorrhoids; possibly increased risk of colon cancer	Legumes, whole-grain breads and cereals, vegetables, fruits
Fiber, soluble: Delay gastric emptying, slow glucose absorption, inhibit cholesterol absorption	Hyperglycemia; hypercholesterolemia	Citrus fruits, oat bran, legumes
Amino Acids/Nitrogen‡ Constituents of structural proteins (muscles, bones), enzymes, antibodies, hormones, chromosomes; transport oxygen, nutrients, and wastes in the blood; acid-base balance; energy (provide 4 kcal/g)	Hypoalbuminemia, edema, lymphopenia, hair easily pluckable, skin lesions, poor wound healing *At risk:* Serious acute or chronic disease, elderly	Meats, poultry, fish, eggs, milk, yogurt, cheese, legumes, nuts, grain products

*IV, Intravenous. Protein sparing refers to the fact that protein can be used for glucose formation via gluconeogenesis (formation of glucose from noncarbohydrates). Adequate carbohydrate intake spares protein to be used for vital functions, rather than energy production.

†Insoluble fiber does not dissolve in water; soluble fiber forms a gel or swells when combined with water.

‡We usually speak of a requirement for protein, but the requirement is actually for nitrogen in the form of amino acids. Proteins are made up of amino acids, which are essential (needed in the diet because the body does not produce a sufficient amount) or nonessential (not necessary in the diet because the body synthesizes it). Essential amino acids are histidine, isoleucine, leucine, lysine, methionine, phenylalanine, threonine, tryptophan, valine, and possibly glutamine. In addition, infants require dietary arginine, cysteine (cystine), and taurine.

Continued

Appendix A Functions and Dietary Sources of Some Important Nutrients—cont'd

Function	Signs and Symptoms of Deficiencies/ Individuals at Increased Risk of Deficiencies (if applicable)	Food Sources
Lipids (Fats and Oils)		
Energy (9 kcal/g); insulation and protection of body organs; essential fatty acids (EFA): precursors of eicosanoids (hormonelike compounds)—prostaglandins, thromboxanes, prostacyclins, and leukotrienes; linoleic acid, an "omega-6" fatty acid, is the primary EFA; "omega-3" fatty acids are also involved in eicosanoid formation and are being intensively studied at present	Essential fatty acid deficiency: dry scaly skin, poor wound healing, delayed growth in children *At risk:* Premature infants, individuals receiving total parenteral nutrition	Nuts, seeds, and their oils; meat, poultry, fish, eggs, whole milk, cream, and their products—butter, yogurt, ice cream, cheese Essential fatty acids: safflower, sunflower, corn, cottonseed, and soybean oils "Omega-3" fatty acids: canola and soybean oils, fatty fish such as salmon, tuna, sardines

Continued

Fat-Soluble Vitamins

Vitamin A

Formation and maintenance of epithelial tissue, formation of visual rods and cones, antioxidant (a substance that prevents damage to cells from "free radicals"—oxygen-containing compounds that can disrupt proteins and lipids in cells, possibly contributing to aging and development of cancers)

Night blindness, growth retardation, Bitot's spots, corneal drying and damage (xerophthalmia), follicular hyperkeratosis

At risk: Individuals with fat malabsorption, poor vegetable intake

Liver, fortified milk; Beta-carotene (vitamin A precursor): deep yellow vegetables and fruits, e.g., carrot, sweet potato, butternut squash, apricot, cantaloupe; deep green leafy vegetables, e.g., spinach, broccoli, greens

Vitamin D

Forms the hormone calcitriol, which increases calcium and phosphorus absorption in the intestine, decreases urinary loss of calcium, and regulates bone calcium

Rickets (children): bowed legs, enlarged joints, knobby deformities on rib cage

Osteomalacia (adults): weakening of bones, bony pain

At risk: People with little sun exposure (institutionalized elderly or children, cultural clothing practices that cover most skin, dark-skinned individuals

Nondiet source: sun exposure

Fortified milk, fatty fish (tuna, salmon, sardines), fortified cereals

Appendix A   Functions and Dietary Sources of Some Important Nutrients—cont'd

Function	Signs and Symptoms of Deficiencies/Individuals at Increased Risk of Deficiencies (if applicable)	Food Sources
Fat-Soluble Vitamins—cont'd		
Vitamin E		
Antioxidant, protects cell membranes from free radical damage	Anemia due to red blood cell hemolysis, neuropathy, and myopathy *At risk*: Premature infants, individuals with fat malabsorption	Plant oils and margarine made from them, whole grains, wheat germ, nuts, peanuts, sweet potato, avocado
Vitamin K		
Activation of clotting factors II (prothrombin), VII, IX, and X	Increased prothrombin time, ecchymoses, bleeding *At risk*: Newborns, individuals receiving prolonged courses of antibiotics (rare)	Egg yolk, liver, green leafy vegetables, synthesized by gut bacteria

Water-Soluble Vitamins (Vitamin C and the B Complex)

Vitamin C (ascorbic acid)

Formation of collagen, thyroxine, epinephrine, norepinephrine, steroid hormones; antioxidant

Scurvy: petechiae, easy bruising, bleeding gums, painful joints, poor wound healing

At risk: Smokers, individuals with poor fruit and vegetable intake, oral contraceptive users, alcoholism, increased stress of illness, surgery, trauma

Citrus fruits, strawberries, kiwifruit, broccoli, peppers (red, green, or chili), cantaloupe, Brussels sprouts, cauliflower, papaya, tomatoes, potatoes

Thiamin (B_1)

Component of coenzyme (thiamin pyrophosphate or TPP) in carbohydrate metabolism

Beriberi: weakness, irritability, peripheral neuropathy, deep muscle pain; wet beriberi: enlarged heart, tachycardia, congestive heart failure; Wernicke-Korsakoff syndrome: confusion, ataxia, eye muscle paralysis

At risk: Alcoholics

Pork, whole-grain and enriched breads and cereals, legumes, liver, nuts

Continued

Appendix A   Functions and Dietary Sources of Some Important Nutrients—cont'd

Function	Signs and Symptoms of Deficiencies/ Individuals at Increased Risk of Deficiencies (if applicable)	Food Sources
Water-Soluble Vitamins (Vitamin C and the B Complex)—cont'd		
Riboflavin (B₂)		
Component of coenzymes (flavin mononucleotide [FMN] and flavin adenine dinucleotide [FAD]) in carbohydrate, protein, and fat metabolism	Cheilosis (cracking at mouth corners), glossitis (inflamed tongue), seborrheic dermatitis (scaly, greasy skin) *At risk:* Alcoholics	Milk, yogurt, enriched breads and cereals, liver
Niacin (B₃)		
Components of coenzymes (nicotinamide adenine dinucleotide [NAD] and nicotinamide adenine dinucleotide phosphate [NADP]) in energy production from carbohydrates, fats, and protein and fat synthesis	Pellagra: anorexia, skin lesions in areas exposed to sunlight, confusion; classic symptoms, "4 Ds," are dermatitis, diarrhea, dementia, death *At risk:* Alcoholics, poverty causing corn and rice to be major protein sources in the diet	Meats, peanuts, enriched breads and cereals, potato with skin

Vitamin	Function	Deficiency/At Risk	Sources
Pantothenic acid	Component of coenzyme A, involved in fatty acid and cholesterol synthesis and lipid, protein, and carbohydrate synthesis	Rarely seen; occurs only experimentally or with other B vitamin deficiencies: burning sensation in feet, fatigue *At risk:* Alcoholics	Widespread, especially in organ meats, meat, poultry, fish, mushrooms, avocado, milk
Pyridoxine (B6)	Component of coenzyme (pyridoxal phosphate [PLP]) involved in transamination reactions, synthesis of hemoglobin	Neuropathy, microcytic anemia *At risk:* Alcoholics, oral contraceptive users, pregnant women, people receiving isoniazid (for tuberculosis)	Whole grains, meat, poultry, fish, bananas, potatoes
Biotin	Cofactor for enzymes in synthesis of fat and purines (DNA, RNA), glucose metabolism	Rarely seen; dermatitis, atrophy of papillae on tongue, hypercholesterolemia *At risk:* Unusually high regular intake of raw egg white, alcoholics, prolonged use of antibiotics	Liver, egg yolk, cauliflower, cheese, whole grains, synthesized by gut bacteria

Continued

Appendix A   Functions and Dietary Sources of Some Important Nutrients—cont'd

Function	Signs and Symptoms of Deficiencies/ Individuals at Increased Risk of Deficiencies (if applicable)	Food Sources
Water-Soluble Vitamins (Vitamin C and the B Complex)—cont'd		
Folic acid (Folacin, Folate)		
One-carbon transfer reactions, e.g., DNA and RNA synthesis, amino acid synthesis	Megaloblastic (macrocytic) anemia, glossitis, diarrhea *At risk:* Alcoholics, pregnant women	Green leafy vegetables, liver, orange juice, legumes
Cobalamin (B_{12})		
Methylation reactions, e.g., synthesis of DNA and RNA, folic acid metabolism	Megaloblastic (macrocytic) anemia, especially pernicious anemia caused by lack of intrinsic factor produced in the stomach, neuropathy, glossitis *At risk:* Elderly, postgastrectomy patients, strict vegetarians, individuals taking >10 times the RDA of vitamin C	Animal products only: liver, meat, fish, poultry, milk, egg, cheese

Major Minerals (More than 100 mg Needed/Day)

Calcium

Component of bones and teeth, blood clotting, nerve transmission, muscle contraction, enzyme activation

Osteoporosis (thinning of bones with long-term deficiency), tetany (muscle excitability because of decreased serum calcium, usually caused by hypoparathyroidism, not dietary Ca deficiency)

At risk: White and Asian women with poor calcium intake, people with fat malabsorption

Milk, yogurt, cheese, canned fish with bones eaten, green leafy vegetables except spinach and Swiss chard, fortified juices, foods made with milk (e.g., pancakes)

Phosphorus

Component of bones, teeth, cell membranes; involved in all energy-producing reactions as ATP

Muscle weakness, cardiorespiratory failure, red blood cell hemolysis

At risk: Individuals with rapid tissue synthesis after starvation (refeeding syndrome)

Milk, cheese, yogurt, meats, whole grains, legumes, nuts, food additives, carbonated beverages

Continued

Appendix A   Functions and Dietary Sources of Some Important Nutrients—cont'd

Function	Signs and Symptoms of Deficiencies/ Individuals at Increased Risk of Deficiencies (if applicable)	Food Sources
Major Minerals (More than 100 mg Needed/Day)—cont'd		
Magnesium (Mg)		
Component of bones, cofactor in many enzyme systems (glucose, fat, nucleic acid metabolism), involved in nerve transmission and muscle contraction	Paresthesias, tremor, muscle spasms, tetany, seizures, coma *At risk:* Alcoholics, those using diuretic therapy	Nuts, legumes, whole grains, dried fruits
Sodium (Na)		
Major cation in extracellular fluid, water balance, nerve transmission	Muscle cramps, nausea, vomiting, dizziness, shock, coma *At risk:* People with excessive perspiration or other fluid loss replaced with plain water	Table salt, processed foods, salted snack foods, condiments, meats, milk, cheese, breads

	Functions	Deficiency/At Risk	Food Sources
Potassium (K)	Major cation in intracellular fluid, water balance, nerve transmission, protein synthesis	Weakness, diminished reflexes, confusion, ileus, cardiac dysrhythmia (heart block) *At risk:* Severe diarrhea or vomiting; thiazide diuretics, diabetic ketoacidosis treated with insulin and glucose	Fruits, vegetables, legumes, nuts, whole grains, meats, milk
Chloride (Cl)	Major anion in extracellular fluid, water balance, hydrochloric acid in stomach	Hypochloremic alkalosis *At risk:* Prolonged vomiting, nasogastric suction	Table salt, salt added in food processing
Trace Minerals or Elements (Less than 100 mg Needed/Day)			
Chromium (Cr)	Cofactor for insulin in glucose metabolism	Glucose intolerance, neuropathy, weight loss, hypercholesterolemia and hypertriglyceridemia *At risk:* Heavy users of highly processed foods	Whole grains, brewer's yeast, meats

Continued

Appendix A Functions and Dietary Sources of Some Important Nutrients—cont'd

Function	Signs and Symptoms of Deficiencies/ Individuals at Increased Risk of Deficiencies (if applicable)	Food Sources
Trace Minerals or Elements (Less than 100 mg Needed/Day)—cont'd		
Copper (Cu)		
Hemoglobin synthesis, cofactor for many enzymes (e.g., in protein synthesis)	Microcytic anemia, low neutrophil count *At risk:* Excessive supplementation with Zn	Liver, meat, shellfish, legumes, nuts, cocoa, copper cookware or water pipes
Fluoride (F)		
Makes tooth enamel resistant to decay	Dental caries *At risk:* People not receiving fluoridated water or dental treatments	Fluoridated water, toothpaste, dental treatments, tea
Iodine (I)		
Component of thyroid hormones	Goiter: enlarged thyroid, hypothyroidism Cretinism: infant with short stature and mental retardation born to woman I-deficient during pregnancy *At risk:* None in U.S.	Iodized salt, seafood, food colorings, bread (from dough conditioner), milk (from cleaning agent in dairies)

Iron (Fe)		
Oxygen transport in hemoglobin and myoglobin, cytochrome enzyme system	Microcytic anemia *At risk:* Infants, children, adolescents, pregnant women, some endurance athletes, individuals with blood loss, postgastrectomy, vegetarians	Liver, meats, eggs, whole and enriched grains, legumes, dark green leafy vegetables, iron cookware
Manganese (Mn)		
Cofactor in protein, carbohydrate, and fat metabolism	Rare and symptoms uncertain: weight loss, hypocholesterolemia, dermatitis *At risk:* Long-term TPN without supplementation	Whole grains, legumes, nuts, leafy vegetables
Molybdenum (Mo)		
Cofactor in oxidase enzymes	Very rare: tachycardia, stupor, central scotomas (loss of vision), coma *At risk:* Long-term TPN without supplementation	Legumes, whole grains

Continued

Appendix A   Functions and Dietary Sources of Some Important Nutrients—cont'd

Function	Signs and Symptoms of Deficiencies/ Individuals at Increased Risk of Deficiencies (if applicable)	Food Sources
Trace Minerals or Elements (Less than 100 mg Needed/Day)—cont'd		
Selenium (Se)		
Component of glutathione peroxidase, an antioxidant	Cardiomyopathy, sudden death *At risk:* People eating food grown in Se-deficient soil (Keshan province of China, New Zealand), long-term TPN without supplementation	Seafoods, whole grains, meats, legumes, milk (meat, milk, and plant Se depend on soil content)
Zinc (Zn)		
Cofactor in more than 70 enzyme systems involved in growth, sexual maturation, reproduction, taste acuity, immune function	Impaired sense of taste and smell, anorexia, dermatitis, growth retardation, delayed sexual maturity, poor wound healing, impaired immune function *At risk:* Excessive Fe supplementation or Cu intake, vegetarian diet, severe diarrhea, intestinal drainage	Shellfish, meats, liver, milk, cheese, eggs, whole grains, legumes

Appendix B
Dietary Fiber in
Common Foods

Recommended intakes
Adults: 25 to 30 g/day
Children: no. of g daily = age in years + 5

Appendix B   Dietary Fiber in Common Foods

		Food		
Dietary Fiber (g per Serving)	Grain Products	Fruits	Dried Beans and Peas	Vegetables
10 or more	All Bran (⅓ c) Fiber One (½ c) Wheat bran (½ c)	Figs, dried (10) Peaches, dried (10 halves)		
5 to 9	Bran Buds (⅓ c) Bran flakes (¾ c) Raisin bran (¾ c)	Prunes, dried (10) Prunes, dried, cooked (½ c)	Beans, cooked: great northern, kidney, lima, red, or refried (½ c) Bean soup (1 c)	
3 to 5	English muffin, whole grain or bran (1) Crackling Oat Bran (⅓ c) Fruit & Fibre (½ c) Mueslix (⅔ c) Muffin, bran (1) Nutri-Grain (⅔ c) Ry-Krisp (2)	Apple with skin (1 med) Apricots, dried (10 halves) Avocado (1 med) Blackberries (½ c) Dates, dried (10) Orange (1 med) Papaya (1 med) Pear, raw (1)	Beans, baked (½ c) Beans or peas, cooked: garbanzos, lentils, navy, pinto, white, black-eye (½ c) Pea soup (1 c)	Brussels sprouts, cooked (½ c) Corn, cooked (½ c) Peas, green, canned or frozen (½ c)

1 to 2	Waffle, frozen (2) Wheat Chex (⅔ c) Wheat germ (¼ c) Bread: cracked wheat, whole-wheat, mixed grain, rye, oat bran, oatmeal (1 slice) Brown rice, cooked (1 c) Cornbread (1 piece) Cornflakes (1 c) Cheerios (1¼ c) French toast (2 slices) Granola (¼ c) Grape-Nuts (¼ c) Muffin, all except bran (1) Pancakes (2) Ry-Krisp (1)	Applesauce (½ c) Apricots (3 med) Blueberries, raw (½ c) Cantaloupe (1 c) Cherries, sweet, raw (10) Grapes (1 c) Kiwifruit (1 med) Mango (1 med) Nectarine (1 med) Peaches, canned (1 c) Peach, raw (1 med) Pear, canned (½ c) Pineapple, raw or canned (1 c) Raisins (2 tbsp) Strawberries, raw or frozen (½ c)	Broccoli, raw or cooked (½ c) Carrot, cooked (½ c) Carrot, raw (1 med) Cauliflower, raw or cooked (½ c) Green beans, frozen, canned, or fresh (½ c) Mushrooms, raw or canned (1 c) Olives (10) Onions, raw (½ c) Peppers, sweet, raw (½ c) Potato, baked or boiled without skin (1 med) Potato salad (½ c)

Continued

Appendix B   Dietary Fiber in Common Foods—cont'd

Dietary Fiber (g per Serving)	Food			
	Grain Products	Fruits	Dried Beans and Peas	Vegetables
1 to 2— cont'd	Shredded wheat (1 large biscuit)	Watermelon, raw (1½ C)		Soups: minestrone or vegetable (1 c) Spinach, cooked (½ c) Squash, summer or winter, cooked (½ c) Sweet potatoes, cooked, (½ c) Tomato, raw (1 med) Turnip, cooked (½ c)

Appendix C
Healthy Weight Ranges for Men and Women of All Ages

Height (ft-in)	Weight Range (lb)	Height (cm)	Weight Range (kg)
4'10"	90-120	147	41-54
4'11"	96-125	150	44-57
5'0"	97-128	152	44-58
5'1"	101-133	155	46-60
5'2"	105-136	157	48-62
5'3"	108-141	160	49-64
5'4"	111-145	162	50-66
5'5"	114-150	165	52-68
5'6"	117-155	168	53-70
5'7"	120-160	170	54-73
5'8"	125-164	173	57-75
5'9"	129-169	175	59-77
5'10"	132-174	178	60-79
5'11"	136-179	180	62-81
6'0"	140-184	183	64-84
6'1"	144-189	185	65-86
6'2"	148-195	188	67-89
6'3"	152-200	191	69-91
6'4"	156-205	193	71-93
6'5"	160-211	196	73-96
6'6"	164-216	198	75-98

Adapted from *Nutrition and your health: dietary guidelines for Americans,* ed 5, Washington, DC, 2000, U.S. Dept of Agriculture, U.S. Department of Health and Human Services.

Appendix D
Growth Charts
(United States)

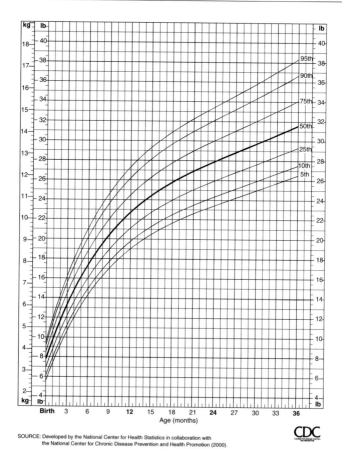

SOURCE: Developed by the National Center for Health Statistics in collaboration with
the National Center for Chronic Disease Prevention and Health Promotion (2000).

Figure D-1
Boys: weight-for-age percentiles; birth to 36 months.

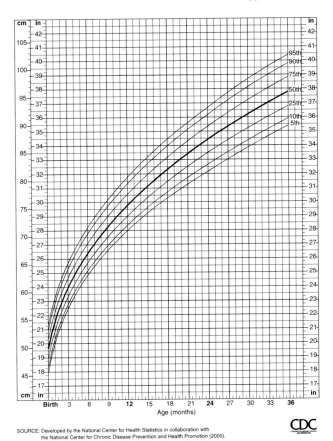

SOURCE: Developed by the National Center for Health Statistics in collaboration with
the National Center for Chronic Disease Prevention and Health Promotion (2000).

CDC

Figure D-2
Boys: length-for-age percentiles, birth to 36 months.

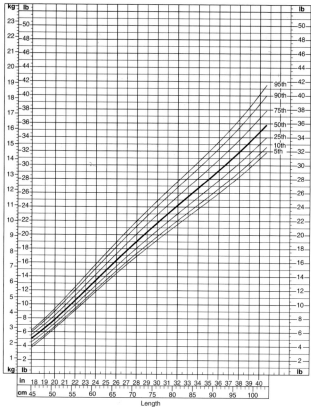

Revised and corrected June 8, 2000.

SOURCE: Developed by the National Center for Health Statistics in collaboration with
the National Center for Chronic Disease Prevention and Health Promotion (2000).

Figure D-3
Boys: weight-for-length percentiles, birth to 36 months.

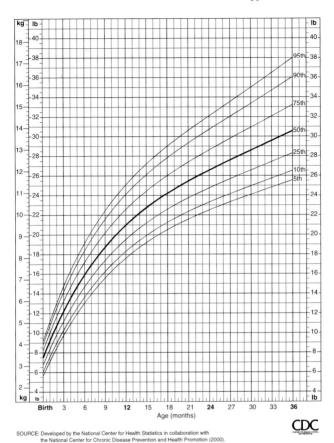

SOURCE: Developed by the National Center for Health Statistics in collaboration with
the National Center for Chronic Disease Prevention and Health Promotion (2000).

Figure D-4
Girls: weight-for-age percentiles, birth to 36 months.

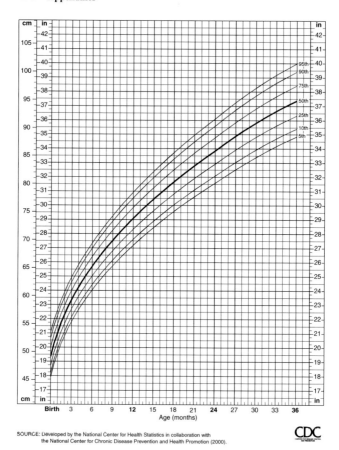

SOURCE: Developed by the National Center for Health Statistics in collaboration with
the National Center for Chronic Disease Prevention and Health Promotion (2000).

Figure D-5
Girls: length-for-age percentiles, birth to 36 months.

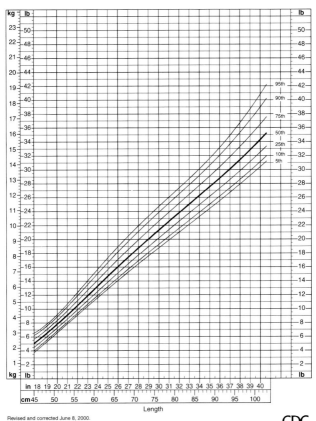

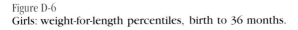

Revised and corrected June 8, 2000.

SOURCE: Developed by the National Center for Health Statistics in collaboration with

Figure D-6
Girls: weight-for-length percentiles, birth to 36 months.

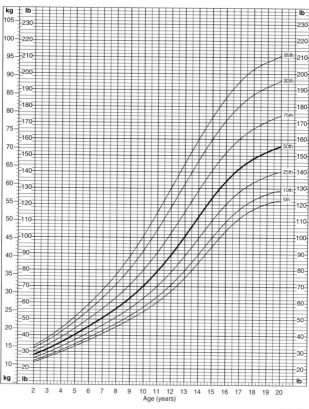

SOURCE: Developed by the National Center for Health Statistics in collaboration with the National Center for Chronic Disease Prevention and Health Promotion (2000).

Figure D-7
Boys: weight-for-age percentiles, 2 to 20 years.

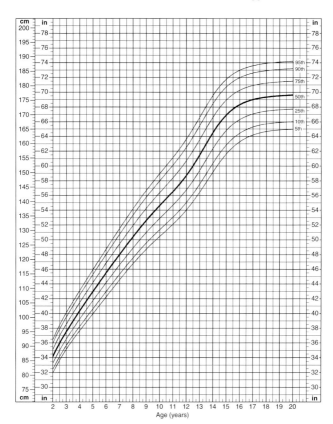

SOURCE: Developed by the National Center for Health Statistics in collaboration with
the National Center for Chronic Disease Prevention and Health Promotion (2000).

Figure D-8
Boys: stature-for-age percentiles, 2 to 20 years.

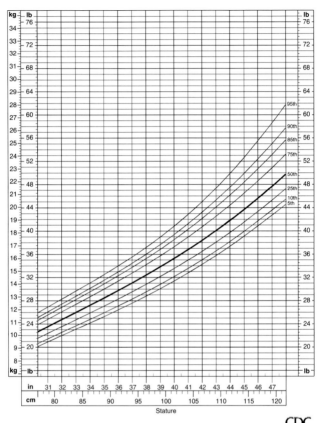

SOURCE: Developed by the National Center for Health Statistics in collaboration with
the National Center for Chronic Disease Prevention and Health Promotion (2000).

Figure D-9
Boys: weight-for-stature percentiles, 2 to 20 years.

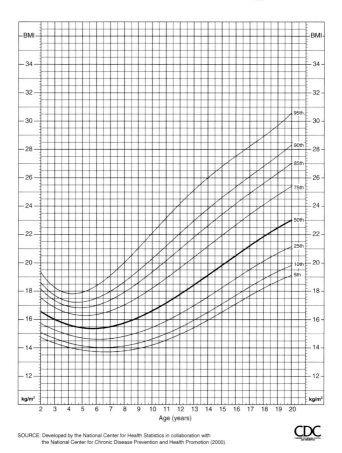

SOURCE: Developed by the National Center for Health Statistics in collaboration with
the National Center for Chronic Disease Prevention and Health Promotion (2000).

Figure D-10
Boys: body mass index-for-age percentiles, 2 to 20 years.

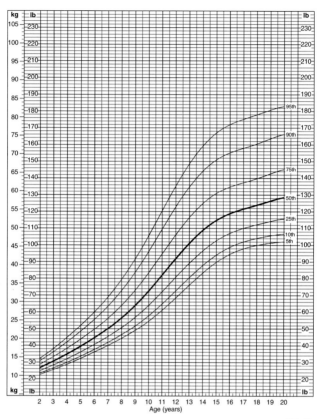

SOURCE: Developed by the National Center for Health Statistics in collaboration with the National Center for Chronic Disease Prevention and Health Promotion (2000).

Figure D-11

Girls: weight-for-age percentiles, 2 to 20 years.

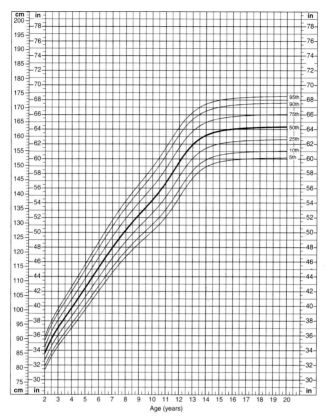

SOURCE: Developed by the National Center for Health Statistics in collaboration with
         the National Center for Chronic Disease Prevention and Health Promotion (2000).

Figure D-12
Girls: stature-for-age percentiles, 2 to 20 years.

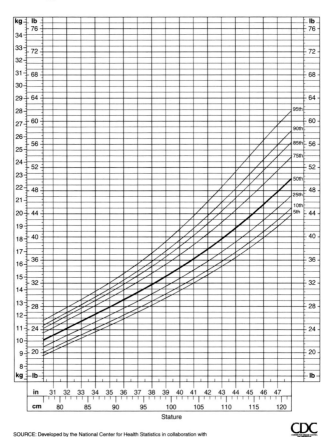

SOURCE: Developed by the National Center for Health Statistics in collaboration with
the National Center for Chronic Disease Prevention and Health Promotion (2000).

CDC

Figure D-13
Girls: weight-for-stature percentiles, 2 to 20 years.

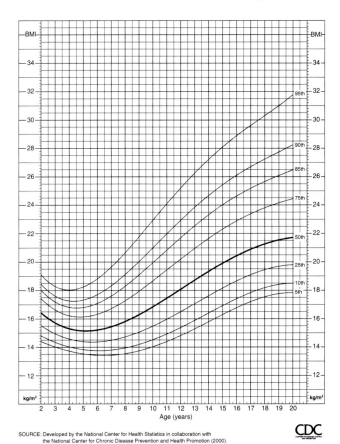

SOURCE: Developed by the National Center for Health Statistics in collaboration with
the National Center for Chronic Disease Prevention and Health Promotion (2000).

Figure D-14
Girls: body mass index-for-age percentiles, 2 to 20 years.

Appendix E
TSF and AMC
Percentiles

Table E-1 Triceps Skinfold (TSF) Measurements
for Whites and Blacks (W/B) in Millimeters

Age (Yr)	Percentiles for Females (W/B)			Percentiles for Males (W/B)		
	5th	85th	95th	5th	85th	95th
6	6/4	13/11	16/19	5/4	12/9	16/13
7	6/4	14/13	19/21	5/4	12/8	18/15
8	6/4	16/16	21/23	5/4	13/10	20/17
9	7/4	17/17	24/25	5/4	13/11	21/19
10	7/5	18/18	26/27	5/4	16/12	22/20
11	8/5	20/21	28/29	5/4	18/13	23/22
12	8/6	22/23	29/30	5/4	18/14	24/23
13	8/6	24/25	31/32	5/4	18/14	24/24
14	8/7	24/26	31/33	5/4	18/16	24/25
15	9/7	25/27	32/34	5/4	18/18	24/25
16	9/7	26/27	32/34	5/4	17/17	24/26
17	9/7	26/27	33/34	5/4	17/17	23/26
18-20	10/7	27/30	24/35	4/3	17/17	22/23
21-29	10/8	29/33	35/37	5/3	20/17	23/23
30-35	11/9	33/36	38/42	5/4	19/18	24/25
36-41	12/10	33/37	38/45	5/4	19/19	23/24
42-50	12/12	35/38	40/44	5/4	19/18	24/26
50-59	13/13	32/35	39/42	5/4	18/15	24/23
60-69	12/12	31/33	36/39	5/4	17/15	23/23

Note: Because overweight is increasing in prevalence in the USA and other industrialized nations, the 95th percentile is likely to be a very conservative indicator
of the presence of overweight/obesity. Therefore, the 85th percentile is
included; individuals with skinfolds at the 85th percentile or greater should
be carefully assessed for other signs of overweight/obesity. The triceps skinfold
measurement correlates more closely with overweight in women than in men.

Table E-2   Arm Muscle Circumference (AMC) in Centimeters

Age (Yr)	Percentiles for Females		Percentiles for Males	
	5th	95th	5th	95th
6	13	17	13	18
7	13	18	14	19
8	14	19	14	20
9	15	20	15	20
10	15	20	16	22
11	15	22	16	23
12	16	22	17	24
13	17	24	17	24
14	17	25	19	26
15	18	24	20	27
16	17	25	21	30
17	18	26	22	31
18-20	18	25	23	32
21-29	18	26	24	32
30-35	18	26	24	33
36-41	19	27	25	33
42-50	19	27	24	33
50-59	19	28	24	32
60-69	18	18	22	32

Sources: Cronk CE, Roche AF: Race- and sex-specific reference data for triceps and subscapular skinfolds and weight/stature,[2] *Am J Clin Nutr* 35:347, 1982; Frisancho AR: New norms of upper limb fat and muscle areas for assessment of nutritional status, *Am J Clin Nutr* 34:2540, 1981; Must A, Dallal GE, Dietz WH: Reference data for obesity: 85th and 95th percentiles of body mass index (wt/ht^2) and triceps skinfold thickness, *Am J Clin Nutr* 53:839, 1991.

Appendix F
Laboratory
Reference Values

Appendix F   **Laboratory Reference Values**

Test	Reference Range	
	Adult	Pediatric
Albumin, serum (g/dl)	3.5-5.0	4 day-14 yr: 3.8-5.4
Calcium, serum (mg/dl)		
Total	8.5-10.5	10 day-24 mo: 9.0-11.0; 2-12 yr: 8.8-10.8
Ionized or free	4.6-5.3	4.8-5.5
β-Carotene, serum (μg/dl)	10-85	
Ceruloplasmin, serum (mg/dl)	18-45; ↑ in preg	24-56
Chloride, serum (mmol/L)	98-107	
Cholesterol, total, serum (mg/dl)	<200	110-200
Chromium		
Blood (μg/L)	2.8-45	
Serum (μg/L)	0.12-2	
Urine (μg/day)	0.1-2	
Copper, serum (μg/dl)	M: 70-140 F: 80-155 Preg: 118-302	<6 mo: 20-70; >6 mo: 80-190
C-peptide, serum (ng/ml)	0.78-1.89	

Values compiled from Burtis CA, Ashwood ER: *Tietz textbook of clinical chemistry*, ed 2, Philadelphia, 1994, WB Saunders; Meites S, ed: *Pediatric clinical chemistry*, ed 3, Washington, DC, 1989, American Association for Clinical Chemistry; and Pagana KD, Pagana TJ: *Mosby's diagnostic and laboratory reference*, ed 2, St Louis, 1995, Mosby.

Continued

Appendix F Laboratory Reference Values—cont'd

Test	Reference Range		
	Adult	Pediatric
Creatinine		
Serum (mg/dl)	M: 0.7-1.3 F: 0.6-1.1	Infant: 0.2-0.4; child: 0.3-0.7; adolescent: 0.5-1.0
Urine (mg/kg/day)	M: 14-26 F: 11-20 Elderly: >10	Infant and child: 8-22; adolescent: 8-30
Fat, fecal (g/day)	<7 g excreted (on 100 g fat diet) or >93% retention of dietary fat	>93% retention of dietary fat
Ferritin, serum (ng/ml)	M: 12-300 F: 10-150	6 mo-15 yr: 7-140
FIGLU (Formiminoglutamic acid), urine (mg/day)	<35 (>35 indicates folic acid deficiency)	
Folic acid (ng/ml)		
Serum	3-16	5-21
RBC	130-628	>160
Glucose, plasma (mg/dl)		
Fasting	70-110	60-100
2 h postprandial	<125	

Glucose tolerance test (GTT), plasma (mg/dl)	Fasting: 70-110; 30 min: <190; 1 h: <170; 2 h: <140; 3 h: 70-110	
Glycated or glycosylated hemoglobin, blood (% total hemoglobin)		
HbA_{1c}	<6.5	<4
Glycerol, free, plasma (mg/dl)	0.29-1.72	0.56-2.14
Hematocrit (% whole blood volume)	M: 39-50 F: 35-47	Infant: >32; 2-12 yr: 32-42; adolescent: 34-48
Hemoglobin, total, blood (g/dl)	M: 12.6-17 F: 11.7-16	11-16
Insulin, fasting, serum (μU/ml)	2-25	
Iron, serum (μg/dl)	M: 65-170 F: 50-170	50-120
Iron-binding capacity, total, serum (μg/dl)	250-450	
Ketones (mg/dl)		
Serum	Negative (<3)	
Urine	Negative	
LDL-cholesterol, serum or plasma (mg/dl)	<130	
Magnesium, serum (mEq/L)	1.3-2.1	1.2-2.0

Values compiled from Burtis CA, Ashwood ER: *Tietz textbook of clinical chemistry,* ed 2, Philadelphia, 1994, WB Saunders; Meites S, ed: *Pediatric clinical chemistry,* ed 3, Washington, DC, 1989, American Association for Clinical Chemistry; and Pagana KD, Pagana TJ: *Mosby's diagnostic and laboratory reference,* ed 2, St Louis, 1995, Mosby.

Continued

Appendix F   Laboratory Reference Values—cont'd

Test	Reference Range		
	Adult	Pediatric	
Niacin, urine (mg/day)	2.4-6.4		
Nitrogen, total, fecal (g/day)	<2		
Pantothenic acid, blood or serum (µg/ml)	1.03-1.83	Infants: 0.1-0.5	
Prealbumin or transthyretin or thyroxine-binding prealbumin, serum (mg/dl)	10-40, ↑ in preg		
Osmolality, serum (mOsm/kg H₂O)	275-295	275-290	
Phosphorus, serum (mg/dl)	2.7-4.5	10 day-2 yr: 4.5-6.7; >2 yr: 4.5-5.5	
Potassium, serum (mEq/L)	3.5-5.1	4.1-5.3	
Prothrombin time, blood (seconds)	11-15		
Riboflavin			
Serum (µg/dl)	4-24		
RBC (µg/dl)	10-50		
Urine (µg/day)	>120		
Schilling test (intrinsic factor test), urine (% of test dose)	>7.5		
Selenium (µg/dl)			
Blood	58-234		
Serum	46-143		

Test		
Sodium, serum or plasma (mEq/L)	136-145	138-145
Transferrin, serum (mg/dl)	200-400	200-360
Transthyretin, see Prealbumin		
Triglycerides, serum, fasting (mg/dl)	M: 40-160 F: 35-135	<150
Urea nitrogen, urine (g/day)	12-20	
Vitamin A, serum (µg/dl)	30-80	
Vitamin B$_6$, plasma (ng/ml)	5-30	20-72
Vitamin B$_{12}$, true, serum (pg/ml)	100-700	
Vitamin C		
Plasma (mg/dl)	0.5-1.5	
Leukocyte (µg/10^3 WBC)	20-53	
Vitamin D$_3$, 1,25-dihydroxy, serum (pg/ml)	18-64	
Vitamin E, serum (µg/ml)	5-18	
Vitamin K (phylloquinone), serum (ng/ml)	0.13-1.19	
Xylose absorption test		
Blood (mg/dl)	>25 (25 g dose)	>30 (5 g dose)
Urine (g/5 h)	>4	16-33% of dose ingested
Zinc, serum (µg/dl)	70-150	

Values compiled from Burtis CA, Ashwood ER: *Tietz textbook of clinical chemistry*, ed 2, Philadelphia, 1994, WB Saunders; Meites S, ed: *Pediatric clinical chemistry*, ed 3, Washington, DC, 1989, American Association for Clinical Chemistry; and Pagana KD, Pagana TJ: *Mosby's diagnostic and laboratory reference*, ed 2, St Louis, 1995, Mosby.

Appendix G
Caffeine Content
of Selected Beverages
and Foods*

Beverage or Food	Caffeine (mg)
Coffees, 240 ml (8 oz) Servings	
Coffee, brewed	135
Orange Cappuccino†	102
Coffee, instant	95
Café Vienna†	90
Mocha‡ or Swiss mocha†	55-60
Amaretto‡	30
Coffee, decaffeinated	5
Teas, 240 ml (8 oz) Servings Unless Otherwise Specified	
Bigelow Raspberry Royale	83
Tea, leaf or bag; black, pekoe or oolong	50
Snapple iced tea, all varieties, 480 ml (16 oz)	48
Nestea Pure Sweetened Iced Tea, 480 ml (16 oz)	34

Information from *Caffeine content of foods and drugs,* press release from the Center for Science in the Public Interest, July 31, 1997 (www.scpinet.org); Barone JJ, Roberts HR: Caffeine consumption, *Food Chem Toxicol* 34:119, 1996; and beverage and food manufacturers.

*Many over-the-counter and some prescription medications contain higher levels of caffeine than these beverages and foods. Consult the product label or a pharmacist about the caffeine content of drugs.

†General Foods International Coffee

‡Maxwell House Cappuccino

Beverage or Food	Caffeine (mg)
Teas, 240 ml (8 oz) Servings Unless Otherwise Specified—cont'd	
Tea, green	30
Arizona iced tea, assorted varieties, 480 ml (16 oz)	15-30
Tea, instant	15
Tea, decaffeinated	<5
Tea, herbal	0
Soft Drinks, 360 ml (12 oz) Servings	
Jolt	72
Mountain Dew, Surge	51-55
Coca-Cola, Diet Coke	45-47
Dr. Pepper, regular or diet; Sunkist Orange Soda; Pepsi-Cola	37-41
Barq's Root Beer	23
7-Up or Diet 7-Up, Barq's Diet Root Beer, caffeine-free colas (all types, regular or diet), Minute Maid Orange Soda, Mug Root Beer, Sprite or Diet Sprite	0
Caffeinated Waters, 0.5 Liter (16.9 oz)	
Java Water	125
Aqua Blast	90
Water Joe, Aqua Java	50-70
Other	
Ben & Jerry's No Fat Coffee Fudge Frozen Yogurt, 1 cup	85
Coffee ice creams, 240 ml (1 cup)	30-60
Dannon coffee yogurt, 240 ml (1 cup)	45
Cappuccino or café au lait yogurts, 180-240 ml (6-8 oz)	<5
Hershey's Special Dark Chocolate Bar, 1 bar (1.5 oz)	31
Hershey Bar (milk chocolate), 1 bar (1.5 oz)	10
Cocoa, hot chocolate, or chocolate milk, 240 ml (8 oz)	5

Appendix H
Drug-Nutrient
Interactions

Box H-1   Drugs Affecting Appetite

Appetite Depressants

Amphetamines and related compounds
  Benzphetamine (Didrex)
  Fenfluramine (Pondimin)
  Phenylpropanolamine (Dexatrim, Dimetapp, Triaminic)
Antibiotics
  Amphotericin B (Fungizone)
  Gentamicin (Garamycin)
  Metronidazole (Flagyl)
  Zidovudine (AZT)
Carbonic anhydrase inhibitors
  Acetazolamide (Diamox)
  Dichlorphenamide (Daranide)
Digitalis preparations
Methylphenidate (Ritalin)

Appetite Stimulants

Antidepressants
  Amitriptyline (Elavil)
Antihistamines
  Astemizole (Hismanal)
  Cyproheptadine (Periactin)
Tranquilizers
  Lithium carbonate (Lithane)
  Benzodiazepines: all, including
  Prazepam (Centrax)
  Diazepam (Valium)
  Phenothiazines: all, including
  Chlorpromazine (Thorazine)
  Promethazine (Phenergan)

Box H-1   Drugs Affecting Appetite—cont'd

Appetite Stimulants—cont'd

Steroids
Anabolic steroids
Oxandrolone (Anavar)
Glucocorticoids
Dexamethasone (Decadron)
Methylprednisolone (Medrol)
Tetrahydrocannabinol (marijuana, THC)
Dronabinol (synthetic THC)

Box H-2   Drugs Whose Absorption is Significantly Affected by Food

Absorption Increased	Absorption Reduced
Atovaquone (high-fat meals)	Astemizole
Carbamazepine	Azithromycin (not tablet)
Cyclosporin	Captopril
Griseofulvin	Ciprofloxacin*†
Lovostatin	Delavirdine
Metropolol	Didanosine
Nelfinavir	Digoxin (bran fiber)
Nitrofurantoin	Levodopa
Ritonavir (high-fat meals)	(high-protein meals)
Saquinavir	Penicillins
Theophylline (extended-release form; do not take less than 1 hour before a high-fat meal; do not take after the evening meal)	Phenytoin†
	Tetracyclines*
	Warfarin†
	Zalcitabine
	Zidovudine

For drugs whose absorption is improved by food, take with a meal, except as noted. For drugs whose absorption is decreased by food, take at least 1 hour before or 2 hours after a meal.
*Especially dairy products
†Enteral tube feedings

Table H-1   Nutritional Effects of Selected Drugs

Drug	Effect on Nutrition
Alcohol	$\uparrow$ Excretion of Mg, K^+, Zn; impaired folic acid utilization
Antacids	
All	$\downarrow$ Fe absorption caused by $\uparrow$ gastric pH
Antibiotics/Antifungals/Antitubercular Agents	
Amphotericin B	Hypokalemia; $\uparrow$ urinary excretion of Mg
Chloramphenicol	$\downarrow$ Hgb synthesis (interferes with response to Fe, folic acid, or vitamin B_{12} therapy)
Cycloserine	$\downarrow$ Serum levels of vitamins B_{12}, B_6, folic acid
Gentamicin	$\uparrow$ Urinary excretion of Mg, K^+, Ca (>10 g cumulative dose)
Isoniazid	Depletion of vitamin B_6; supplement should be given
Neomycin	Diarrhea and mucosal injury; $\downarrow$ absorption of fat, lactose, protein, vitamins A, D, K, B_{12}, Ca, Fe, K^+
Paraaminosalicylic acid	$\downarrow$ Absorption of fat, folic acid, vitamin B_{12}
Anticonvulsants	
Phenytoin	$\downarrow$ Absorption of Ca
Phenobarbital	$\downarrow$ Absorption of Ca
Primidone	$\downarrow$ Absorption of Ca
Antidiarrheal Agent	
Sulfasalazine	$\downarrow$ Absorption of folic acid; megaloblastic anemia
Antihypertensive Agents	
Diazoxide	Hyperglycemia
Hydralazine	$\uparrow$ Excretion of vitamin B_6
Nitroprusside	$\downarrow$ Serum vitamin B_{12}

Table H-1   Nutritional Effects of Selected Drugs—cont'd

Drug	Effect on Nutrition
Antiinflammatory Agents	
Aspirin	$\uparrow$ Urinary loss of vitamin C; Fe deficiency caused by GI blood loss
Colchicine	$\downarrow$ Absorption of vitamin B_{12}, fat, carotene, lactose, protein, Na, K^+
Indomethacin	$\uparrow$ Urinary loss of vitamin C; Fe deficiency caused by GI blood loss
Antineoplastic drugs	See Chapter 13
Carbonic Anhydrase Inhibitors	
All	Hyperglycemia; $\uparrow$ excretion of K^+
Cardiac Drugs	
Digitalis, digoxin, digitoxin, etc.	Diarrhea, malabsorption of all nutrients
Chelating Agents	
Penicillamine	$\downarrow$ Absorption of Cu, Zn, Fe
Corticosteroids	
All	$\uparrow$ Protein catabolism; $\downarrow$ protein synthesis; hyperglycemia; $\uparrow$ serum triglycerides and cholesterol; $\downarrow$ absorption of Ca, P, K^+; $\uparrow$ requirement for vitamins C, B_6, D, folic acid, Zn; osteopenia

Continued

Table H-1   Nutritional Effects of Selected Drugs—cont'd

Drug	Effect on Nutrition
Diuretics	
All	↑ Urinary excretion of Mg, Zn, K^+, thiamin (some greater than others)
Ethacrynic acid	Hypomagnesemia, hypokalemia; ↑ loss of urinary Ca
Furosemide	↓ Glucose tolerance; hyperglycemia; ↑ loss of urinary Ca
Thiazides	↓ Glucose tolerance; hyperglycemia; hypokalemia
H_2-Receptor Antagonists	
All (cimetidine, famotidine, nizatidine, ranitidine)	↓ Fe and Ca absorption caused by ↑ gastric pH
Hypocholesterolemics	
Cholestyramine, clofibrate, colestipol	↓ Absorption of fat, carotene, vitamins A, E, D, K, B_{12}, Fe
Laxatives	
Cathartics (e.g., senna, cascara, phenolphthalein)	↑ Fecal loss of Ca and K^+ (clinically significant only with laxative abuse)
Mineral oil	Potential for ↓ absorption of vitamins A, D, E, K, Ca^{2+}; recent evidence indicates that effects on vitamin absorption are probably not clinically significant
Levodopa	↑ Requirement for vitamin B_6
Lipid emulsions	↑ Requirement for vitamin E
Opiates	
Heroin	↓ Glucose tolerance, ↓ K^+

Table H-1   Nutritional Effects of Selected Drugs—cont'd

Drug	Effect on Nutrition
Oral Contraceptive Agents	↓ Serum vitamin C; possible ↓ serum vitamin B_{12}, B_6, B_2, folic acid, Mg, Zn; ↑ Hct, Hgb, serum Fe, Cu, vitamins A, E
Parasympatholytic Agents	
Atropine	↓ Fe absorption caused by ↑ gastric pH
Uricosuric Agents (for gout)	↑ Excretion of Ca, Mg, Na, K^+, P, Cl, vitamin B_2, amino acids
Urinary Antiseptics	
Nitrofurantoin	↓ Serum folic acid; megaloblastic anemia

Table H-2   Foods, Food Components, or Nutrients with Specific Effects on Drug Action

Food, Food Component, or Nutrient	Drugs Affected
Diet Factors That Decrease Drug Effectiveness	
Vitamin K sources: liver, cabbage, spinach, kale, olive oil, soybean oil and margarines and salad dressings made with it	Coumarin
Caffeine	Guanadrel
Folic acid supplement	Methotrexate
High-protein diet	Levodopa
Pyridoxine (vitamin B_6) supplement*	Levodopa
Supplements of Fe, Mg, Zn, and Ca	Fluoroquinolones

*>5 mg/day   *Continued*

Food, Food Component, or Nutrient	Drugs Affected
Diet Factors That Increase Risk of Drug Toxicity	
Caffeine	Lithium
Sodium-restricted diet	Lithium
Folic acid deficiency	Methotrexate
Potassium deficit	Digitalis and related drugs
Diet Factors with Other Drug Interactions	
Grapefruit juice—decreases first pass extraction and causes elevated blood drug levels; avoid taking grapefruit juice with these drugs	Many drugs, including cyclosporine; felodipine, nifedipine, nimodipine, and other calcium antagonists (calcium channel blockers); saquinavir; triazolam
Imported (natural) licorice—can cause excessive potassium losses, cardiac dysrhythmia, sodium and water retention	Thiazides: chlorothiazide, hydrochlorothiazide, chlorthalidone
Salt substitutes (potassium-containing)—drug can elevate potassium levels	ACE (angiotensin converting enzyme) inhibitors
Tyramine and dopamine sources: liver, hard salami and other dry sausages; any pickled, aged, fermented, or smoked protein foods such as pickled herring, aged cheese, yogurt; commercial gravies; meat extracts; alcoholic beverages; sour cream; soy sauce; Italian broad (fava) beans; raisins; figs; bananas—can cause headache, hypertensive crisis, potential intracranial hemorrhage	Monoamine oxidase (MAO) inhibitors: phenelzine, isocarboxazid, tranylcypromine, procarbazine

SELECTED BIBLIOGRAPHY

Fuhr U: Drug interactions with grapefruit juice. Extent, probable mechanism and clinical relevance, *Drug Safety* 18:251, 1998.

Gauthier I, Malone M: Drug-food interactions in hospitalised patients. Methods of prevention, *Drug Safety* 18:383, 1998.

Livingston MG, Livingston HM: Monoamine oxidase inhibitors. An update of drug interactions, *Drug Safety* 14:219, 1996.

Thomas JA, Burns RA: Important drug-nutrient interactions in the elderly, *Drugs Aging* 13:199, 1998.

Varella L, Jones E, Meguid MM: Drug-nutrient interactions in enteral feeding: a primary care focus, *Nurse Pract* 22:98, 1997.

Appendix I
Resources for Planning Interventions, Referrals, and Teaching

Because of space limitations, this list cannot be complete; however, it provides some of the major sources of nutrition information and a starting point for finding additional resources.

General Information About Nutrition and Food Safety

American Dietetic Association
216 West Jackson Blvd., Suite 800
Chicago, IL 60606-6995
Consumer hotline: (800) 366-1655
www.eatright.org

American Medical Association
Dept. of Foods and Nutrition
515 North State St.
Chicago, IL 60610
(312) 464-5000
www.ama-assn.org

Center for Food Safety and Applied Nutrition
U.S. Food and Drug Administration
200 C Street, SW
HFS-555, Room 5809
Washington, DC 20204
(800) FDA-4010
vm.cfsan.fda.gov/

Center for Nutrition Policy and Promotion
U.S. Dept. of Agriculture
1120 20th St., NW
Suite 200, North Lobby
Washington, DC 20036
(202) 418-2312
www.usda.gov/cnpp/

Center for Science in the Public Interest
1875 Connecticut Avenue, NW
Suite 300
Washington, DC 20009-5728
(202) 322-9110
www.cspinet.org

Food and Nutrition Information Center,
U.S. Dept. of Agriculture
10301 Baltimore Avenue
Room 304
Beltsville, MD 20705-2351
(301) 504-4719
www.nal.usda.gov/fnic/

Gateway to government food safety information online
www.foodsafety.gov

Local dietitians or nutritionists
(registered dietitians or RDs)

National Center for Chronic Disease Prevention and Health
    Promotion
Centers for Disease Control and Prevention
Technical Information and Editorial Services Branch
4770 Buford Highway NE
Mailstop K13
Atlanta, GA 30341-3724
www.cdc.gov/nccdphp/nccdhome.htm

National Institutes of Health Center for Complementary and
    Alternative Medicine
NCCAM Clearinghouse
P.O. Box 8218
Silver Spring, MD 20907-8218
(888) 644-6226
nccam.nih.gov

Society for Nutrition Education
7101 Wisconsin Ave, Suite 901
Bethesda, MD 20814
(800) 235-6690
pitt.ces.state.nc.us/sne/

Aging
Alzheimer's Disease Education and Referral (ADEAR) Center
National Institutes on Aging
P.O. Box 8250
Silver Spring, MD 20907-8250
(800) 438-4380
www.alzheimers.org

Nutrition Screening Initiative
1010 Wisconsin Ave., NW
Suite 800
Washington, DC 20007
www.aafp.org/nsi/

AIDS and HIV Infection
Centers for Disease Control and Prevention National AIDS
    Prevention Information Network
P.O. Box 6003
Rockville, MD 20849
(800) 458-5231
cdcnpin.gov

Anorexia Nervosa and Bulimia
American Anorexia/Bulimia Association
293 Central Park W, Ste. 1R
New York, NY 10024
(212) 501-8351
members@aol.com/anambu

National Association of Anorexia Nervosa and Associated
    Disorders
P.O. Box 7
Highland Park, IL 60035
(847) 831-3438
www.anred.com

Cancer
American Cancer Society
1599 Clifton Rd., NE
Atlanta, GA 30329-4251
(800) ACS-2345
www.cancer.org

Cancer Information Service
National Cancer Institute
Bldg. 31, Rm. 10A-03
Bethesda, MD 20892
(800) 4-CANCER
cis.nci.nih.gov

Diabetes
American Diabetes Association
1660 Duke St.
P.O. Box 25757
Alexandria, VA 22314
(800) ADA-DISC
www.diabetes.org

Juvenile Diabetes Foundation International
120 Wall St.
New York, NY 10005-3904
(800) JDF-CURE
www.jdf.org

National Diabetes Information Clearinghouse
1 Information Way
Bethesda, MD 20892-3560
www.niddk.nih.gov/health/diabetes/diabetes.htm

Fraud and Quackery
Center for Food Safety and Applied Nutrition
U.S. Food and Drug Administration
200 C Street, SW
HFS-555, Room 5809
Washington, DC 20204
(800) FDA-4010
vm.cfsan.fda.gov/

National Council for Reliable Health Information
P.O. Box 1276
Loma Linda, CA 92354
(909) 824-4690
www.ncrhi.org

Quackwatch
P.O. Box 1747
Allentown, PA 18105
www.quackwatch.com

Gastrointestinal Diseases
Celiac Sprue Association
P.O. Box 31700
Omaha, NE 68131-0700
(402) 558-0600
www.csaceliacs.org

Crohn's and Colitis Foundation of America
386 Park Ave. S.
New York, NY 10016-8804
(800) 932-2423
www.healthy.net/pan/cso/cioi/CCFA.HTM

Cystic Fibrosis Foundation
6931 Arlington Rd.
Bethesda, MD 20814
(800) 344-4823
www.cff.org

National Digestive Diseases Information Clearinghouse
2 Information Way
Bethesda, MD 20892
(301) 654-3810
www.niddk.nih.gov/health/digest/digest.htm

Heart Disease
American Heart Association
7272 Greenville Ave.
Dallas, TX 75231-4596
(800) 242-4596
www.americanheart.org

National Center for Cardiac Information
8080 Greensboro Dr., #1070
McLean, VA 22102
(703) 356-6568
www.cardiacinfo.org

National Heart, Lung, and Blood Institute Information Center
P.O. Box 30105
Bethesda, MD 20824-0105
(301) 496-8573
e-mail: NHLBIinfo@rover.nhlbi.nih.gov
www.nhlbi.nih.gov/nhlbi/nhlbi.htm

Kidney Disease
National Kidney and Urologic Disease Information Clearinghouse
3 Information Way
Bethesda, MD 20892
(301) 654-4415
www.niddk.nih.gov

National Kidney Foundation, Inc.
30 East 33rd St., #1100
New York, NY 10016
(212) 889-2210
www.kidney.org

Nutrition Support
American Society for Parenteral and Enteral Nutrition
8630 Fenton St., Suite 412
Silver Spring, MD 20910
(301) 587-6315
www.nutritioncare.org

Oley Foundation for Home Parenteral and Enteral Nutrition
Albany Medical Center
214 Hun Memorial, A-23
Albany, NY 12208
(800) 776-OLEY

Obesity and Overweight
Overeaters Anonymous
6075 Zenith Ct. NE
Rio Rancho, NM 87214-6424
(505) 891-2664
www.overeatersanonymous.org

Weight-Control Information Network
National Institute of Diabetes, Digestive, and Kidney Disease
6101 Executive Blvd, Suite 300
Rockville, MD 20852
(800) WIN-8098
www.niddk.nih.gov/nutrit/nutrit.htm

Pregnancy, Lactation, and Women's Health
La Leche League International
1400 N. Meacham Rd.
Schaumburg, IL 60173
(847) 519-7730
www.lalecheleague.org

March of Dimes Birth Defects Foundation
1275 Mamaroneck Ave.
White Plains, NY 10605
(914) 428-7100

National Maternal and Child Health Clearinghouse
Health Resources and Services Administration
Information Specialist
2070 Chain Bridge Rd., Suite 450
Vienna, VA 22182-2536
www.nmchc.org/

National Women's Health Information Center
U.S. Public Health Service Office on Women's Health
(800) 994-WOMAN
www.4women.org

National Women's Health Resource Center
5255 Loughboro Rd., NW
Washington, DC 20016
(202) 537-4015
www.healthywomen.org

Pulmonary Disease
Cystic Fibrosis Foundation
6931 Arlington Rd., #200
Bethesda, MD 20814
(800) 344-4823
www.cff.org

National Heart, Lung, and Blood Institute Information Center
P.O. Box 30105
Bethesda, MD 20824-0105
(301) 496-8573
e-mail: NHLBIinfo@rover.nhlbi.nih.gov
www.nhlbi.nih.gov/nhlbi/nhlbi.htm

Reliable Journals and Newsletters

American Journal of Clinical Nutrition
Consumer Reports on Health
Diabetes
Diabetes Care
Diabetes Forecast
FDA Consumer
Journal of the American Dietetic Association
Journal of the American Medical Association
Journal of Nutrition Education (especially good source of teaching
    tools and techniques)
Journal of Parenteral and Enteral Nutrition
Nutrition and the MD
Nutrition in Clinical Practice
Nutrition Reviews
Nutrition Today

Appendix J
Modified Diets*

Modified Diets*

Diets Modified in Texture or Consistency

Clear liquid diet

Common uses/rationale:

Early postoperative period; provides fluids and some electrolytes with little residue (indigestible food)

Diet modification/comments:

Includes only broth, gelatin, clear fruit juices, popsicles, tea and other clear beverages, low-residue supplements; usually does not provide the RDA for any nutrients except perhaps vitamin C and should not be used more than 2 to 3 days without supplementation

Full liquid diet

Common uses/rationale:

Facial trauma or mandibular fractures, esophageal stricture, postoperative patients; supplies protein and carbohydrate for healing and energy in an easily swallowed form

Diet modification/comments:

Foods that are liquid at room temperature; milk, ice cream, strained soups, pudding, all juices, enteral feeding products; many allowed foods contain lactose and are not well tolerated by lactose-intolerant individuals; low in iron unless commercial liquid supplements are used

---

*In some instances, the rationale for using the diet is not well supported by empirical evidence; nevertheless, these diets are often used in clinical practice. Certain modified diets are thoroughly described in the text; consult the appropriate chapters for more information. These include the diabetic or "ADA" (American Diabetes Association) diets (see Chapter 18); low-sodium diets (see Chapter 15); low-protein diets (see Chapters 12 and 17); low-fat and/or low-cholesterol diets (see Chapters 12 and 15); and gluten-free diet (see Chapter 12).

Modified Diets—cont'd

Diets Modified in Texture or Consistency—cont'd
Soft diet
Common uses/rationale:
Postoperative period, dental problems, hiatal hernia; avoids foods that are difficult to chew and digest; low in residue
Diet modification/comments:
Includes tender, low-fiber foods: cooked vegetables, cooked or canned fruits, tender meats, no fried foods or coarse whole grains; can be nutritionally complete, except perhaps for fiber

Mechanical soft, pureed, or ground diet
Common uses/rationale:
Dysphagia or dental problems; little chewing required
Diet modification/comments:
Same as soft diet except meats, fruits, and vegetables are ground or pureed

Bland diet
Common uses/rationale:
Peptic ulcer disease, eliminates foods suspected of being gastric irritants; foods served in several small meals and snacks a day to buffer gastric secretions
Diet modification/comments:
Alcohol, caffeine, black pepper, and meat extractives (e.g., gravy and soup bases); nutritionally complete

Low-fiber or low-residue diet
Common uses/rationale:
Acute exacerbations of inflammatory bowel disease, diverticulitis; avoids mechanical irritation of GI mucosal lining
Diet modification/comments:
Excludes alcohol, fried foods, nuts, dried fruits, whole grains, raw fruits or vegetables except banana and avocado, pepper, spicy foods; milk limited to one or two servings a day; can be nutritionally complete except for fiber; calcium intake must be assessed

Continued

Modified Diets—cont'd

Diets Modified in Texture or Consistency—cont'd
High-fiber diet
Common uses/rationale:
Constipation, diverticulosis, hemorrhoids; increases stool bulk and stimulates intestinal elimination
Diet modification/comments:
No food excluded; emphasize whole grains (oatmeal, whole-wheat breads and cereals, brown rice), raw or lightly cooked vegetables; raw or dried fruits, legumes; bran may be added; encourage at least 8 cups of fluid a day to hydrate fiber and create soft stool; nutritionally complete

Diets with Protein or Amino Acid Modifications
High-protein diet
Common uses/rationale:
Burns, trauma, major surgery, corticosteroid therapy, hepatitis; provides protein for healing or tissue formation; steroids increase conversion of protein to glucose, which creates increased needs
Diet modification/comments:
Increased serving sizes of meat, dairy products, eggs, legumes; ensure that carbohydrate and fat intake is adequate for protein sparing (providing kcal so that protein is not used to meet energy needs); nutritionally adequate
Low-protein diet
Common uses/rationale:
Liver or renal failure, when there is limited ability to metabolize or excrete the nitrogen released by breakdown of protein
Diet modification/comments:
Intake of meats, poultry, fish, eggs, nuts, dry beans, dairy products, grain products, and starchy vegetables is limited; see Chapters 12 and 17; nutritional status must be carefully monitored

Modified Diets—cont'd

Diets with Protein or Amino Acid Modifications—cont'd

Gluten-free diet

Common uses/rationale:

Celiac disease (gluten-sensitive enteropathy or nontropical sprue); intake of gluten, a protein in most grains, causes damage to the intestinal mucosa in individuals with this disorder

Diet modification/comments:

Eliminate wheat, rye, barley, oats, and buckwheat from the diet; see Table 12-3

Low-phenylalanine diet

Common uses/rationale:

Phenylketonuria (PKU), an inborn error of metabolism affecting the conversion of phenylalanine to tyrosine, results in severe retardation if a low-phenylalanine diet is not begun in infancy; intellectual function is best if the individual continues on the diet at least through adolescence (possibly longer); women with PKU should follow a low-phenylalanine diet before conception (optimally) and throughout pregnancy to avoid damage to the fetus

Diet modification/comments:

Restrict meat, milk, eggs, breads, and other sources of dietary protein; low-phenylalanine infant formulas (Lofenalac [Mead Johnson] or PKU 1 [Milupa]) and milk replacements (Phenyl-free [Mead Johnson] or PKU 2 [Milupa]) are available; blood levels of phenylalanine are monitored to determine the amount of phenylalanine allowed in the diet and the success of dietary restrictions

Low-tyramine diet or monoamine oxidase inhibitor (MAOI) diet

Common uses/rationale:

Used for as long as an individual is receiving an MAOI, a class of antidepressant medication including phenelzine, isocarboxazid, tranylcypromine; tyramine and dopamine formed by aging, protein breakdown, and putrefaction in foods could cause headache and hypertensive crisis

Continued

Modified Diets—cont'd

Diets with Protein or Amino Acid Modifications—cont'd
Low-tyramine diet or monoamine oxidase inhibitor (MAOI) diet—cont'd
Diet modification/comments:
Avoid liver; alcohol; any aged, pickled, fermented, or smoked protein foods (all cheese, smoked or dried meats, salted dried or smoked fish, pickled herring, aged game); meat extracts; commercial gravies; yeast extracts; sour cream; yogurt; soy sauce, chocolate; homemade yeast bread; bananas; avocados; figs; raisins; Italian broad (fava) beans; eggplant; limit to 1 small orange/day; limit to ½ cup tomato/day; nutritionally adequate

Diets with Carbohydrate Modifications
Diabetic diet
Common uses/rationale:
Diabetes, controls hyperglycemia by regulating the amount of dietary carbohydrate consumed at any time and spacing the carbohydrate throughout the day
Diet modifications/comments:
Amount of carbohydrate, protein, and fat in diet is calculated and is divided into 3 to 6 (or more) meals and snacks during the day; diet is also low in cholesterol and saturated fat to reduce the risk of heart disease, a common complication in diabetes; nutritionally adequate
Low-sugar diet
Common uses/rationale:
Corticosteroid therapy, which can cause glucose intolerance
Diet modification/comments:
Restrict simple sugars (sweets and fruits); nutritionally adequate
Lactose-restricted or lactose-free diet
Common uses/rationale:
Lactase deficiency (which may be either primary or genetically determined, or secondary to intestinal mucosal damage in gastroenteritis, radiation therapy of the bowel, celiac disease, etc.); deficiency of lactase, the enzyme that digests milk sugar (lactose), results in cramping, bloating, and diarrhea after lactose consumption

Modified Diets—cont'd

Diets with Carbohydrate Modifications—cont'd

Lactose-restricted or lactose-free diet—cont'd

Diet modification/comments:

Restrict milk and milk products except hard cheeses; some individuals tolerate small amounts of milk, ice cream, and cultured milk products (e.g., yogurt, buttermilk, acidophilus milk); lactase is available for addition to milk products; can be nutritionally adequate; assess calcium intake

Galactose-free diet

Common uses/rationale:

Galactosemia, an inborn error of metabolism, results from inability to metabolize galactose to glucose; sequelae of galactosemia include cataracts (in galactokinase deficiency) and vomiting, failure to thrive, hepatomegaly, jaundice, cataracts, learning disorders, and ovarian dysfunction in deficiencies of galactose-1-phosphate uridyltransferase. Galactose and lactose (which is composed of galactose and glucose) must be omitted from the diet permanently

Diet modification/comments:

Avoid all dairy products, commercial products to which lactose is added (frankfurters, margarine, instant mashed potatoes, etc.), medications containing lactose as a filler; soy formula, soy milk fortified with calcium, or a calcium supplement should be used daily

Diets with Fat or Cholesterol Modifications

Low-fat diet

Common uses/rationale:

Decrease discomfort or pain in steatorrhea or gallbladder disease

Diet modification/comments:

Limit intake of fats (oils, margarine, butter, bacon, avocado, olives, salad dressings, egg yolks) to no more than 5 servings/day; use lean cuts of meat, poultry without skin, and skim milk and dairy products made with skim milk; avoid chocolate candy, coconut, breads made with fat, peanut butter, pastry; see Table 12-2; nutritionally adequate

Continued

Modified Diets—cont'd

Diets with Fat or Cholesterol Modifications—cont'd
Low-cholesterol, low-saturated fat diet
Common uses/rationale:
Decrease risk or progression of arteriosclerotic heart disease
Diet modification/comments:
Limit intake of egg yolks to 2/week; limit meat intake to about 6 oz/day; use lean meats, poultry without skin, skim milk, and dairy products made with skim milk; use corn, cottonseed, soybean, canola, olive, sunflower, and safflower oils; avoid coconut and palm oils and butter or foods containing these products; avoid organ meats (liver, kidney, brains, sweetbreads); see Chapter 15; nutritionally adequate

Diets Used in Diagnostic Testing
5-hydroxyindoleacetic acid (5-HIAA) test diet
Common uses/rationale:
Used for ~3 days before and during 24-hr urine collection for 5-HIAA. Used in diagnosis and monitoring of carcinoid tumors, which secrete serotonin (metabolized in the liver to 5-HIAA).
Diet modification/comments:
Omit foods containing serotonin; avocado, banana, eggplant, pineapple, plums, tomatoes, and walnuts
300 g carbohydrate diet
Common uses/rationale:
Used for approximately 3 days before a glucose tolerance test, since low-carbohydrate diet can result in a falsely abnormal result
Diet modification/comments:
Includes 300 g or more of carbohydrate/day in a balanced diet

Modified Diets—cont'd

Diets Used in Diagnostic Testing—cont'd

Vanillylmandelic acid (VMA) test diet

Common uses/rationale:
Used for 2 to 3 days before and during 24-hour urine collection for VMA; the test is used in diagnosis of pheochromocytoma, an adrenal tumor that secretes high levels of epinephrine and/or norepinephrine; VMA is a metabolic product of these substances, and some foods increase VMA levels

Diet modification/comments:
Eliminate caffeine (coffee, tea, cola beverages, chocolate), apples, bananas, citrus fruits, vanilla and vanilla-containing foods, tomatoes, and squash

100 g Fat Diet

Common uses/rationale:
Used for ~3 days before and 3 days during 72-hour stool collection for fat analysis; used in assessing steatorrhea and malabsorption; adults should not excrete more than 5 g fat/day in feces; children should not excrete more than 5% to 7% of fat consumed

Diet modification/comments:
Include 100 g fat/day in diet by consumption of margarine, butter, oil, meats, whole milk, eggs, etc.; most young children cannot consume 100 g fat/day; a record of their intake is kept, and fecal fat is expressed as a proportion of the intake

Appendix K
Food Safety Guidelines

Box K-1   Common or Especially Serious Foodborne Illnesses

Campylobacteriosis *(Campylobacter jejuni)*

Symptoms: Abdominal pain, diarrhea, nausea, headache, muscle pain, and fever; rare: Guillain-Barré syndrome (acute paralysis)

People most at risk: This is the most common foodborne illness, but children under 5 years and individuals 15-29 years of age are most frequently affected. Arthritis, a rare complication, occurs primarily in people who have the human lymphocyte antigen B27.

Common food sources: Raw and undercooked meat and poultry, unpasteurized milk, untreated water

Prevention: Cook food thoroughly; use pasteurized milk and cheese; use water from a safe source

Botulism (Toxin from *Clostridium botulinum*)

Symptoms: Generalized muscle paralysis—double vision, inability to swallow, speech difficulty, respiratory insufficiency

People most at risk: All are at risk from disease caused by ingesting the toxin; infants less than 12 months may develop infant botulinism from ingesting *C. botulinism* spores in honey.

Common food sources of toxin: Home-canned or prepared low-acid foods (e.g., corn, green beans, soup, spinach, chicken, mushrooms, peppers, low-acid tomatoes, garlic-in-oil mixtures); bulging or leaking commercial canned foods; smoked or dried fish

Botulism (Toxin from *Clostridium botulinum*)—cont'd

Prevention: Use proper canning methods for low-acid foods (consult U.S. Department of Agriculture or state agricultural extension service publications); garlic-in-oil mixtures must be acidified or treated with antimicrobials; avoid commercially canned foods from bulging or leaking cans. *Discard any food that is suspect; never taste it.* Never let infants less than 12 months old eat honey.

Enterohemorrhagic *Escherichia coli* Infection (*E. coli*)

Symptoms: Abdominal cramping, diarrhea (watery progressing to bloody)

People most at risk: All

Common food sources: Meat, especially raw or undercooked ground meat; unpasteurized milk, apple cider, or apple juice; vegetable sprouts

Prevention: Cook all meat to an interior temperature of 160° F (72° C); use pasteurized milk, cider, and juice and cheese made with pasteurized milk; wash uncooked raw fruits and vegetables in clean drinking water; avoid raw sprouts even if they have been washed

Listeriosis (*Listeria monocytogenes*)

Symptoms: Flulike symptoms initially—chills, fever, headache, and sometimes nausea and vomiting; can progress to bacteremia, meningitis, and encephalitis, and these complications may occur as much as 3 weeks after initial infection; spontaneous abortion or stillbirth

People most at risk: Pregnant women, newborns, people with impaired immunity, and people taking cimetidine or antacids

Common food sources: Unpasteurized milk and cheese; raw or undercooked meat, poultry, and fish

Prevention: Use pasteurized milk and cheese made from pasteurized milk; use hard cheeses rather than soft cheeses (soft cheeses include Mexican queso blanco, fresco, de hoya, de crema or asadero; brie; Camembert; feta; Roquefort and other blue-veined cheese) or cook soft cheeses until bubbling if pregnant or immunosuppressed; if unpasteurized hard cheeses are consumed, choose those aged at least 60 days; cook all meat, fish, and poultry thoroughly

Continued

Box K-1 Common or Especially Serious Foodborne Illnesses—cont'd

Salmonellosis (*Salmonella* Bacteria)

Symptoms: Abdominal cramping, nausea, vomiting, diarrhea, fever, headache; chronic: arthritic symptoms

People most at risk: Elderly, infants, and individuals with immune suppression; AIDS patients are ~20 times more likely than the general population to contract salmonellosis.

Common food sources: Raw or undercooked eggs, poultry, and meat; seafood; dairy products; salad dressing; cream-filled desserts and toppings; dried gelatin

Prevention: Cook eggs, poultry, meats, and seafoods thoroughly; avoid foods made with raw or undercooked eggs (Caesar salad, "chiffon"-type pies, some meringues, royal icing); use pasteurized milk and cheese; avoid cross-contamination of foods or cooking utensils (see below)

Shigellosis or Bacillary Dysentery (*Shigella* Bacteria)

Symptoms: Abdominal pain; cramps; diarrhea; fever; vomiting; blood, pus, or mucus in stools

People most at risk: Infants, elderly, and immunosuppressed; especially those with AIDS and AIDS-related complex

Common food sources: Salads (potato, tuna, shrimp, macaroni, and chicken), raw vegetables, milk and dairy products, poultry

Prevention: Refrigerate salads as soon as they are prepared; use pasteurized dairy products; wash raw produce thoroughly; cook poultry thoroughly

Staphylococcal Food Poisoning (*Staphylococcus aureus*)

Symptoms: Nausea, vomiting, abdominal cramping, and prostration

People most at risk: All

Common food sources: Raw or undercooked meat, poultry, and egg products; salads such as egg, tuna, chicken, potato, and macaroni; bakery products such as cream-filled pastries and cream pies; sandwich fillings; milk and dairy products

Prevention: Cook meats, poultry and eggs thoroughly; refrigerate salads and susceptible bakery products; keep sandwiches cool until serving

Box K-1 Common or Especially Serious Foodborne Illnesses—cont'd

Toxoplasmosis *(Toxoplasma gondii)*

Symptoms: Central nervous system disorders, particularly mental retardation and visual impairment
> *People most at risk:* Young children
> *Common food sources:* Meat, especially pork
> *Prevention:* Cook all meats thoroughly

Vibrio vulnificus Infection

Symptoms: Gastroenteritis—abdominal cramping, diarrhea, nausea; primary septicemia—septic shock, bulbous skin lesions
> *People most at risk:* Gastroenteritis—all; primary septicemia—individuals with diabetes, cirrhosis, leukemia, AIDS, or those who take immunosuppressive drugs or steroids
> *Common food sources:* Raw or undercooked shellfish
> *Prevention:* Cook all shellfish thoroughly

Yersiniosis *(Yersinia Bacteria, Especially Y. enterocolitica)*

Symptoms: Fever, abdominal pain, diarrhea, and/or vomiting; symptoms may mimic appendicitis; the bacteria may also cause infections of wounds, joints, and the urinary tract
> *People most at risk:* Young children, debilitated people, elderly, those with AIDS, and persons undergoing immunosuppressive therapy
> *Common food sources:* Meats (pork, beef, lamb, etc.), oysters, fish, raw milk and produce
> *Prevention:* Cook all meats and fish thoroughly; use pasteurized milk; wash produce well especially if eaten raw

Many food manufacturers and processors are now incorporating into their manufacturing processes Hazard Analysis Critical Control Point (HACCP), a new food safety procedure. This means that they identify points at which hazardous materials can be introduced into the food and then monitor and correct these potential problem areas. This same type of process can be followed during the purchasing, storage, preparation, and serving of foods by individuals and families. Some of the likely problem areas are food selection, storage conditions, length of storage, and potential for cross-contamination of foods. The information in Box K-2 is designed to reduce the risk of problems in any of these areas.

Box K-2   Reducing the Risk of Foodborne Illness

Purchasing Food

- Choose only pasteurized milk and dairy products and hard cheeses. If hard cheese made with unpasteurized milk is consumed, be sure that it was aged at least 60 days. If soft cheeses are purchased, plan to cook them until they are bubbling.
- Make sure that any "sell by" or "use by" date on the food label has not passed.
- Avoid purchasing any cans that are bulging, severely dented, or rusted.
- Avoid purchasing any food that shows evidence of cross-contamination by another product (e.g., cooked seafood displayed on the same bed of ice with raw seafood), and bag fresh or frozen meats, poultry, and fish separately from produce or other foods that could become contaminated.
- Quickly get foods that need refrigeration into the freezer or refrigerator. On hot days, an ice chest may be needed during transport of foods.
- Some foods (e.g., produce, spices) are irradiated. This process is approved by the Food and Drug Administration as a method for reducing or eliminating pathogenic bacteria, insects, and parasites from foods. It does not leave any radioactivity in the food.
- Avoid cracked eggs.

Box K-2   Reducing the Risk of Foodborne Illness—cont'd

Food Storage

- Keep refrigerator set at 40° F (4° C) or less. This is sufficient to halt the growth of most common bacteria.
- Use fresh shell eggs within 4 to 5 weeks and eggs cooked in the shell within 1 week.
- Use fresh refrigerated poultry, seafood, and ground meat within 1 to 2 days or freeze at 32° F (0° C) indefinitely. Use refrigerated fresh whole cuts of meat (beef, pork, lamb, etc.) within 3 to 5 days or freeze at 32° F (0° C) indefinitely.
- Refrigerate leftovers as soon as possible (within 2 hours or less). If there is a large amount, divide it into smaller units so that they will chill quickly. Use leftovers within 3 to 4 days. When in doubt, throw it out.

Food Handling and Preparation

- Wash hands before preparing any food.
- Wash hands and any used utensils after preparing one food and before starting preparation of another. This reduces the risk of cross-contamination (e.g., contamination of raw salad vegetables from raw meat cut on the same cutting board).
- A bleach solution (5 ml [1 teaspoon] bleach in 1 liter of water) is effective in cleaning countertops and cutting boards used in food preparations. It can be kept in a spray bottle in the kitchen for convenience.
- Thaw frozen foods in the refrigerator, in cold water, or in the microwave.
- Marinate foods in the refrigerator, not out on the counter.
- When taking foods off the grill, do not put the cooked items on the same platter that held the raw meat. Raw meat juices can contain bacteria that could cross-contaminate cooked foods.
- Use a meat thermometer to check the internal temperature of meats, fish, and poultry for doneness (145° F [63° C] for 15 seconds for seafood, 160° F [72° C] for meats, and 180° F [82° C] for the interior of the thigh on whole poultry). Internal color is not an accurate guide to doneness of meats.

Continued

Food Handling and Preparation—cont'd

- Avoid raw or undercooked eggs, which may be found in items such as Caesar salad, homemade ice cream, eggnog, some meringues, and chiffon-type pies. Undercooked eggs have runny, rather than firm, yolks or whites.

- Wash fresh fruits and vegetables thoroughly with drinking water. Use of detergent may leave a residue on the food, and detergents are not approved for human consumption by the Food and Drug Administration.

- Clean cutting boards thoroughly with hot soapy water after use and rinse well; sanitize with dilute bleach solution (15 ml [1 tablespoon] in 4 liters [1 gallon] water) or by washing in a dishwasher. Avoid cross-contamination of foods; for example, do not use the same knife and cutting board to cut up meat and to dice raw vegetables without cleaning the utensils between the foods. Plastic cutting boards are easier to clean than wooden ones.

- Cook stuffing in a separate dish, outside the bird. If you choose to cook a stuffed bird, use a meat thermometer and be sure that the middle of the stuffing reaches 165° F (74° C). Do not buy prestuffed birds or prestuff them for later cooking; stuff them immediately before cooking.

- Reheat leftovers until they reach at least 165° F (74° C).

Serving Foods

- Keep hot foods above 140° F (61° C) and cold foods below 40° F (4° C).

- Serve cooked foods on clean dishes with clean hands and clean utensils. Never put cooked foods on a dish that has held raw products unless the dish is first washed with soap and water.

- Perishable foods used for picnics should be kept in an ice chest chilled with ice or frozen gel packs to a temperature of 40° F (4° C) or less until they are consumed. Keep the ice chest closed as much as possible to keep the temperature from rising. Leftovers should be discarded if they cannot be maintained at 40° F (4° C) or less until they reach home.

- Perishable items packed in lunches for school or lunch should be kept chilled with a frozen juice box or frozen gel pack until lunch. Any perishable items not eaten at lunch should be discarded and not brought home and reused.

Glossary

achalasia: incomplete relaxation of the lower esophageal sphincter after swallowing.

Adequate Intake (AI): a recommendation for the level of intake of a nutrient. The AI is assigned, rather than a Recommended Dietary Allowance (RDA), when the nutrient intake recommended is believed to cover the needs of almost all of the population, but nutrient needs cannot be quantified as precisely as those for an RDA.

alcohol abuse: heavy drinking with an increasing tolerance for ethanol but no withdrawal symptoms when drinking stops.

alcoholism: a strong craving for ethanol, associated with increasing tolerance to alcohol's intoxicating effects and symptoms of withdrawal when drinking is discontinued.

alternative medical therapies: treatments that are not usually part of traditional Western medical practice, e.g., use of acupuncture rather than medications for control of pain.

anabolism: formation of new body tissue.

anemia of chronic disease: an anemia observed in some patients affected by cancer, renal failure, and other chronic illnesses in which the bone marrow fails to produce adequate red blood cells, even though iron stores may be normal. The anemia is often normocytic (normal-sized cells), rather than microcytic, as in iron deficiency.

anorexia nervosa: a psychiatric eating disorder often resulting in extreme thinness. The affected person usually has a strong aversion to food intake and a distorted body image (perceiving him or herself as fat when the opposite is the case).

anthropometric measurements: measurements of the designated aspects of the human body, such as height and weight.

antioxidant: a substance that reduces the formation of free radicals from oxygen in the cells and protects unsaturated fatty acids from oxidation. Antioxidant nutrients include (but are not limited to) vitamins A, C, and E; β-carotene; and selenium.

Attention Deficit/Hyperactivity Disorders (ADHDs): a set of related disorders characterized by focusing on irrelevant stimuli, impulsive behavior, inconsistency, and lack of persistence. Overactivity may be a feature of the disorder in some children.

basal energy expenditure: amount of energy required to maintain the critical life processes (e.g., breathing, beating of the heart) in an individual at rest, in a comfortable thermal environment, and after an overnight fast. Usually used as a synonym for basal metabolic rate and resting metabolic rate.

body mass index (BMI): an indication of the appropriateness of a person's weight for height, which correlates relatively well with measures of body fat. BMI is usually calculated as the person's weight (in kg) divided by the height (in meters) squared.

bronchopulmonary dysplasia (BPD): lung damage almost always found in infants who have required oxygen therapy and mechanical ventilation. BPD is characterized by a persistent requirement for supplemental oxygen beyond 36 weeks of gestational age.

bulimia nervosa: a psychiatric eating disorder characterized by repeated episodes of bingeing on large amounts of foods, followed by efforts to rid the body of the food by self-induced vomiting or abuse of laxatives and diuretics. Also known as the binge-purge syndrome.

cancer cachexia: a severe form of cancer-related malnutrition associated with a poor prognosis and characterized by anorexia, early satiety, weight loss, anemia, weakness, and muscle wasting.

carbohydrate counting: a technique for planning the diet in diabetes that focuses on the carbohydrate content of foods consumed.

carotenoids: a group of pigments (yellow, orange, or red) found in fruits and vegetables. β-carotene, lutein, cryptoxanthin, and zeaxanthin are examples of carotenoids. All carotenoids have some vitamin A activity, but β-carotene is the primary vitamin A precursor.

catabolism: breakdown of body tissues.

celiac disease (nontropical sprue or gluten-sensitive enteropathy): a disorder characterized by impaired absorption and steatorrhea. It results from intestinal mucosal damage caused by an immune reaction to the gliadin fraction of the gluten protein.

chylomicron: a lipoprotein formed in the intestine after consumption of fat. It transports the fat from the intestinal cell into the lymph and from there into the blood.

colostrum: the milk produced for about the first 3 to 5 days after birth. Colostrum is yellowish, rich in immunoglobulins and lymphocytes, and higher in protein than mature human milk.

complementary medical therapies: treatments that are often not part of traditional Western medical practice but that may be used as adjuncts to that practice. Use of herbal therapies (e.g., gingko biloba to improve memory) is one example.

complete protein: a protein that contains all of the essential amino acids in sufficient amounts and in proportion to one another so that it can support growth and maintenance of tissues.

Crohn's disease: a form of inflammatory bowel disease that can affect any portion of the gastrointestinal tract and can extend through all layers of the bowel. It is often associated with severe chronic diarrhea, nutritional deficits, and weight loss.

cystic fibrosis (CF): a disease resulting from a defect in the cystic fibrosis transmembrane conductance regulator (CFTR) gene. This defect prevents the formation of CFTR, a protein involved in chloride transport across cell membranes in the body. It results in several problems, including thickened mucous secretions in the lungs, interfering with lung function and promoting respiratory infections, and pancreatic insufficiency.

Daily Value (DV): a reference value used in nutrition labeling of foods. The DV, which is based on the Recommended Dietary Allowances (RDA), provides a guideline to the amount of a particular nutrient that the daily diet should contain. On the label, information for most nutrients is expressed in both units of weight (g or mg) and %Daily Value (DV).

dehydration: a deficit of body fluid.

Dietary Guidelines for Americans: guidelines written in lay language that are intended to help Americans optimize their health and reduce nutrition-related health risks.

Dietary Reference Intakes (DRIs): guidelines for nutrient intake for the healthy population. The DRIs contain two types of measures, the Recommended Dietary Allowances (RDAs) and Tolerable Upper Intake Levels. The DRIs do not focus merely on preventing deficiency diseases but quantify the relationship between nutrients and risk of disease, e.g., calcium and osteoporosis. The DRIs include important nonnutrients found in food, such as fiber.

dumping syndrome: a common side effect of gastric bypass or gastrectomy. It occurs because stomach contents pass into the small bowel rapidly. Nutrients that raise the osmotic concentration within the small bowel substantially, such as simple carbohydrates, draw fluid into the bowel and cause a reduction in the circulating blood volume. The symptoms include dizziness, sweating, nausea, weakness, tachycardia, and diarrhea.

dysphagia: difficulty in swallowing.

elemental formulas: liquid diets containing predigested nutrients (e.g., hydrolyzed protein and/or free amino acids). These are commonly used for individuals with digestive or absorptive disorders. Also known as oligomeric formulas.

energy balance: the match between energy (calorie) intake and energy expenditure in any individual. Neutral energy balance (consuming the amount of energy that is expended) results in maintenance of body weight. Being in positive energy balance, or consuming more calories than expended, results in weight gain and can lead to overweight and obesity. Negative energy balance—consuming fewer calories than expended or increasing the amount of physical activity to use more energy—results in weight loss.

enteral feedings: feedings delivered into any part of the gastrointestinal tract. Enteral feedings are given either by mouth or by tube.

erythropoietin: a hormone produced by the kidney that stimulates red blood cell formation.

essential amino acids (EAAs): amino acids that cannot be synthesized in the body in the amounts needed for the building of tissues and therefore must be provided by the diet.

extremely low birth weight (ELBW): weighing less than 1000 g at birth.

failure to thrive: failure of an infant to regain his or her birth weight by 3 weeks of age, or continuous weight loss or failure to gain weight at the appropriate rate during infancy or childhood.

fetal alcohol syndrome (FAS): a constellation of congenital abnormalities that results from alcohol intake during pregnancy. Features of FAS may include microcephaly (abnormally small head circumference), prenatal and postnatal growth failure, mental retardation, facial abnormalities, cleft palate, skeletal-joint abnormalities, abnormal palmar creases, cardiac defects, and behavioral abnormalities. The only known preventive measure is to avoid drinking alcohol during pregnancy.

Food Guide Pyramid: a schematic tool to help individuals plan a varied diet. The pyramid has six components. The base is made up of the grain group, emphasizing the importance of this group as a foundation to good nutrition. The next layer is composed of two groups, vegetables and fruits. The third layer from the bottom is composed of milk products and meat, poultry, fish, eggs, and nuts. The apex of the pyramid, the smallest part, is devoted to fats and sweets, as a reminder to use these products only sparingly.

food hypersensitivity: an immunologic (allergic) reaction to ingestion of a food or food additive. Symptoms can include anaphylaxis, failure to thrive (in infants and children), vomiting, abdominal pain, diarrhea, rhinitis, sinusitis, otitis media, cough, wheezing, rash, urticaria, and atopic dermatitis.

food jags: periods during which young children consume only one or two foods for several days. This behavior is normal unless it lasts more than a few days.

gastroesophageal reflux disease (GERD): reflux of stomach contents into the esophagus.

gastroparesis: delayed gastric emptying.

gestational diabetes mellitus: diabetes that first becomes evident during pregnancy.

gliadin: a part of the gluten protein, found in wheat, barley, rye, and possibly oats.

gluten: a protein found in wheat, barley, and rye and possibly oats.

glycemic index: ratio between the change in the blood glucose concentration produced by consuming some food, compared with the change produced by some reference carbohydrate (usually white bread or glucose).

glycosylated hemoglobin (HbA_{1c}): hemoglobin with glucose molecules attached; it is increased by elevated blood glucose over the lifespan of the red blood cells and serves as an indicator of blood glucose concentrations over a period of several weeks to a few months.

hemochromatosis: a genetic disorder in which excessive iron is stored in various organs, especially the liver, pancreas, heart, gonad, skin, and joints, disrupting organ function.

hepatic encephalopathy: a disorder resulting from accumulation of toxic substances in the blood as a result of liver failure. It is characterized by memory loss, personality change, tremors, and a decrease in the level of consciousness. The affected person may progress to stupor and coma.

hepatitis: an inflammation of the liver caused by a virus, toxin, obstruction, parasite, or drug.

high biologic value proteins (HBV): proteins of high quality that promote positive nitrogen balance; believed to be effective in maintenance and synthesis of tissues.

high-density lipoprotein (HDL): a lipoprotein formed in the liver to transport cholesterol from the tissues to the liver for metabolism. This function makes HDL protective against heart disease, and thus the HDL-cholesterol is considered "good" cholesterol.

hydrogenation: addition of hydrogen atoms to unsaturated fats to saturate the double bonds with hydrogen. This process converts the fats from liquids to solids (e.g., shortening or margarine).

hyperemesis gravidarum: severe nausea and vomiting that may continue throughout pregnancy.

hyperkalemia: elevated circulating potassium concentrations.

hypermetabolism: abnormally increased energy expenditure, as occurs in sepsis or following injuries such as burns.

hyperoxaluria: excessive loss of oxalates in the urine.

impaired glucose tolerance (IGT): having a glucose concentration ≥ 140 mg/dl (7.8 mmol/l) and <200 mg/dl (11.1 mmol/l) 2 hours after ingestion of a 75 g glucose load; a risk factor for later development of diabetes mellitus.

incomplete protein: a protein lacking in one or more essential amino acids and therefore lacking in the ability to maintain normal growth and maintenance of tissues.

inflammatory bowel disease (IBD): two types of inflammatory processes, Crohn's disease and ulcerative colitis, that affect the gastrointestinal tract. Crohn's disease can affect any part of the gastrointestinal tract and can extend through all layers of the bowel. Ulcerative colitis is primarily a disease of the large bowel, and it affects only the intestinal mucosa and the submucosal layer. The most common symptom is chronic bloody diarrhea. Nutritional deficits are common, especially in Crohn's disease, where malabsorption and weight loss may be severe.

insulin resistance: impaired response of cells (primarily those in the skeletal muscle and adipose tissue) to insulin.

isoflavones: compounds found in soy that appear to lower low-density lipoprotein (LDL) cholesterol concentrations.

ketogenic diet: a high-fat diet that stimulates ketone production.

kwashiorkor: a form of protein-calorie malnutrition characterized by low levels of visceral proteins such as serum albumin, transferrin, or prealbumin; edema; poor wound healing; and impaired immune function. It often develops rapidly in people experiencing trauma, surgery, or infection and receiving inadequate protein or calories.

leptin: the product of the *ob* gene. Leptin is released by adipose (fat) tissue, and it appears to provide a mechanism for the adipose tissue to communicate with the central nervous system and contribute to the control of food intake and energy metabolism.

lipoproteins: the major carriers of lipids (fats) in the plasma. They are formed of lipids bound to proteins.

low birth weight (LBW): weighing less than 2500 g (5.5 lb) at birth.

low-density lipoproteins (LDLs): lipoproteins that have a very high content of cholesterol, which the LDL deposit in the tissues. The cholesterol in LDL is considered to be the main cause of elevated cholesterol levels, making LDL-cholesterol the so-called "bad" cholesterol in causation of heart disease.

malnutrition: poor nutritional status (either undernutrition or overnutrition). It can result from inadequate intake, disorders of digestion or absorption, or excessive intake of nutrients.

marasmus: a form of protein-calorie malnutrition resulting from an inadequate intake of energy over a period of months or even years. The individual experiences loss of subcutaneous fat and muscle and appears thin and wasted, but levels of visceral proteins such as serum albumin, transferrin, or prealbumin are often normal.

medium-chain triglyceride (MCT): a triglyceride (consisting of glycerol bound to three fatty acids) in which the fatty acids are 8 to 12 carbons in length. MCTs are most often used in the nutritional care of people with limited digestive and absorptive ability.

micelle: a combination of bile salts and fat in which the bile emulsifies fat into very small particles to increase its exposure to digestive enzymes and to enhance its solubility so that it can be absorbed by the intestinal mucosa.

monounsaturated fat: a fatty acid with one carbon-carbon double bond.

necrotizing enterocolitis (NEC): an intestinal disorder most often occurring in preterm infants. On x-ray, gas can be seen between the layers of the intestine; in severe cases, intestinal perforation and peritonitis are present.

nephrolithiasis: formation of calculi (stones) in the kidney.

nephrotic syndrome: a condition in which there is damage to the basement membrane of the nephrons. The syndrome is characterized by loss of protein in the urine, edema, and decreased serum albumin concentrations.

nitrogen balance: the relationship between the amount of nitrogen (from proteins or amino acids) consumed and the amount excreted. Balance is positive if more nitrogen is consumed than excreted and negative if more nitrogen is excreted than consumed.

nonessential amino acid: an amino acid that can be synthesized in the body in amounts sufficient to maintain tissue and sustain growth.

nonnutritive feeding: sucking a pacifier. It develops muscle tone needed for feeding by nipple and may be soothing for infants in stressful situations.

nutrition assessment: the process used to evaluate nutritional status, identify malnutrition, and determine which individuals need aggressive nutritional support.

nutrition support: the provision of specially formulated and/or delivered parenteral or enteral nutrients to maintain or restore optimal nutritional status.

nutritional quackery: promotion of misconceptions about food and nutrition. Examples include the idea that certain foods or dietary supplements have "fat-burning" properties and the belief that nutritional supplements are necessary to maintain health.

omega-3 fatty acid (n-3 fatty acid): a fatty acid with a carbon-carbon double bond three carbons from the omega (methyl group) end of its chain. These fatty acids have been reported to reduce serum triglyceride concentrations and to reduce the aggregation of platelets, resulting in a reduced risk of myocardial infarction (heart attack). Fish from cold waters are generally rich in omega-3 fatty acids; canola oil is another source.

osmolality: the property of a solution that depends on the concentration of solute (the number of osmotically active particles) per kilogram of solvent (usually water).

parenteral feedings: delivery of nutrients via the intravenous route.

phytochemicals: nonnutrients in plant foods that have health-protective effects.

pancreatitis: inflammation, edema, and necrosis of the pancreas as a result of digestion of the organ by pancreatic enzymes.

pica: the consumption of substances usually considered nonfoods (e.g., clay) or of excessive amounts of food products low in nutrients (e.g., ice, cornstarch).

polymeric formulas: liquid diets used for oral supplementation or enteral tube feeding. Polymeric formulas contain intact (not predigested) carbohydrates, proteins, and fats.

polyunsaturated fat: a fatty acid containing more than one carbon-carbon double bond.

pregnancy-induced hypertension (PIH): a syndrome character-ized by hypertension, albuminuria, and excessive edema. Also called preeclampsia or toxemia.

protein-calorie malnutrition (PCM): undernutrition resulting from inadequate intake, digestion, or absorption of protein or calories. There are two forms, kwashiorkor and marasmus, and it is possible to have a combined form, referred to as marasmic kwashiorkor.

Recommended Dietary Allowances (RDAs): an amount of a nutrient estimated to meet the biological needs of almost all (97% to 98%) of the healthy population. The RDA is one of the measures included in the Dietary Reference Intakes (DRIs).

refeeding syndrome: a potential complication of refeeding of the severely malnourished individual. During refeeding, especially with high-carbohydrate feedings, insulin levels rise and cellular uptake of glucose, water, phosphorus, potassium, and other nutrients is stimulated. Serum levels of phosphorus, potassium, magnesium, and other minerals or electrolytes subsequently fall, if close attention is not paid to their replacement. Refeeding syndrome is characterized by cardiac dysrhythmias, congestive heart failure, hemolysis, muscular weakness, seizures, acute respiratory failure, and a variety of other complications, including sudden death.

respiratory quotient (RQ): the ratio of the carbon dioxide produced to the oxygen consumed in a given unit of time.

resting energy expenditure (REE): amount of energy required to maintain the vital life processes (e.g., breathing, circulation) at rest in an overnight-fasted condition and in a comfortable environmental temperature.

short-bowel syndrome: varying degrees of impaired digestion and absorption resulting from surgical removal of parts of the intestines.

small-for-gestational age (SGA): exhibiting intrauterine growth failure; low birth weight and length for the infant's gestational age.

steatorrhea: loss of fat in the stools.

Step-One Diet: a diet recommended as a first step in treatment of elevated serum cholesterol in the person with risk from heart disease; the same diet is recommended by the American Heart Association as a means of reducing the risk of heart disease for adults in the general population. Dietary fat intake is limited to no more than 30% of the energy (calorie) intake, and saturated fat intake is limited to no more than 10% of total calories. Cholesterol intake is limited to 300 mg daily.

Step-Two Diet: a diet recommended for individuals that do not respond to the Step-One Diet with adequate lowering of their serum cholesterol. It is similar to the Step-One Diet except that saturated fat intake is further limited to no more than 7% of total calories and cholesterol intake to no more than 200 mg/day.

Syndrome X: also known as the metabolic syndrome; refers to the combination of obesity, hypertension, and diabetes. Hyperinsulinemia (increased pancreatic release of insulin) is believed to be the common factor linking the three conditions.

thermic effect of food (TEF): production of body heat as a result of food intake; the energy required to digest and absorb food and transport nutrients to the cells. TEF accounts for approximately 10% of daily energy needs. Also referred to as diet-induced thermogenesis.

Tolerable Upper Intake Level (UL): the upper limit of intake associated with a low risk of adverse effects in almost all members of a given population. The UL is one of the measures included in the Dietary Reference Intakes (DRIs).

trans **fatty acid:** a fatty acid (component of fats) formed when unsaturated oils are partially hydrogenated to make them harder. The fatty acid molecules usually bend at the remaining carbon-carbon double bonds, and in the *trans* fatty acid the two ends of the fatty acid are arranged so that they are on opposite sides of the double bond. (In naturally occurring *cis* fatty acids, the two ends are on the same side of the double bond.)

type 1 diabetes mellitus: previously known as insulin-dependent diabetes; characterized by insulin deficiency, which results from destruction of the beta cells of the pancreas, usually by an autoimmune process. Classic symptoms include excessive hunger and thirst and weight loss.

type 2 diabetes mellitus: previously known as non–insulin-dependent diabetes; characterized by insulin resistance, or decreased tissue uptake of glucose in response to insulin.

ulcerative colitis: a form of inflammatory bowel disease that usually involves only the large bowel and primarily affects the mucosal and submucosal layers of the intestine.

ultrafiltration: filtration of fluid through a semipermeable membrane that holds back large molecules (e.g., proteins) contained in the fluid.

unsaturated fat: a fatty acid (component of fats) that does not contain the maximum possible number of hydrogen atoms, allowing it to have carbon-carbon double bonds. There are two types of unsaturated fatty acids, monounsaturated (having one double bond) and polyunsaturated (having more than one double bond).

very low birth weight (VLBW): weighing less than 1500 g at birth.

very low-density lipoprotein (VLDL): lipoprotein formed in the liver to transport lipids made in the liver to other body cells. Most of their lipid content is in the form of triglycerides, but they also transport cholesterol.

villi: small projections from the surface of a membrane, especially the small fingerlike projections of the intestinal mucosa. Villi greatly increase the surface area of a membrane.

weight cycling: also known as "yo-yo" dieting, occurs when individuals repeatedly lose and regain weight.

Wernicke-Korsakoff syndrome: a serious disorder of the central nervous system that can occur in alcoholism and other thiamin deficient states. Symptoms are mental confusion, memory loss, confabulation, ataxia, abnormal ocular motility (ophthalmoplegia and nystagmus), and peripheral neuropathy.

Index

Page numbers in italics indicate illustrations; t indicates tables.

521